YOU

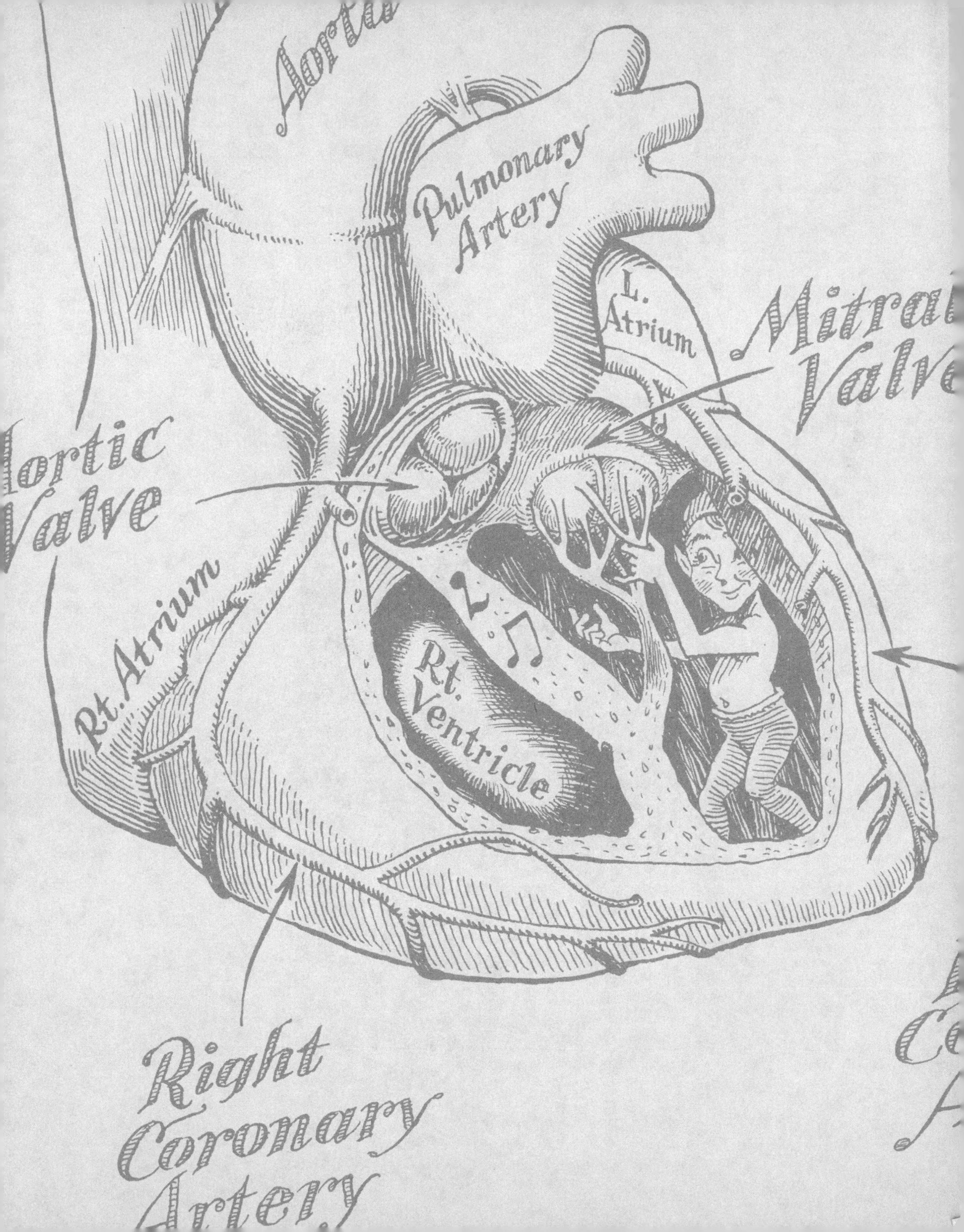
Aorta
Pulmonary Artery
L. Atrium
Mitral Valve
Aortic Valve
Rt. Atrium
Rt. Ventricle
Right Coronary Artery

YOU

The Owner's Manual, Updated and Expanded Edition

An Insider's Guide to the Body That Will Make You Healthier and Younger

MICHAEL F. ROIZEN, M.D.,
AND MEHMET C. OZ, M.D.

WITH LISA OZ AND TED SPIKER

ILLUSTRATIONS BY GARY HALLGREN

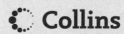

Collins

An Imprint of HarperCollinsPublishers

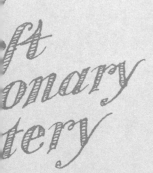

YOU: THE OWNER'S MANUAL. Copyright © 2005, 2008 by Michael F. Roizen, MD, and Mehmet C. Oz, MD Illustrations copyright © 2005, 2008 by Gary Hallgren, Michael F. Roizen, MD, and Mehmet C. Oz, MD Adaptation of Mensa test on page 100 copyright © 1992 by Abbie Salny, American MENSA Ltd. All rights reserved. Printed in the United States of America. No part of this book may be used or reproduced in any manner whatsoever without written permission except in the case of brief quotations embodied in critical articles and reviews. For information, address HarperCollins Publishers, 10 East 53rd Street, New York, NY 10022.

HarperCollins books may be purchased for educational, business, or sales promotional use. For information please write: Special Markets Department, HarperCollins Publishers, 10 East 53rd Street, New York, NY 10022.

The first hardcover edition was published by HarperResource © 2005.

FIRST COLLINS EDITION 2008

Designed by William Ruoto

The Library of Congress Cataloging-in-Publication has been applied for.

ISBN 978-0-06-147367-8

08   09   10   11   12   DIX/RRD   10   9   8   7   6   5   4   3   2   1

To our children: Alex, Arabella, Daphne, Jeffrey, Jennifer, Oliver, Thad, and Zoe

Contents

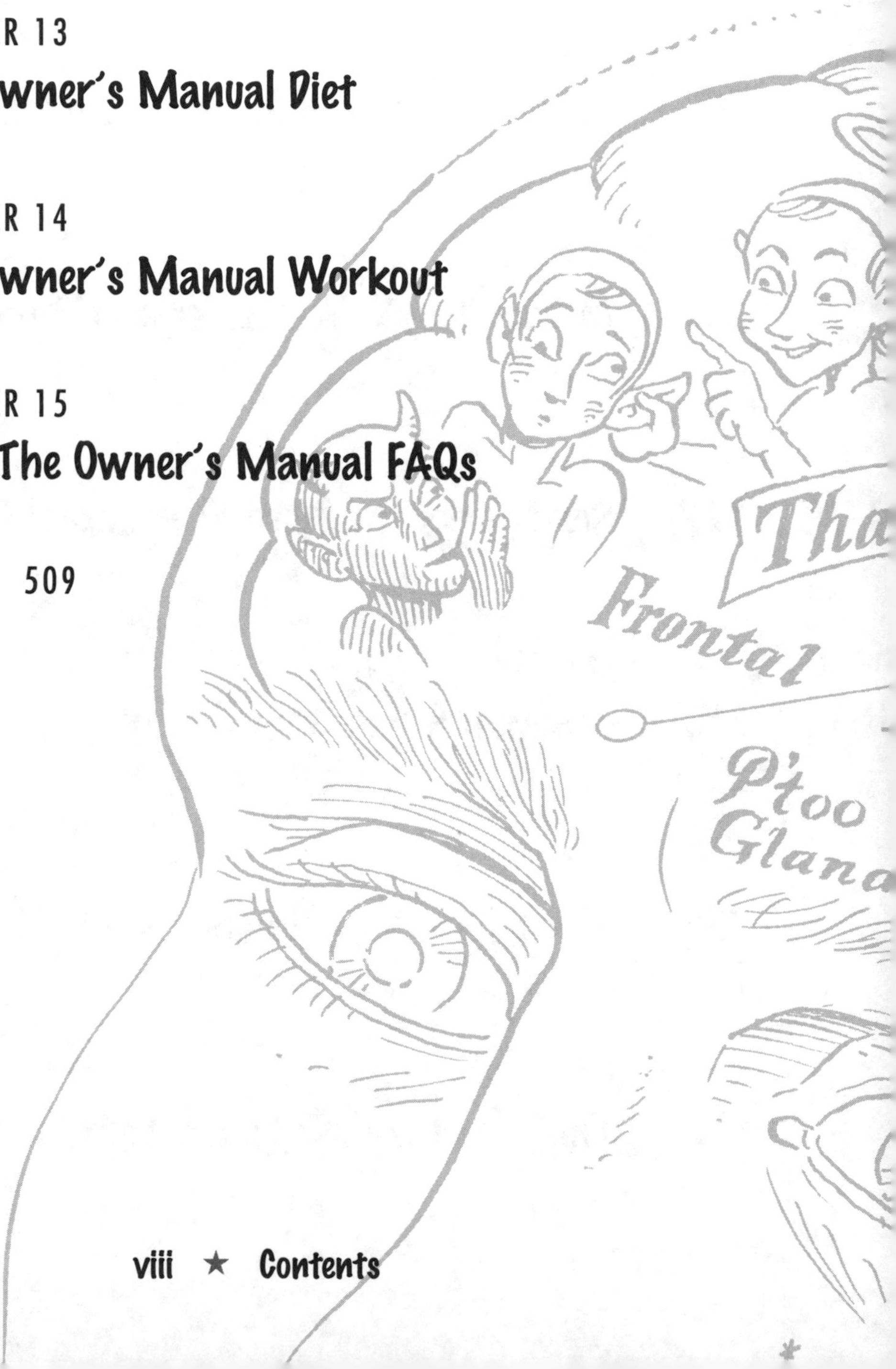
Frontal

Acknowledgments

Lisa, Gary, and Ted made this book possible—and much more fun. While it may be unusual to say that the hours of book research and writing were as much fun as a party, we often felt that they were. Each delivered what they promised, when they promised it. Lisa always made us remember the stronger gender, helped redirect us toward a more upbeat, hip book, and pushed for Ted as our collaborator. Ted has a remarkable ability to embrace complex medical topics and make them fun; when he said something would be done, it was. We could not be bigger fans and admirers of his remarkable talents. Gary's off-the-beaten-track genius came to life with stunning pictures that made us work even harder to match his creativity. Our agent Candice Fuhrman's level head and insightful comments and negotiations brought this book to life.

We also want to thank the group at HarperCollins who keep believing in us, and who are just great to work with: Shelby Meizlik and especially Kathryn Huck—she made herself available and is clearly a rising star.

We also want to thank the many patients and the thousands of people who sent questions, notes, cards, and e-mails that inspired many of the thoughts in this book, and, of course, the FAQs. We now receive eight hundred thank-you e-mails a day on our Web site (www.RealAge.com/youdocs). Nothing could motivate us more. Thank you.

Joel Harper provided the inspiration and perspiration for the new workouts added in this edition—we are appreciative and younger due to his additions.

Finally, we wish to express our gratitude for the many hours of work he created, the great friend who brought us together—Craig Wynett. Besides being a world-class wit, Craig has a remarkable grasp of what the world needs that made him the mentor of many others before us. He took the time to connect the dots that we could not envision and provided advice that helped shape the direction of our book. Please blame him if you are unhappy with your purchase.

Mike's Acknowledgments

I am grateful to the many other people who did not discard the e-mails asking them for help. Dr. Jon Walters, a physician who doubles as a home makeover expert, seemed to find time to read as he drove from Pittsburgh to Cleveland and back again to teach us how to make the metaphors appropriate for both the home repairman and the health care professional (if you were driven off the road between Pittsburgh and Cleveland, blame us). He also contributed significantly to the science, especially in the sex chapter. The family trio of Dr. Axel Goetz, Anka Goetz, and Margarthe Goetz also merits special thanks for their critical review of the science, the artistry, and the style of the book chapter by chapter. I also want to thank Debbie Schwinn, MD, PhD, of UW, Seattle; Jeff Watson, DDS; John Hoepner, MD; John Campodonico; Sydney Unobskey; Jim Graham; Chas Brendler, MD; Roz Wattell; Marcie Anthone; Kandi Amelon; Jennifer Plant; Linda DeFrancisco; and Irwin Davis, who each took red pen to more than one chapter. Ruth Klein made the diet chapter easier to follow with her revisions. I also need to thank Tracy Hafen, who taught me a magnificent amount about exercise; Sukie Miller and Anita Shreve, for saying the early chapters were just what they wanted to read; the many gerontologists and internists who read sections of the book for accuracy; others on the RealAge team who validate and verify the content and contributed their expertise to the book, including the many who contributed recipes, such as Rich Tramonte and Gale Gand of Tru in Chicago; John La Puma, who taught me an amazing amount about cooking and nutrition, and collaboration; the staff of Rick Bayless's restaurants; Dan Zakri, and the chefs at the Kendall College of Nutrition in Chicago, who created many of the recipes; Shivani Chadha and Kate Poneta, the research associates who worked tirelessly to analyze the nutrients and calculate the RealAge effect of each recipe; especially Donna Szymanski (she must have incredible patience—she taught me how to cook, and she cooked every recipe we tested—over 350—at least three times); and our tasters, especially the Wattels of Lettuce Entertain You.

I also want to acknowledge the passion and tough love from the staff of the Center for Partnership Medicine at Northwestern Memorial Hospital in Chicago, who encouraged the goals of RealAge and *You: The Owner's Manual,* especially Dan Dermann, MD; Drew Palumbo; and Dean Harrison. And my partners, who allowed me the time to complete the work: Aaron Gerber, MD, Mike Kessel, and Jane Spinner; and others who encouraged the work, including Enrico Camporesi, Chris Fey, Laura Hand, Joel Delmonico, Jessie Dylan, Peter Uva, and Donna Gould.

I want to especially acknowledge my colleagues at the Cleveland Clinic: Drs. Toby Cosgrove, Joe Hahn, Bridget Duffy, and Richard Lang. It is no accident that the clinic has been rated number one in cardiac care for thirteen years in a row (even Mehmet trained here). Eileen Sheil, Mike O'Donnell, David Strand, Claire and Jim Young, Jim Blazer, and Paul Matsen make wellness a priority every day.

Anne-Marie Ruthrauff, Michelle Lewis, Candy Lawrence, and Beth Grubb each deserves special thanks, as do some RealAge partners: Martin Rom and Charlie Silver; Arline McDonald, Tate Erlinger, Linda Van Horne, Carl Peck, Sally Kim, Mark Rudberg, Mike Parzen, and especially Keith Roach; and Harriet Imrey, the scientific partners (in addition to Axel Goetz) in the process of evaluating the data and scientific content of RealAge. I would feel as if I needed to do forty-eight minutes more on an exercise bike every day if I didn't acknowledge that Diane Reverand told me "not to worry about offending medical colleagues—as long as the science was solid, they would understand you were trying to motivate the readers to understand they could control their own health and were responsible for doing so and for enjoying the extra energy and vitality."

I cannot thank my wife, Nancy, enough for her constant love, encouragement, and support, and our children, Jeffrey and Jennifer, for their help, understanding, and patience. They read this book and used their scientific expertise in critical reading to ensure the content was an accurate representation of what we intended.

I hope and believe this book will help YOU to take control of your body. That would be the best reward any physician could want.

Mehmet's Acknowledgments

Some of the concepts for the book came from *Second Opinion with Dr. Oz*, a Discovery Channel series that helped viewers become world experts on their bodies. The vision and opportunity for this program came from my lifelong friend Billy Campbell. Together with his wonderful team, including Clark "Bust Through the Clutter" Bunting, Tomi Landis, Jim Berger, Janice Jensen, Lisa Tucker, and of course my executive producer wife, Lisa, we created content that became worthy of this book. Many of the finer concepts have been matured with the Discovery Health team, including Eileen O'Neil, Donald Thoms, John Grassie, Erica Green, and John Greco. Mark Twain quipped, "If I had more time, I would have made it shorter." My colleagues at New York–Presbyterian Columbia University Medical Center helped me carve out the time needed to write as efficiently as needed for this "owner's manual," especially Eric Rose, Craig Smith, Yoshifuma Naka, Mike Argenziano, Henry Spotnitz, Barry Esrig, Alan Stewart, and the other superb surgeons on our team. The physician's assistants, especially Laura Baer, and nurses in the OR led by Flora Wang, ICU led by Majella Venturanza, and floor led by Eumne Shim show me frontline healing daily. Lidia Nieves, Michelle Washburn, and Diane Amato either organized my schedule so that no moment could be wasted or advised me wisely so I could slave over the book.

Thanks to all my physician colleagues in other specialties who provided content either through the show or by providing feedback on our writing: Herb Pardes, Paul Simonelli, Silviu Itescu, Jay Lombard, Scott Forman, Bill Levine, Ian Storper, Joel Fuhrman, Stephen Halpert, Jonathan LaPook, Rob Abel, Benjamin Lewis, Eric Seamon, Hilda Hutcherson, Mitch Gaynor, Pam Peeke, Dean Ornish, Nancy Snyderman, Ridwan Shapsig, McHenry Lee, Ernie April, Linda Vahdat, Christy Mack, Jane Buckle, Jeffrey Ahn, Alan and Vincent Chow, Joel Ernst, Lisa Saiman, and Jim Garza.

Thanks also to the very supportive public affairs group at New York-Presbyterian, including Bryan Dotson, Alicia Park, and Myna Manners, who have taught me to stay on message. Ivan Kronenfeld provided sage advice to focus our efforts.

My parents-in-law, Gerald and Emily Jane Lemole, bring wisdom into our family's life daily and are role models to me. Their insights into medicine and healing, especially in the micronutrient and dietary recommendations, brought this book into focus. Finally, thanks to Mustafa and Suna Oz for making and inspiring me.

Preface

Welcome to *YOU: The Owner's Manual*, version 2.0 (we call it YOU2; you can, too). As is the case with any second edition, version, or sequel, we hope that this one motivates you more and is even better than the first. In this book, you'll find plenty of updated information and loads of new material—some of which is sprinkled sneakily throughout the chapters and some of which stands out like a punk rocker's hair.

What are some of those highlights? For one, we've added another entire chapter on an organ that got very little play in the first version: the liver. It was a terrible omission on our part, considering it's probably the most powerful and least understood organ in our bodies (terrible publicist the liver has). We've also included new recipes for those of you who are always looking to add more spice to your life. And we've included a great, new workout to help improve your body.

Perhaps our favorite part of this new edition comes in the form of our interaction with you, the readers and viewers who have written in to ask us about their health problems, concerns, and mysteries. (After all, this book is about you, right?) At the end of the book, you'll find more than 100 FAQs that have come directly from your curious brains and often frustrated bodies. In that chapter, we'll answer everything from how to make your brain better to how to stop the noxious release of gas that happens to find its way from your intestines into your living room.

We appreciate that you've joined us in our journey of exploration of the human body. We've always found the body to be the most fascinating, marvelous, and wondrous thing in the world. And we hope that you agree.

Here's to you.

Michael F. Roizen, MD, and Mehmet C. Oz, MD

Chapter 1

Your Body, Your Home: Super Health

Beautiful bodies sell magazines. Tattooed bodies attract gawkers. Well-trained bodies win championships (and lucrative endorsement contracts). Celebrity bodies get stalked by paparazzi, chronicled by tabloids, and lampooned by late-night talk-show hosts. Infomercials promise better bodies (*Lose 700 pounds with this revolutionary belly button cream!*). And now, even so-called flawed bodies star as the protagonists in one form of pop culture: plastic-surgery reality shows.

There's no doubt that corporate America has capitalized on the fact that a beautiful body stimulates the economy as well as the hormones. We're all for admiring the body for its curves, angles, and ability to make Nielsen ratings soar. But maybe our obsession with skin belies the importance of everything that chugs, churns, and pounds underneath it. Because many people have developed a view of the human body that's more superficial than a paper cut, we want to step back and look deeper—into places where only surgeons, MRI machines, and the occasional tapeworm can see:

Inside your body.

Why? Because what goes on inside of your body is what gives you the ability to see, run, smell, have wild sex on the beach, feed babies, create dinosaurs out of Legos, surf, solve algebra problems, tie shoelaces, hum "Margaritaville," and do the thousands of different things you do every day. Your body gives you life. Your body *is* life.

But even if you understand your body's many functions, you may not really know how it functions—and, more important, how you can make it stronger, healthier, and younger.

Maybe that's because complex medical issues and scientific jargon race through our brains like cars on an interstate—reports, data, and recommendations stream by so fast that you barely have time to notice them, let alone figure out what they all mean. The result of this information inundation is that spotting important health news is about as easy as finding a kernel of corn in a landfill. Then, to figure out which kernel of information you can apply to your own life, it takes digging, persistence, and time, not to mention some waders to protect yourself from all the junk that's out there. But it's vital for your health—and your life—that you own a pair of informational waders. With this book, we've strapped on our waders and have pulled out the kernels for you.

So you can live a healthier life.

So you can become the world expert on your body.

To do that, we want you to think of your body as a home—as your home. When we started thinking about the similarities between bodies and homes, we realized that the two have a more striking resemblance than the Olsen twins. Your house and body are both important investments. They both provide shelter to invaluable personal property. And they're both places you want to protect with all your power. That's the big picture. But if we explore the comparison even more—

and we will throughout this book—you'll understand the relationship even better. Your bones are the two-by-fours that support and protect the inner structure of your home; your eyes are the windows; your lungs are the ventilation ducts; your brain is the fuse box; your intestines are the plumbing system; your mouth is the food processor; your heart is the water main; your hair is the lawn (some of us have more grass than others); and your fat is all the unnecessary junk you've stored in the attic that your spouse has been nagging you to get rid of. If you can get past the fact that your forehead doesn't have a street number and that a two-story brick Colonial doesn't look all that good in a bathing suit, the similarities are remarkable—so remarkable, in fact, that we believe you can learn about how your body works by thinking about how your house does.

And that's really the, uh, foundation for this book: Knowing your body gives you the power to change it, maintain it, decorate it, and strengthen it. In each chapter, we'll start by explaining the anatomy of your body's major organs. To do that, we'll take you inside—and show you how your body's organs operate and interact with each other. We won't do it in doctor-speak, but we also won't treat you like you're a fourth-grader. We're not going to make the science simplistic; we're going to make it simple. From there, we're going to tell you how to make your organs function better—so you can prevent disease and live a younger, healthier life. We'll show you how disease starts, how it affects your body, and how you can learn to fend off and beat problems and conditions that can threaten not only your life but also your quality of life.

To return to the house analogy, we want you to take the same approach to basic body maintenance and repairs as you do in your home. You don't call the plumber if you have a little backup in your pipes. You try a plunger, lift the back off the toilet and fiddle with the floating ball, and try to remedy the problem yourself. You don't call the exterminator when you spot a fly in the kitchen. You don't call the electrician if a lightbulb burns out. You rely on yourself for maintaining control over how your house ages—because you know that it's less expensive to prevent problems and treat minor ones than let everything deteriorate to the point where your house needs a major overhaul to continue functioning properly.

Ultimately, we want you to get comfortable enough with your own body so that you'll feel confident with basic body maintenance, so that you'll avoid the things that cause the most wear and tear and do the things that best maintain the long-term value of your body.

To do that, we'll show you such things as how your arteries clog, why you can't remember where you put your keys, how to have a more satisfying sex life, how to exercise your heart and bones, why your immune cells fight some diseases and not others, and what you can see on a tour inside your intestines (we told you we had waders). We'll explore your whole body so you can see how it works, as well as how to make it work better.

As you read this book, we hope that you learn a lot, laugh a little, and find the things in your life that you can change to take complete control of your health. Before we start, we think it's important to know a little bit more about the major principles and goals of *YOU: The Owner's Manual*. Here, we want to outline the most important things about health—about super health—that we want to pass along to you in this journey through the body.

YOU Control Your Health Destiny

If this world didn't have doctors, there'd probably be no such thing as quadruple bypasses, laser eye surgery, or illegible handwriting. But for all the wonderful things that organized medicine provides—from amazingly advanced treatments to cutting-edge research that will someday cure incurable diseases—this book isn't about organized medicine. It's not a guide to treatments, and it's not a textbook or encyclopedia. Think of it as a manual for prevention. *Your* manual for preventing the effects of aging—by keeping you feeling, looking, and being younger than your calendar age. Doctors will be the first ones to tell you that they can't keep you from getting heart disease, or put sunblock on your nose before a noontime run, or snatch the third Twinkie out of your paw before you torpedo it down your throat.

But you can.

You can control your health destiny. While you can't always control what happens to you (no matter how fit you are), there are some things you can control: your attitude, your determination, and—what serves as the crux of this book—your willingness to take your health into your own hands and know as much about your body as possible.

Now, in no way are we endorsing that you order a box of scalpels and remove suspect-looking moles from your arm or schedule a self-performed colonoscopy after the kids go to bed. (Even we don't do *that*.) We all need doctors. The point is that the power you have to control your health destiny is real—and it's in your hands, not someone else's.

In this book, we're going to give you dozens of recommendations that you can use to make yourself healthier; but to prove a point, we want to boil down the issue of personal control to one fact: If you make five—just five—adjustments to your life, you can have a dramatic effect on your life expectancy and the quality of your life. The five things are: controlling your blood pressure; avoiding cigarettes; exercising thirty minutes a day; controlling stress; and following an easy-to-love, healthy diet. (That last one is the basis of a major part of this book—The Owner's Manual Diet, which we'll discuss later in this chapter and in Chapter 13.) But if you can do those five things, in the next ten years you will have just a 10 percent chance of dying or having to suffer disability compared to a typical person your age. We'll take that bet.

YOU Can Choose Your Age

Whether you look at clocks, calendars, or hourglasses, time doesn't stop. It ticks and tocks at the same pace day after day, minute after minute, second after second. Everyone ages at the same rate with birthdays every year—that's your calendar age. But you have the power to turn your clock faster or slower with the lifestyle choices you make regarding what you do with your body and what you put into it. For example, a fifty-year-old who douses her lungs with nicotine and builds her food pyramid with chopped liver and sausage actually may have the body of a sixty-five-year-old because of the destruction she's doing, while a fifty-year-old who eats well, stays away from toxins, and takes care of her body with moderate physical activity could have the body and health of a thirty-six-year-old. Throughout the book, we'll refer to the RealAge effect that certain lifestyle choices have on your health. This is the basis of the RealAge concept. While some of you may be familiar with it, for those who aren't, it's the system that shows you how large an effect the choices you make can have on making yourself younger or accelerating your aging.

To show you the power you have, consider this: You control more than 70 percent of how well and how long you live. By the time you reach fifty, your lifestyle dictates 80 percent of how you age; the rest is controlled by inherited genetics.

Of course, we can't stop aging. That's because our bodies are continually aged by the environment through oxidation or other processes within your body. Oxidation, which is a lot like the rusting of your house's foundation or pillars, is a natural, important process that's a by-product of the proper functioning of your body. But when too much oxidation occurs, it puts you at a higher risk of aging—or rusting—of your body. It's why so many foods that are good for us are antioxidants—foods that slow the oxidation process. We do not know that the antioxidant property of these foods is responsible for the health benefits you get from them. But what we do know is that there are three main factors in age-related disease that you can control—and by controlling them, you slow the aging process. From a purely scientific perspective, we don't really know what causes aging, but we do know what makes us feel old before age one hundred, and that's age-related disease. So we can tell you 80 percent of how to stop these three factors in age-related disease. They are:

★   aging of your heart and blood vessels (responsible for things like strokes, heart attacks, memory loss, and impotence, when arteries cut off nutrient-rich blood to important organs)

★   aging of your immune system (which leads to autoimmune diseases, infection, and cancer)

★   aging caused by environmental or social issues (accidents and social factors like stress are very powerful factors that contribute to aging)

Of course, we're going to show you how all of these systems work and what you can do to keep everything young, but the important concept to remember is that the RealAge effects you'll see in the book help put a value on all of these factors. It's almost like longevity currency.

One way to make the body come alive is to show real anatomy, so we have fun illustrations with our mascot elf helping you understand the subtle elements of your organs. The pictures are medically accurate, even though subtle humor slips into the drawings. The devil is in the details, so spend some time with the anatomy.

And as a bonus, we even give you crib sheets (Table 1.1, page 30) to make it easy to manage your own health.

YOU Are on Your Way to Living with More Vitality

Flipping through the newspaper, you can read about all kinds of news—whether it's about international conflicts or another celebrity breakup. But sometimes, at least to us, it seems that the only health news that gets attention is the bad news. Every time you turn the page, you read a stat or a story that is depressing: There's another famous case of Alzheimer's. Diabetes rates are skyrocketing. Americans are fatter than an A-lister's wallet. The effect? Eventually, it seems so depressing that you avoid health news and information the way polar bears avoid Fiji. Yes, we have some serious health problems to address, but they are only one side of the story.

For starters, look at the average life expectancy: forty-seven in 1900, and nearly eighty in 2000. A lot of credit for these extra thirty-three years goes to public health and organized medicine. So statistics show that we're going to live long. Maybe the most impressive statistics are these: While the rest of the world thinks we have the corner on obesity, there may be signs we're changing. From 1966 to 1996, the number of Americans who engaged in regular physical activity decreased by 1 percent every year. But from 1996 to 2006, the amount of physical activity grew by 1 percent every year. Smoking prevalence decreased from 50 percent of the adult population in 1970 to 23 percent in 2004. And the people with high blood pressure who went untreated fell from 80 percent in 1970 to 37 percent in 2005.

Even corporate America is catching on: General Mills stopped selling cereal that isn't whole grain, and Wal-Mart no longer distributes foods with evil trans fats or sells fish with toxins—important signals to food manufacturers that we can demand healthier products.

What does this all mean? Although we're not perfect, we are making progress—by increasing activity, squashing cigarettes, and changing our diets. And that points to the fact that the person who has the most say over how well you age isn't us or even your regular doctors. It's the one who has five fingers on either side of this book.

YOU Should Think of Medicine as Part Science, Part Art

Sometimes people think medicine is a connect-the-dots kind of field. Symptom A plus symptom B must equal disease C. In some ways, the body is a logical, mechanical factory that works by doing the same routine over and over and over again. While researchers have certainly figured out many of the idiosyncrasies about the way the body works, sometimes the workers in the factory take a break, or decide they want to do something else, or even go on a rampage and mess up the whole assembly line. We don't always know why these problems happen—or even what they mean. That's why there are thousands of researchers who dedicate their lives to exploring cell behavior in humans and animals to get a better understanding of the body.

To that end, there's a lot the scientific community knows about your body, and we hope to relay some of the most important elements to you. Medicine has an intricate process of proof that helps us move past myths to recommendations supported by hard science. This works for many treatments and prevention methods. For others, medicine hasn't gone though the full range of research, but there's enough anecdotal and preliminary scientific evidence for us to make recommendations to our family and friends, and that's also what we'll tell you.

Ultimately, we're going to concentrate on the organs and conditions most important in the aging process, as well as the conditions that are the most preventable. So don't expect that we'll cover every type of disease; instead, we'll concentrate on the ones that science has helped prove that we can prevent.

Food Is Fuel: The Owner's Manual Diet

We all know what happens when the power lines outside your house go down. The electricity is low, and you can't generate enough power to work the toaster, turn on the TV, or power the hair dryer. Just in the way that low electricity levels can change many things about the way you live, so does your diet. The factors from the outside change the way you work on the inside. Depending on what you put into your body—as well as in what amounts and how often—it affects how you feel and how you live.

Now, of course, there are lots of reasons to eat—you're bored, you're at a party, your kid left seventeen fries on the plate. The ultimate reason to eat is to provide fuel for your body—not only to keep you lean, energetic, and strong, but also to feed your organs with the foods and nutrients that they crave to keep your entire internal infrastructure running smoothly. If you don't understand how the body processes food—as well as all of the inner workings of your body—you can't understand why and how food is important. Once you see how certain foods function, you'll understand how eating them will make you feel better and be healthier—and even lose weight in the process.

A major part of this book will be our discussion about what foods play a role in the livelihood of different organs and anatomical processes, so we'll arm you with the Owner's Manual Diet, explained in detail in Chapter 13. We'll provide you a ten-day, thirty-recipe plan that shows you a way of eating that's designed for optimum health. It's not a calorie-restricted weight-loss diet per se, though one of the side effects will be that you lose weight. Within each chapter, we'll provide the nutrients that are best for that part of the body and the foods that contain those nutrients so you can tailor your diet to your specific health needs. Two of the differences between our diet and so many others is that it's great tasting and it's easy—no induction phases, no counting or weighing, no maintenance dieting. What we want to emphasize is that you can change the way your body works—and the way you feel—with the food you eat. The diet focuses on foods like healthy fats, whole-grain foods, fruits and vegetables, protein, and the many other nutrients that your body is meant to have. By following the great-tasting Owner's Manual Diet, you'll feed your organs the nutrients they need to function better, to stave off disease, and to keep your body healthy.

Two other important points to consider when thinking about food is how the nutrients you put into you mouth are processed—and why your body processes them in a certain way. In order to understand nutrition, you'll need to know a little about metabolism—and the way your body digests food for energy. See, when most people diet, they don't eat enough—and they actually slow their metabolism; they go into a pseudo-starvation mode in which their bodies stop burning calories as fast because they sense they need to preserve them. That's why exercise is so important. Physical activity helps keep the metabolic rate moving quickly, because exercise is what gives your body approval to burn calories. So you essentially have to exercise in order to keep your body from panicking and going into starvation mode. Together, exercise and eating make the Owner's Manual Diet a way of life.

Testing Your BQ: The Body-Quotient Quiz

Everyone knows that IQ (intelligence quotient) measures your smarts. There's also such a thing as EQ (emotional quotient), which measures traits linked to personality and character. Though some people may live and die by DQ (Dairy Queen), our favorite acronym is BQ: body quotient. How much do you know about your body? Sure, you know your legs make you run, your liver cleans up your happy-hour shenanigans, and your gut makes a nice ledge for your bottle of Bud, but we want to give you a little test—to introduce your to how cool your body is and to challenge your preconceived notions about how your body works and ages.

Though you've lived in yours for thirty, forty, fifty, sixty, maybe seventy or more years, our contention is that you probably don't know your body as intimately as you think. By knowing your body, you develop a base of knowledge that gives you the power and authority to preserve and strengthen your life.

Don't worry if you fail this Body-Quotient Quiz because we'll answer everything throughout the book. Remember, too, that after you're finished with our book, you have ready tutors: your doctors. And you should use your doctors for more than just signing prescriptions. Use them as teachers; after all, that's what the word *doctor* means in Latin. Most want to be used this way—it is their fun, let them have it. Ask them questions. Use their knowledge to learn more about how *your* body works.

So now pluck that pencil from your kid's backpack, and take a guess at these questions. At the end, flip to the back pages in this chapter, check out the answers, and find out how well you know your body.

The BQ Quiz: How Body Smart Are You?

1. Which of the following ages you the least?
    a. Smoking one pack of cigarettes a day
    b. A HDL (good) cholesterol level of 29 mg/dl
    c. Consistently avoiding "cleaning grout" on your to-do list
    d. Eating steak twice a week

2. What is the ideal blood pressure?
    a. 115/76
    b. Anything less than 140/90
    c. Whatever the heck made George Burns live to one hundred
    d. Depends on your family history

3. Which of the following is the best advice about diets?
    a. The less you eat, the more weight you'll lose
    b. The best diet is one you can follow forever
    c. A good weight-loss diet include foods with little or no fat
    d. Would somebody please pass the bacon?

4. What is the greatest threat to your arteries?
    a. An elevated blood pressure of 160/90
    b. An elevated LDL (bad) cholesterol of 200
    c. An elevated helping of fried zucchini sticks
    d. An elevated amount of time spent on the couch

5. Which of the following conditions is not primarily caused by the deterioration of arteries?

   a. Strokes

   b. Wrinkles

   c. Diabetes

   d. Impotence

6. What's the best Valentine's Day gift you can give your partner to make him/her healthier?

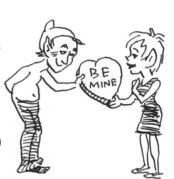

   a. A little real chocolate candy for its nutritional effects

   b. Schedule a warm massage for loosening up muscles

   c. Flowers, for their therapeutic and aromatic effects

   d. I'll be more than happy to take a spin through the Victoria's Secret catalog to get a few ideas

7. What is the ideal amount of aspirin you should take to decrease arterial aging?

   a. Whatever it takes to cure a hangover

   b. Two or more baby aspirins or half a regular aspirin

   c. One baby aspirin

   d. None; ibuprofen is better

8. What is the most revealing sign that you might have Alzheimer's-related dementia?

   a. You constantly forget where you put your keys

   b. You can't recognize information that someone told you five minutes ago

   c. You forget that you told the same story to your coworkers last week

   d. What was the question again?

9. *What food has qualities least similar to that of an addictive drug?*
   a.   No. 2 with a large Coke and a chocolate shake
   b.   Peanuts
   c.   Potatoes
   d.   Sugary cereals

10. *Which of the following is true about the gender differences in brains?*
    a.   Men are able to solve problems faster while women analyze complex issues better
    b.   Women have more emotional intelligence than men
    c.   Men's brains have a neural substation hiding under their Calvin Kleins
    d.   Men and women have the same brain system

11. *What's the best kind of crossword puzzle you can do for your brain?*
    a.   Whatever's available on the back of the toilet at the time
    b.   One you can finish
    c.   One you can't finish
    d.   I don't know, but I'm looking for an eight-letter insulin secretor starting with a *p* and ending with an *s*

12. *What size particles are most hazardous to your lungs?*
    a.   Size of the peanut, since they can block your windpipe
    b.   Size of small pieces of tobacco
    c.   Size of the stuff that causes smog
    d.   Size so small that you'd need more than the usual light-powered microscope to see them

13. *Fill in the blank with the most appropriate comparison. Sleep is like _____.*
    a. Sex, because you can never get too much
    b. Seat belts, because it helps your body come to a stop
    c. Your boss, because it's most agreeable when it's uninterrupted
    d. Church, because it's always so quiet and peaceful

14. *What is excessive snoring the sign of?*
    a. That you stopped breathing
    b. That there's some kind of obstruction in your throat
    c. That you haven't had enough sleep
    d. Imminent divorce

15. *What's the equivalent risk of an hour's exposure to secondhand smoke?*
    a. Smoking four cigarettes yourself
    b. Driving without a seat belt
    c. Sunning yourself for an hour without sunscreen
    d. Having a cholesterol level of 240

16. *Which of the following is not an inherited taste?*
    a. Sweet
    b. Sour
    c. Adam Sandler movies
    d. Fat

17. *Your intestines are most similar to what other organ?*
    a. Your heart, because it pumps nutrients through the body
    b. Your brain, because it releases the same chemicals
    c. Your vocal cords, because they growl when you're hungry
    d. The big one at the back of the church, because it makes all kinds of majestic sounds

18. *Who is most likely to give you a stomach ulcer?*
    a.   Your boss (from stress)
    b.   Your chef (from bad food)
    c.   Your spouse (from kissing)
    d.   Yourself (from overeating)

19. *What is the major function of the colon?*
    a.   To signal your brain that you're full
    b.   To suck fluid into your body
    c.   To digest food and get rid of gas
    d.   To separate an independent clause from a dependent one

20. *Which trick has been shown scientifically to help you eat less at a meal?*
    a.   Eating a lot at your previous meal
    b.   Eating fat at the start of every meal
    c.   Duct tape
    d.   Drinking a nondiet soft drink before your meal

21. *What is the reason that men can drink more alcohol than women?*
    a.   Two words: *Animal House*
    b.   Men have more testosterone
    c.   Men are bigger physically
    d.   Men's blood gets less of what they consume

22. *Where does conception take place?*
    a.   Uterus
    b.   Fallopian tubes
    c.   Cervix
    d.   The Holiday Inn

23. *Complete the following sentence. The size of a man's sex organ _____ .*
   a.   Has got to make you wonder what Speedo was thinking
   b.   Is based on the need to attract members of the opposite sex
   c.   Is important for proper prostate function and sexual satisfaction
   d.   Doesn't matter

24. *Which of these substances is most responsible for sex drive in both men and women?*
   a.   Tequila
   b.   Estrogen
   c.   Testosterone
   d.   Nicotine

25. *What is the best test to measure if you have the cardiovascular stamina to have sex?*
   a.   Do ten push-ups without stopping
   b.   Climb two flights of stairs without stopping
   c.   Run on a treadmill for ten minutes
   d.   Practice by yourself

26. *In menopause, what is the major thing that happens?*
   a.   The ovaries signal they have only a few eggs left
   b.   A woman loses her ability to have sustained levels of growth hormone and estrogen
   c.   A woman's sexual desire decreases
   d.   Husbands seek shelter from pan flinging

27. *What does a Pap smear detect?*
   a.   Herpes
   b.   Cervical cancer
   c.   Fertility
   d.   Nasty gossip from old friends

28. What foods increase fertility rates?
    a. Walnuts
    b. Oysters
    c. Calcium-rich foods
    d. Anything, as long as it includes flowers, a couple bottles of wine, and a nice night of dancing

29. What are the most active muscles in the body?
    a. The ones used in your back
    b. The ones used around your jaw
    c. The ones used around your eyes
    d. The ones used during your honeymoon

30. Why should you avoid using Q-tips to clean your ears?
    a. It breaks most of Emily Post's major rules about dinner-table manners
    b. It can tear your eardrum
    c. It can push the wax into position to block sound waves
    d. Cleaning ear wax just increases the amount you produce

31. What is an indication that you're legally blind?
    a. You wear pink pants with a red shirt
    b. Your loved ones accuse you of having no insight
    c. You can't see the big letters on a vision chart from a distance of twenty feet
    d. You can't read this, Mr. Magoo

32. What part of the body is least likely to be damaged by the sun?
    a. Your eyes, because they're not skin
    b. Your scalp, because it's covered by hair
    c. Your butt, because it's covered by clothes (or hair)
    d. The backs of your ears, because they're such a small area

33. *What is the main purpose of skin?*
    a.   To keep Hef in business
    b.   To protect your insides from the outside world
    c.   To keep salt and potassium inside your cells
    d.   To hold hair follicles

34. *What is the most likely effect of training for and running a marathon?*
    a.   You will develop the cardiovascular endurance of elite athletes
    b.   You will do long-term damage to your bones and joints
    c.   You will breathe in a lethal amount of toxins if you race in a large city
    d.   You'll win a role as Bond's girl

35. *Which of the following is true about joints?*
    a.   They're almost all constructed with just two bones and a hinge in between
    b.   Most link bones with a hinge that is lubricated better when you eat fish oils or nuts
    c.   They're all composed of muscles, tendons, ligaments, cartilage, nerves, and bones
    d.   They're illegal in at least forty-eight states

36. *Which of the following is true about the bone condition osteoporosis?*
    a.   It's the leading cause of most hip fractures in women but not men
    b.   Its risks are reduced with lunges, squats, vitamin D, and calcium in both men and women
    c.   It causes aches and pains
    d.   It's more common in larger people because they have more bone mass

37. *Which of the following is true about the joint condition osteoarthritis?*
    a.   It's found in 85 percent of people over age eighty-five
    b.   It's something you don't need to worry about until you're eighty-five

     c.   It's made worse by cracking your knuckles

     d.   It's made better by swimming

38.   *Which of the following is true about your bones?*

     a.   They're fully formed by the age twenty-three

     b.   They have a matrix structure like the Eiffel Tower

     c.   They weaken in women, but not men

     d.   They're the hardest substance in your body

39.   *What's the primary role of your muscles?*

     a.   To sell jeans on Times Square billboards

     b.   To help us move, think, breathe, and urinate

     c.   To justify a gym membership

     d.   To store carbohydrates and sugars that your body digests

40.   *Which of the following is true about back pain?*

     a.   It originates in your pelvic muscles

     b.   It gets more common as you get older

     c.   It's reduced by those weight belts often worn by people who exercise or work in warehouses

     d.   It can be largely prevented by doing exercise that centers around the pelvis and abdomen

41.   *What are the three best forms of physical activity?*

     a.   Cardiovascular exercise, weight training, any other

     b.   Walking, running, swimming

     c.   Morning sex, afternoon sex, evening sex

     d.   Does taking a shower count as physical activity?

42. *Which of the following is most important when training with weights?*
    a.   That you do enough repetitions and weight so that your muscles fatigue
    b.   That you use exercise machines
    c.   That you have a good view of the mirror
    d.   That you follow the form of other people in the gym

43. *Walking with "little" three-pound dumbbells in your hands is . . . :*
    a.   A good way to build muscle and get a cardiovascular workout
    b.   An easy way to increase your calorie burn dramatically
    c.   Putting you at risk for shoulder injury
    d.   A heck of a lot better than walking with three-pound ankle weights

44. *What is the first line of defense against infection?*
    a.   A sneeze or cough
    b.   The antibodies in your mouth and nose
    c.   Bathing with antibacterial soap
    d.   Your skin

45. *What is the worst part about untreated low-grade infections that don't have overt symptoms?*
    a.   They can cause you to miss work
    b.   They can cause cancer of the pancreas
    c.   They can cause chronic inflammation in your arteries
    d.   They can make you resistant to antibiotics

46. *What is the safest way to shorten the duration of the common cold?*
    a.   Your mom's chicken soup
    b.   Zinc lozenges
    c.   Vitamin C and bed rest
    d.   Antibiotics

47. *What is the best thing you can do to prevent infections?*
    a.   Use a water filter
    b.   Use condoms
    c.   Wash your hands
    d.   Stop taking antibiotics as soon as the infection is gone

48. *What is the most common hormone abnormality in people older than sixty?*
    a.   Hypothyroidism
    b.   Diabetes
    c.   Testosterone deficiency
    d.   Loss of sex drive (aka Brad-Pittuitary deficiency)

49. *Which of the following is true about hormones?*
    a.   More is better
    b.   Plant hormones are natural
    c.   All decrease as you age
    d.   Most over-the-counter hormone supplements are shams

50. *Which of the following is true about cancer?*
    a.   It is almost never preventable
    b.   You cannot coexist with cancer
    c.   There are no cancers that are 100 percent lethal
    d.   Most cancers are contagious

Answers to The BQ Quiz: How Body Smart Are You?

1. D: Eating steak twice a week makes you less than one year older compared to smoking a pack of cigarettes (eight years older), an inadequate healthy HDL cholesterol of 29 (about four years older), and the stress of avoiding a nagging task makes you eight years older.

2. A: The ideal blood pressure is 115/76, established in fifty-six studies and fifty-two countries and over 20 million people. It is the same in New Delhi as it is in Chicago as it is in Tokyo. A lower blood pressure does not add much to your rate of aging, but higher numbers aren't good—over 50 percent of heart attacks can be attributed to a blood pressure between 125/80 and 140/90.

3. B: The key to a diet is loving it and being able to stay on it. Eating too little will slow your metabolism.

4. A: Blood pressure of 160/90 is more than three times more of a threat to make your arteries dysfunctional than any of the others. That doesn't mean you should avoid physical activity or avoid lowering a lousy cholesterol reading; it just means that your blood pressure may be the most important number you know, other than your spouse's birthday, especially if your blood pressure is over 160/90.

5. C: Diabetes makes disease of the arteries worse but is primarily a genetic disease made more evident by obesity in adults. The others—impotence, wrinkling of the skin, and strokes—are like heart attacks: They are primarily caused by the aging of your arteries.

6. A: The flavonoids and healthier fat in real cocoa-based chocolate make it healthy. Scheduling a massage does not count until you get it.

7.   B: The data show that you get as much benefit for preventing arterial disease and cancer from two or more baby aspirins as from a full aspirin. And two baby aspirins are more than twice as good at preventing arterial disease as is one baby aspirin.

8.   B: While you forget recent information with Alzheimer's, the forgetfulness is so profound that you can't recognize that you forgot.

9.   B: Only peanuts don't cause the direct release of the pleasure neurotransmitter dopamine. Peanuts are actually a healthy substance with both healthy fat and healthy protein.

10. A: Those are the data; nothing more said.

11. C: By consistently challenging yourself, you increase the growth of brain cell dendrites and brain functioning.

12. D: Smaller particles escape your natural defenses of the beating brushes in your trachea and get deep into your lung, where they can cause inflammation, among other problems.

13. C: The more uninterrupted your sleep, the better it is, because you get the rapid eye movement and slow wave sleep patterns that are restorative to functioning.

14. B: Snoring is caused by a narrowed passage for air to move through. It's actually the sound of turbulence in the air movement caused by partial obstruction rather than smooth airflow.

15. A: Secondhand smoke is remarkably similar to firsthand smoke when it comes to its health effects in making your arteries dysfunctional and causing impotence.

16. D: Fat is a learned taste, so you can change what kind of fats you enjoy tasting over an eight-week period.

17. B: Your intestine is very similar to your brain because of its nervous system and chemicals.

18. C: The bacteria that cause most stomach ulcers can be transmitted back and forth from significant others.

19. B: You need to remove the fluid to concentrate your stool and also to maintain a high enough fluid level in the rest of your body.

20. B: Eating a little fat first at the start of every meal slows your stomach from emptying; you feel full sooner and stay full longer, so you don't want to eat as much.

21. D: Men have more of the acid alcohol dehydrogenase in their gut lining, which metabolizes about half of the alcohol before it gets into their blood.

22. B: The fertilized egg implants itself in the uterus. The actual site where the sperm fertilizes the egg is often in the Fallopian tubes but can occur almost anywhere the two get together.

23. B: Yup, that's the reason (from an evolutionary perspective).

24. C: In both genders, testosterone influences sex drive.

25. B: If you can't climb two flights of stairs without stopping, then sex is risky and you need more practice.

26. A: The ovaries apparently help govern the start of menopause rather than the brain just sending signals south.

27. B: This test is important for women to get at least every year if they are sexually active.

28. A: Walnuts actually have the highest quantity of omega-3 fatty acids of all nuts. Omega 3s improve fertility rates in both males and females by improving the functional swimming ability of the sperm and improving the environment implantation in the women. Other reasons may exist as well.

29. C: They are always moving.

30. B: The smallest thing you should put in your ear is your elbow.

31. C: If you can't do this, you may need to listen to this book.

32. C: Ever see a wrinkled butt?

33. B: The skin is a major protection for you.

34. B: Yes, there is such a thing as too much exercise.

35. B: Fish oil and nuts are a great way to reduce pain and to keep your joints functioning for the long term.

36. B: You strengthen your bones by doing exercises that stress the muscles and joints that surround them or connect them. Vitamin D and calcium are important as well for both men and women.

37. A: That's why it is so important to do things to keep your joints acting less than age eighty-five.

38. B: Yes, the Eiffel Tower was designed with your bones in mind and is incredibly sturdy as a result.

39. B: Didn't think they did all that, did you? Muscles do help you move, breathe, and urinate, and they even help you think, since exercise keeps your brain younger.

40. D: Like most things, you can prevent or reduce back pain with just a little consistent effort in advance or after it gets better.

41. A: The three components of physical activity that independently affect your health include any physical activity, strength training, and exercise that makes you sweat in a cool room. But to have the greatest chance of succeeding, do the "any activity" like walking before the weight training, and do the weight training before cardiovascular activity.

42. A: It's only when your muscles are fatiguing within twelve repetitions that you are actually building strength in the muscles rather than just increasing their stamina.

43. C: Walking with little dumbbells should help employ an orthopedic surgeon who concentrates on shoulder repairs.

44. D: Your skin really does the best job.

45. C: Low-grade infections may be much worse than having high cholesterol in making your arteries dysfunctional.

46. A: We don't know any dangers of your mom's chicken soup, and it does shorten the length of time course for the common cold as much as zinc lozenges or vitamin C do.

47. C: Your mom was right.

48. A: Hypothyroidism is present in more than 10 percent of people over the age of sixty, which is one reason why we urge you to get a thyroid test every five years starting at forty-five.

49. D: Well, at least the worst that happens is that there is a transfer of money from you to the person selling, and you most likely won't get sick from it.

50. C: That's right, there's hope with even the worst, and spontaneous recovery as your immune system fights back.

Your Score:
Give yourself one point for each one you got right to get your final BQ score.

45–50:   EXCELLENT. You've either been accepted to medical school or watch way too many *ER* reruns. Prescription: The medical texts are on the next shelf, Doogie.

30–44:   GOOD. You know more about the human body than many people. With a good, strong basis in anatomical knowledge, you'll appreciate the insights and action steps of this book. Prescription: Read one chapter a night for two weeks.

16–29:   AVERAGE. Though you wouldn't break any *Jeopardy* records, you know enough about your body to understand its complexity and artistry. Prescription: Take the next 371 pages and call us in the morning.

0–15:   WHAT, YOU A LIZARD OR SOMETHING? The bad news is that you need to explore the human body a lot more. The good news is that you can become an expert with a strong dose of knowledge, supplemented by a lifelong course of action. Prescription: Turn the page and get crackin'.

TABLE 1.1 **List of Crib Sheets**

The Owner's Manual Workout	Page 446
Yoga Sun Salutation	Page 132
Physical Activity	Page 135
Sleep	Page 156
Diet Activity Plan	Page 364
Diet Basics	Page 367

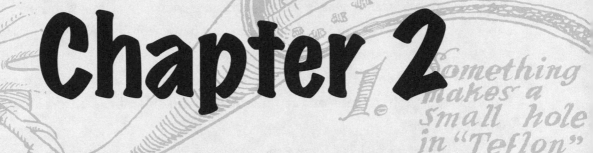

Chapter 2

The Beat Goes On: Your Heart and Arteries

1. Something makes a small hole in "Teflon" lining.

Major Myths About Your Heart

Heart Myth #1   You'll know when you're having a heart attack.

Heart Myth #2   The biggest threat to your arteries is cholesterol.

Heart Myth #3   An artery clogged 90 percent is worse than one clogged 50 percent.

2. Cholesterol fills the hole...but sloppily.

For all the attention that hearts get, you've got to pity your body's other organs. It's not like seventh-grade girls doodle small intestines when they go gaga over a cute boy. Candy makers aren't packaging chocolate caramels in boxes the shape of bladders. The Tin Man didn't plead for a new esophagus. And when was the last time you ever played blackjack with a queen of spleens? All for good reason, too. As the symbol of love and courage, the heart is more than just inspiration for songwriters, poets, tattoo artists, and celebrity stalkers. And it's more than just a symbol for life. It *is* life.

Your heart, which is a lot like the water main of your anatomical house, provides the nutrients you need to live. In your house, clean water lets you drink safely and wash away germs. In your body, your heart pumps blood to every room in your body—to your brain so you can think, to your sex organs so you can procreate, to your digestive system so you can process food, to your muscles so you can help your neighbors move their piano.

The fact is, you feel an intimacy with and awareness of your heart that you probably feel with few other organs (except maybe those we talk about in Chapter 8). We've understood this reality as far back as prehistoric times, because the heart has another advantage over many other organs: It is palpable; we can feel its presence and its work just by pressing on our chest or grabbing our wrist for a few seconds. As our internal metronome, it measures out the music of our lives (and our health), and it keeps us alive. Besides speaking in public and using bus station restrooms, nothing scares us more than this fact: If our heart stops working, so do we.

Coronary artery disease, or CAD, is the leading cause of death in every developed country. Every American, Asian, and European has a 40 percent chance of dying of heart disease and a 50 percent chance that his or her quality of life will be damaged by arterial aging disease. That last part is a real kicker because many people, especially if they're young, worry more about hangnails than they do about death. But when you realize that arterial aging affects a lot more than the arteries going to your heart, the importance of arterial health becomes clearer. Damaged arteries slow down your memory, the ability of your other organs to function, and your sex life. In other words, they slow *you* down.

See, when your heart is working right, it's an astoundingly efficient machine. The blood vessels supplying the muscles in your body are open and supple like rubber bicycle inner tubes that expand as needed. The blood vessels leaving your heart shuttle blood throughout your body from one source to another, no matter how much you need. Your heart is so powerful that it can change pumping levels to whatever situation you're in, whether you're walking on a treadmill or escaping from an angry flock of geese. Imagine clenching your fist sixty to seventy times per minute for your entire life, which is essentially what your heart does—without ever becoming exhausted. That pumping processes five liters of blood per minute when you're resting. When you decide to pop in your Richard Simmons workout tape, you're immediately pumping twenty liters of blood. Your heart is equipped to handle the drastic change, but it can't work alone, and it can't work efficiently if you don't take care of it.

The most important factor in your heart's health and ability to pump more blood is its own blood supply—the efficiency of your coronary arteries to transport blood to your heart. The most common barrier to that supply is coronary artery disease, in which the arteries become narrowed or blocked. When that happens, your heart muscle weakens from lack of blood. Luckily, you—and not some city bureaucracy—act as the water company of your body. You supply the ingredients that dictate what fluids run through your pipes and damage or protect the lining—through what you eat, how you exercise, and how you respond to social and environmental stresses. You have the power to make your heart both stronger and younger—making your heart the most life-giving organ in your body. And if that doesn't deserve a spot on Valentine's Day boxer shorts, we're not sure what does.

Your Heart: The Anatomy

Another way to think about your heart and vascular system is by picturing a subway or train system. Your heart is the main station, the hub, the place through which all trains must travel. The arteries and veins are the tracks and tunnels—the pathways that flow all over your body, dropping passengers (blood) to stations all over the body (the Saturday-evening train toward those Jockeys is especially crowded). Now, if there's a break in the tracks—or some kind of obstruction that won't let the trains through—that's when the customers get irate. If that blockage goes on long enough, it can put some organs right out of a job. In your body, a station without blood is a station that will shut down—and could in turn shut down many stations around it. If that Saturday train doesn't make it to its final destination, for example, impotence occurs. To understand the concept a little better, let's pull out the map and take a ride. Ticket, please.

Your Heart

When we feel our own pulse pressing upward to our skin, we tend to picture the heart beating like a drum or a ball being squeezed, pushing outward on each beat. But the heart really twists or wrings blood out like wringing water from a towel more than thumps. It begins like this: Electricity from special cells (called pacemaker cells)—starting at the top of the heart and moving down—stimulates the heart muscle to wring the blood out through the aortic valve. The wave of blood that has been twisted out of the heart is ejected into the aorta itself, the body's largest artery, which carries oxygen-rich blood to the rest of the body. Once that happens, the heart relaxes—as if your hands had just let go of the towel. As it does, the coronary vessels, which lie on the surface of the heart, also relax. Then the space between the tight muscle cells opens up, and the rich, oxygenated blood that was just ejected from

Myth or Fact?
You'll know when the big one is coming

Half of all people who have heart attacks have never felt a symptom — or at least never recognized what they felt as a symptom. Part of the problem is that a heart attack happens in very different ways — and the discomfort can come and go, which makes it easier to blame it on something else, like digestive upsets. The most common signs are the following:

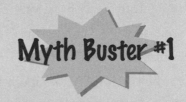

Myth Buster #1

★ chest pain or discomfort (can feel like pressure, fullness, or squeezing)
★ discomfort in upper body (could be one or the other arm, back, neck, jaw, or stomach)
★ shortness of breath
★ cold sweat
★ nausea
★ sudden extreme fatigue (without lack of sleep)

The reason the pain or discomfort can be so unpredictable (the reason, for instance, that Larry King felt intense pain in his right arm, which is not the usual side for heart pain) is that the heart itself does not feel pain; it does not have specific pain fibers. The heart's nerves do not feel pain directly. But when something is going wrong with the heart, its nerves may become electrically unstable. And when they cross the spinal column, they may short-circuit other nerves — nerves that connect with your arm, for example, or your chest. And *those* nerves are the ones that transmit the pain impulses. So your arm aches, or your chest, or your jaw, wherever nerves are being shorted out. The brain sometimes also joins the action by stimulating the vagus nerve to cause stomach upset and a cold sweat. But if these nerve fibers do not cross, you won't have any discomfort, even while having a heart attack, and that's why so many people don't know they are having a heart attack.

the heart fills the arteries on the heart's surface and slips down between those cells and feeds them. Most of the ejected blood goes on to fuel the rest of the body—but not before the heart puts its own tax on it, taking its first cut of the life-sustaining fluid.

Your heart has a very clever way of ensuring its own survival—and, therefore, *your* survival. It takes care of itself first before it takes care of any other organ. Just as a mother eats food for herself before she feeds her baby milk, your heart has to get its fill of blood before it can accomplish its job of pumping elsewhere. It's as if your body had its own little retirement fund for your future welfare: You pay a little bit to

FACTOID

As the heart develops in the unborn child, it takes on several distinct appearances, each resembling other animal hearts and each a step higher on the evolutionary ladder. At first, the tubelike heart is much like a fish heart. When it divides into two chambers, it is similar to a frog heart; with three chambers, a snake or turtle heart. Finally, with four chambers, a fully formed heart looks like what it is: the most highly evolved heart of a mammal. The four-chambered heart has a distinct advantage over simpler structures: It allows us to send our "dirty" blood to the cleaners—the lungs—and our "clean" blood to the rest of the body without having to mix the two, a very efficient system. The blood coming from the left side of the heart is pure, fully oxygenated, ready to fuel the muscles; a fish heart, on the other hand, has to pump blood to the body that is only half as pure, because it doesn't have separate chambers that enable it to clean the blood in one cycle and then distribute it in the next. Our sophisticated ticker allows us to process energy more efficiently and therefore move farther from our energy source—we can do lots of work in between looking for food, while a fish has to live in its energy source, eating all the time. Unfortunately, this efficiency also enables humans to easily store extra energy, especially as dreaded fat.

your heart first with each beat, and the better you are able to do that (by pumping blood through the coronary arteries), the better your life will be as you age. After the process of towel wringing—squeezing blood into the aorta followed by muscle relaxation—and the heart feeding itself—then, sixty or more times a minute, the pacemakers send out their next signal, beginning the process all over again.

Your Arteries

Your arteries have three layers, each one with a unique job. The innermost layer, the one in contact with the blood as it flows through, is called the intima. It's nice and slippery, like Teflon, so the blood can easily flow over it. In a normal state, that interior layer, lined with a layer of cells, is perfectly smooth, keeping the trains moving fast and efficiently. It's also where the initial action of heart disease takes place, as we'll discuss in a moment. This inner lining also helps protect the middle layer, called the media, which supports the structure of the artery. The media is muscular, so it can respond to what's going on in your head or somewhere else in your body: it spasms when you're depressed or anxious, and opens up when you exercise to allow more blood through to supply the individual muscles. The outer layer is the adventitia, and it's like a sausage casing; it holds your artery together from the outside, within a kind of cellophane wrap. Several things, of course, can throw the works off schedule, and you can see how the process functions in Figure 2.1. They are:

NICKS   The smooth lining inside of arteries maintains its integrity with delicate cells that can be injured by subtle abnormalities such as too much sugar or pressure in the bloodstream, or by toxic products like nicotine or homocysteine. When these smooth-lining cells are injured, they pull away from each other and form a gap. The resulting "nick" has to be closed quickly to protect the blood vessel lining. Nicks are caused by a raft of factors that you can largely control: high blood pressure, high blood levels of some compounds like homocysteine, smoking, chronic inflammation from things as diverse as gum (periodontal) disease or sexually transmitted disease, stress, anger, and having a too-high blood sugar level. Most of these you can control, even if your mom and every uncle in your family had them: high blood pressure can be reduced to normal with physical activity or diet (more on this later), or pills, if need be; homocysteine can be genetic or it can occur from too much protein or too little folic acid (folate, a vitamin) in your diet; you can prevent STDs with condoms and gum disease with floss and teeth cleaning. Similarly, you can prevent nicks from each of the other conditions (see the Live Younger action plan below). But the nick itself is the first step. It is then plastered over by a cholesterol patch, which then causes inflammation and attracts more clots.

CLOGS   Your body gets upset when a flaw—a tear or nick—occurs in the artery's inner lining, because then the middle lining is exposed to the blood. So your body, like a handyman hired to patch up your drywall, rushes in with plaster to cover up the wounds in the inner lining. (The plaster itself ends up making the problem worse, which we'll discuss in a moment.) While one type of plaster—the cholesterol—has gotten more bad press than child actors, its bad rep is not really fair. Cholesterol is actually essential to your body's functioning. While the lousy (LDL) cholesterol deserves the bad press, the good or healthy kind of cholesterol is carried through your body by high-density lipoprotein (HDL) and acts as the spatula of your arterial system—so that type of cholesterol

FIGURE 2.1 # Aging Arteries

High blood pressure, high blood sugar, the effects of cigarettes, and other factors can nick the smooth inner layer of your arteries. Your body tries to repair that nick using cholesterol as a plaster. But if the proteins carrying the cholesterol are bad (LDL), an inflammatory reaction is triggered that signals for white cells to invade the area. The resulting plaque becomes irritated and ruptures, which encourages a blood clot to form. That clot can suddenly block the entire artery—and lead to heart attack, stroke, impotence, and memory loss.

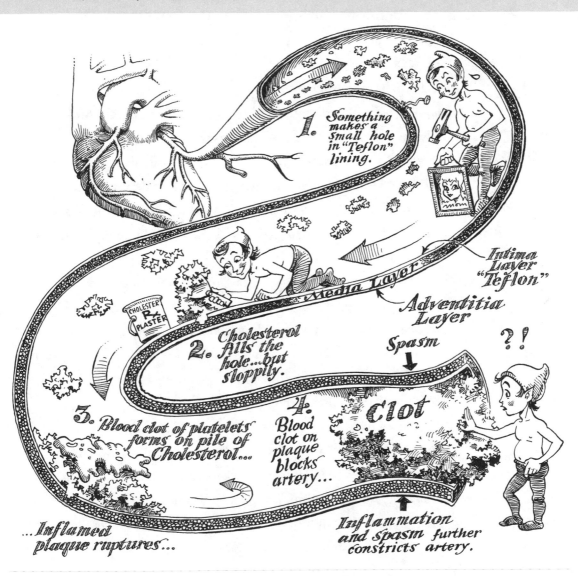

deserves praise. Compact and powerful, it comes in and swoops through your arteries to try to take the extra plaster away. The bad or lousy cholesterol, which is carried by low-density lipoprotein (LDL), is like a defective Macy's Thanksgiving Day balloon. It's big and puffy, unstable, and prone to breaking up and scattering bits of cholesterol when it hits the walls of the artery. Now, when your LDL levels are high to begin with (maybe from your diet, or maybe from heredity), and then you go and damage the inner lining of your arteries, your body gets carried away with plaster. In its zeal to heal, it starts covering up the damage with the "bad" cholesterol, slapping it on like too much plaster over a hole in a wall. And that's only the beginning, since it stimulates the immune system to attract white-cell protectors to try to smooth out and gobble up the rotten cholesterol. Those, in turn, spill some of their toxic contents that normally attack enemy infections, which causes generalized inflammation. The inflammation and cholesterol build up blister-sized spaces in the walls called foam cells, which increases the size of the plaque, or plaster, even more, makes the artery surface rougher, and triggers more inflammation, creating bulges and potholes in the wall. It's like a high school party going on in your arteries when the parents are away for the weekend. The kids are doing a lot of damage, they keep inviting more guests, and nobody's even calling the cops.

Those big, foamy cells get so greedy they outgrow the blood supply. When that happens, some of them begin to starve from lack of blood, and as they die, they become "irritable"—they have an electrical charge to them, similar to the electric shock you get sometimes while combing your hair. That charge attracts even more of the Busch-drinking, sixteen-year-old party crashers: sticky blood platelets, which like to travel in crowds and form clots in your arteries. So the first problem is nicks, the next is too much plaster (the lousy cholesterol) or too little spatula action (the healthy cholesterol), the third is inflammation, and the last is clots on the cholesterol patches.

CLOTS

Platelets, a type of blood cell that look like rumpled sheets from an unmade bed, do good work. For instance, they're the guys who keep you from bleeding to death after cutting yourself with a razor. They're nice and calm until they come up against something rough, like the patch on the inside of an artery that has been plastered over with cholesterol. When they do hit that rough patch, they degranulate and grab onto the lining as if it's a life preserver. (If the roughness were a cut in the skin, you'd be glad they'd arrived on the scene because they'd be there to make a clot at the end of the blood vessel, which would eventually become a scab that would help you stop bleeding and heal.) If the roughness is plaque clinging to the potholes in your arteries, and especially if the plaque is electrically charged with dying cells, the platelets end up forming a big clot on top of the irritated, inflamed plaque, which brings more clotting proteins to the area. This inflammation, and the potholes, attract platelets that pile up, until one day—*Boom!* The walls that have been inflamed and that have grown fatter and fatter suddenly attract so many platelets and clot that they fill the entire artery. The result: The living heart tissue that was fed by that blood vessel is starved of its vital nourishment. It begins to die. Let's leave that cholesterol inflammation party for

Myth Buster #2

a minute and consider one other way clots are unwanted guests in your arteries. Sometimes a clot that has been crowding that party on your arterial wall decides to move on down the road. When that happens, it's more than annoying; it can be downright lethal. If a clot wanders down your arteries, it can catch up to a party in an even smaller space and get completely stuck, so your blood can't get through the door. If that party is taking place in a vital area, all the festivities can be over for good—and in a hurry.

This scenario describes one of the strangest aspects of heart disease: Because of this rude party-hopping habit, sometimes a person with a worse buildup—say, 90 percent of the artery wall is closed off—is better off than a person with only a 50 percent blockage.

Here's how it works: If an artery has spent twenty years throwing parties—that is, growing plaque and becoming increasingly narrow—its host body has spent at least some of those years learning how to do some of the artery's work somewhere else. It's called collateral blood supply. It's as if the bridge you take to work every day has been closing down one lane at a time, causing traffic jams. After swearing like a character on *The Sopranos,* you learn—over weeks or months—new routes to your office. That's your body building new blood vessels to help out the traffic-clogged main vessel—a great adaptive response that humans have developed to survive injury. When vessels close, the sur-

Myth Buster #3

rounding blood-starved tissues release proteins that signal new blood supplies to develop. Staying physically active forces tissues to demand even more blood with resulting increases in collateral blood supply. But if you've become completely reliant on that one bridge, which has always gotten you to work more or less on time every day, and one day you arrive at the tollbooth and the entire bridge is closed down, you're stuck. No amount of %$@*!ing will help you now: You're not going to get to work. Likewise, let's say a big clot has set up shop along your somewhat narrowed arteries. With only a 50 percent clog, your blood may have flowed freely enough that your body didn't find it necessary to build extra highways and an alternate-route bridge. When that clot expands to fill the path, your main bridge is closed, your heart's not getting enough oxygenated blood, and the party's over. The result is the same as the increased inflammation process described above: The living heart tissue that was fed by that blood vessel is starved of its vital nourishment. Without alternate routes, the clot closes the artery and the heart muscle "watered" by that artery begins to die.

FACTOID

If you fly a lot, you should get up and walk around every two hours, or move your feet with exercises at your seat. Doing so will help you prevent a condition called deep vein thrombosis (or clotted leg vein) that occurs when you're sitting in the same position for a long time. The danger is that without movement, a blood clot can form in the leg. That clot can then slip up into the lungs and block off their blood supply (that's a *bad* thing). Walking around or rolling your feet lets your leg veins pump the blood back through your body to prevent clots. You should also take 162 milligrams of aspirin (that's two baby aspirin or half a regular one, and a glass of water) before long flights to make your platelets less sticky and to reduce the risk of deep vein thrombosis occurring.

Your Electrical System

Think for a minute about what keeps your heart going, beat after beat (the answer is not George Clooney). Yes, it needs a constant blood supply (that's why those smooth artery walls are so important), but it also needs the crucial impulse that makes it beat steadily an average of 3.3 billion times in your lifetime. Those parties in your arteries, which are crowding the passage of blood, can also affect the regularity of your heartbeat. In fact, about half of all people who have coronary heart disease also end up developing electrical problems that affect the heart's rhythms (that's partly what went wrong with Vice President Dick Cheney's heart).

The problem is instability or, you might even say, confusion. When parts of your heart muscle have died from lack of blood (because your arteries were blocked), the muscle cells that are perched on the border of those dead areas get unstable and confused, and they stop doing their job right. They start fighting with each other instead of supporting each other. They're so busy wrangling that they stop transmitting the electrical impulses that make your heart beat (see Figure 2.2).

Their fight turns into a crazy kind of dance called fibrillation. Instead of the balletlike grace of a strong muscle moving rhythmically, you have something that looks more like a four A.M. dance floor—everybody moving to different beats with no regard for anything else in their way. It's deadly because none of the wiggles is strong enough to pump blood to your body. It takes a big electrical current to shock the heart back to a regular rhythm (those paddles you see on TV shows provide that shock). The miracle of today's medicine is that people who are prone to rhythm problems can get an implant, called an automatic internal cardiac defibrillator (AICD), put right into their chest. The AICD can sense irregular rhythms and automatically shock the heart back to regularity.

Now, just like your house, your heart also has an atrium, which holds the blood

FIGURE 2.2 **Beating the System**   The SA node rules your heart rhythm with quick conduction to the AV node; that electrical system can be shorted out by rogue cells from other parts of the atrium and cardiovascular system, especially the pulmonary veins. The effect: irregular beats, like atrial fibrillation.

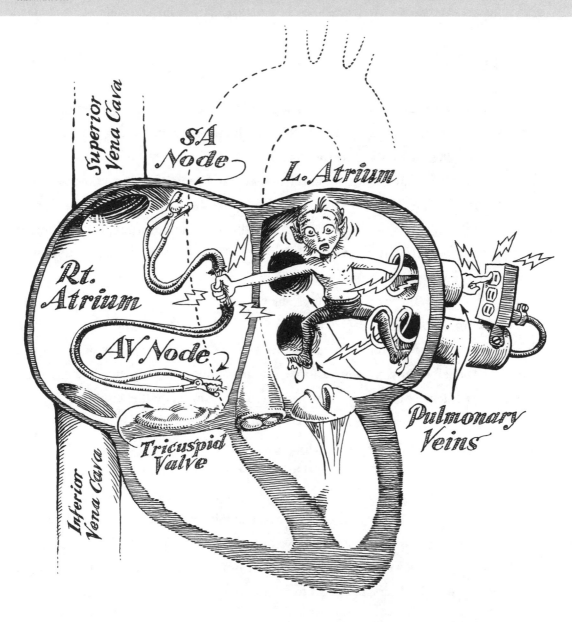

coming into the heart. When fibrillation happens in this less critical chamber, folks feel palpitations. Instead of an AICD, these people sometimes need minimally invasive procedures like a pacemaker insertion, ablation, or medications including a blood thinner to prevent blood clots that accumulate on the quivering atrial walls and can cause strokes.

The Valves

The valves play a key and surprisingly basic role in the never-ending cycle of blood through the heart: They are doormen who keep the blood from retracing its journey, leaking backward into the chambers it has just left. There are valves between each atrium and ventricle, and between each ventricle and the blood vessel that leaves it. As the blood swishes through, the valves slam shut, producing what we hear on TV as a heartbeat. (Doctors listening through the stethoscope are trying to hear how your heart valves are functioning—the "crispness of the sound" describes how well the valves are coming together, and murmurs can indicate the size of the valve openings or any leakage through the valves.)

The most common valve problem is mitral valve prolapse (the name "mitral," by the way, comes from miter, the two-leaved hat worn by popes), in which the valve between the left atrium and left ventricle doesn't slam closed fully, just like in Figure 2.3. Picture the valve as a sail: Normally it should be caught by the wind and snapped into place, but in mitral valve prolapse the sail is a little too big, or its ropes too long, and instead it rattles in the wind, closing kind of sloppily and letting some of the wind (that is, the blood) get past. That faulty process irritates the nerves in the atrium, which in turn can cause palpitations and sweating. Fifteen percent of women are diagnosed with mitral valve prolapse. Although men also have abnormal valves, the syndrome of palpitations, sweating, and panic attacks that is associated with these floppy valves is usually found in young women. It can be treated with drugs called beta-blockers, but most folks end up outgrowing the condition.

FIGURE 2.3 Leaky Valves The coronary arteries, which lie on the heart's surface, drip blood into the heart muscle. With strings attached to that muscle, the mitral valve regulates blood into the left ventricle. If those strings are too long, the valve leaflets slip too far up—allowing blood back into the left atrium. That's a condition called mitral valve prolapse. Aortic valve leaflets can tighten and tear from wear and tear, causing leakage or, conversely, too narrow an opening.

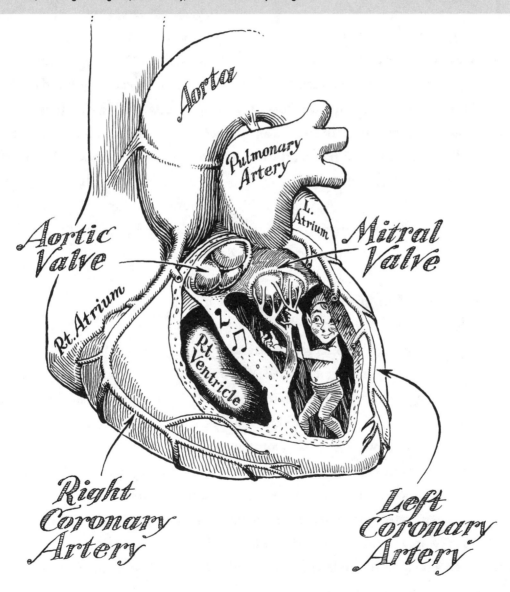

Your Heart: The Live Younger Action Plan

You inherit a lot from your family—looks, political views, meat loaf recipes. Add heart trouble to the list, too. If a parent or other close family member developed coronary artery disease before age sixty, your chances are significantly higher than the average person's of developing it, too. It appears that abnormalities in lipid production can be inherited—that is, a tendency to have higher LDL levels, lower HDL, or other risk factors like high blood pressure. But behaviors can be inherited, too: your father smoked, you might smoke, too; your family ate highly salted foods (which can promote high blood pressure), you might, too; your mother had a stressful job, you might as well. Whatever the mechanism, anyone with a family history of heart disease should be extra vigilant about heart-risky behaviors. That said, Uncle Hank shouldn't take all the blame; lifestyle choices are even more dangerous. Just look at all the cardiovascular poisons around you—cigarettes, pastrami, the couch. If you know your enemy, you can learn how to defeat it.

Action 1: Pump Your Heart

Just through everyday life, your body fries more fat than a fast-food cook. In fact, your body is a natural fat burner. You burn calories all the time—whether you're gardening, reading, or going to the bathroom. For optimum health, you'll do enough physical activity (exercise) to burn between 3,500 and 6,500 calories a week (or from 500 to about 950 a day). Most of that calorie burn comes from everyday activities, without your even trying to do so. But the scientific data shows that in addition to those calories you burn from general physical activities, you also need about sixty minutes a week of stamina training—that is, a cardiovascular activity that elevates your heart rate to 80 percent or more of your age-adjusted maximum (220 minus your age) for an extended period of time. Ultimately, the stamina training nec-

Find the Time

Simply doing physical activity for twenty minutes is enough to make a difference—in your heart, your arteries, your bones, your joints, your attitude, and your whole health. To define that twenty minutes, it's twenty minutes of sustained activity that leads to your being slightly out of breath, or enough for you to sweat consistently during that time. We know that you have responsibilities to jobs, kids, and the three-foot-high weeds in the backyard, but it's a good thing to be selfish when it comes to taking time for exercise— especially when you realize you'll be in better shape to take care of your kids or parents if you yourself are in better shape. If you're in a time crunch, we suggest setting the alarm clock back thirty minutes. The earlier you can do it, the fewer distractions you'll have to overcome.

essary to obtain optimum health (more is needed for getting into *great* shape but not needed for health) comes in the form of only three twenty-minute workouts per week at this heart rate. It's also the level that would make you sweat in a cool room. The funny thing is, once you go over sixty or so minutes, there's no more benefit to your body from a longevity standpoint. And by burning more than 6,500 calories a week, you actually *decrease* your longevity because of the wear and tear your body endures going through the rigors of additional exercise (a fifty-five-year-old man who burns 6,500 calories a week has the body of a forty-seven-year-old man, while a fifty-five-year-old man who burns more than that has the body of a fifty-two-year-old man; see Chapter 4 for more details). Only three twenty-minute workouts might not be the best regimen for someone who needs to lose ninety pounds or who wants to win the Boston Marathon, but it is for living younger and living longer.

There are a couple of reasons why exercise is so important. For one, any amount of physical activity lowers both systolic (the pressure being exerted when the heart contracts; the first or top number) and diastolic (the pressure in the arteries when the heart is at rest; the bottom or second number) blood pressure, which are the most important factors in arterial aging. Even walking just a few extra minutes a day lowers your lousy (LDL) cholesterol, raises your healthy (HDL) cholesterol, and decreases inflammation, among other benefits. Working any muscle to its maximum strengthens it, so we shouldn't be surprised that the heart muscle gets stronger from being periodically stressed. The exercise may also strengthen blood vessels by forcing them to dilate and perhaps making them more elastic. If you haven't exercised in a while, start with walking until you can do weight lifting and then add some kind of activity—cycling, swimming, using an elliptical trainer—to elevate your heart rate (running chronically often stresses your joints too much). By adding strength training, which we'll discuss in Chapter 4, and then stamina training, the average fifty-five-year-old man becomes eight years younger in RealAge, and a fifty-five-year-old woman makes herself 9.1 years younger.

Perhaps the most important reason to exercise is that it can help prevent you from ballooning up to the size of a two-bedroom condo. You increase your risk of heart disease in two ways if you're seriously overweight (a body mass index [BMI] of above 35—for example, being five feet eight inches and 230 pounds) or if your waist size is greater than forty inches for men or thirty-seven inches or greater for women (measure around the belly button while you suck in your gut; see *YOU: On a Diet*). Of course, many people cheat on the latter criterion by measuring the size of their belt, which unfortunately has been hiding under a beer belly for a few years. That waist carries two important risks. First, you're much more likely to have or develop other risky conditions like high blood pressure, diabetes, lipid disorders like high LDL levels, sleep apnea, or arthritis, which will inhibit your desire to exercise. Second, that extra weight that's carried around your waist places you at an even higher risk, because the fat cells in abdominal fat secrete a hormone that directly increases inflammation in your blood vessels. A weight loss of even 5 percent of body weight will significantly improve your overall and cardiovascular health. Another way exercise can help you is by reducing stress, which is one of the greatest agers of your body.

Action 2: Know Your Numbers

For many people, the day they took the SATs was the last time they had to do any type of calculation. But just because you might fear numbers the way adulterers fear Dr. Phil doesn't mean that you should ignore them. The more you have a handle on important levels in your body, the better you'll be able to measure your risk, predict heart problems, and flag danger. Consider these tests and numbers a vital part of your heart health—a stock ticker for your ticker.

BLOOD PRESSURE TEST   Blood pressure is the amount of force exerted by your blood on the walls of your arteries as it passes through. If your blood pressure is high (optimum level is 115/76; the national median is 129/86), that force is literally gouging holes in your arteries, causing the nicks we described earlier. But high blood pressure has no symptoms, which makes it easier to ignore than a dirty air filter in your house. It is also, however, as easily treatable with drugs or lifestyle changes (diet and exercise), which means that everyone should have their blood pressure measured regularly and take immediate steps if it is high. Blood pressure readings can be more variable than trouser sizes at the bus stop—but you always want your blood pressure reading to be low. Have your blood pressure taken in the morning, during the day, and at night when you are doing what you normally do (except *that*, Fabio). If it is high at any of those times, you can make your RealAge younger. If you are fifty-five years old, you are one year older in RealAge for every 5 mmHg increase to the top number or 7 mmHg increase in the bottom number. But drop 160/90 readings down to the ideal, and you make yourself nine years younger. (You can also ask your doctor about a double blood pressure test—called the ankle brachial index test.)

BLOOD TEST   Sure, you'd probably rather slurp liquefied slugs than take a needle. But a yearly blood test will shed insight into your overall heart health. Here's what to look for:

Cholesterol

LDL cholesterol is carried by low-density lipoproteins, and it's the "bad" kind—the kind that breaks apart easily and builds up on the walls of your arteries wherever there is a nick or hole. We've realized in the last few years that the overall cholesterol number isn't nearly as important as breaking it down into LDL and HDL, because the two have such different actions. We remember it by first initials— L for lousy, H for healthy. High LDL levels can be the result of eating a lot of foods like McLard Ribs or croissants— foods laden with cholesterol, simple carbohydrates, and trans and saturated fats. Or it can be partially determined by genetics: a tendency to have high LDL can run in families. Exercising, losing even ten pounds of weight, avoiding simple carbohydrates (most all white foods like white bread, white sugar, and white pasta), and restricting saturated and trans fats to fewer than 20 grams a day will lower your LDL. You don't have to be a calorie-counting addict to benefit: just read labels and be smart enough to know that choices such as roasted pork tenderloin at 4 grams of saturated fat per serving are substantially less than one Bloomin' Onion. (That's 90-plus grams of saturated and trans fat or four days' worth and twelve days of aging itself.) You can have up to five servings of pork tenderloin with its low amount of saturated fat (less than 20 grams a day), although we advocate that you try to eliminate as much as possible. The payoff to being just this smart can be substantial: A fifty-five-year-old with a LDL of 180 mg/dl who lowers it to 100 will make himself three years younger. LDL is more important for men under sixty; getting HDL up is more important for men over sixty and women of all ages (see below).

Avoiding more than 20 grams of saturated and trans fats every day has another benefit—it keeps your arteries able to dilate, providing you with more energy (it is really easy to do; both of us and our wives do it every day). Meals laden with saturated and trans fats lead to blood laden with saturated and trans fats, which in turn paralyzes that muscular middle wall of your arteries. And you want that artery muscle to be functional, so when you ask a leg muscle to move, it gets enough energy to do so. So to be energetic, keep your saturated fat and trans fats to fewer than 20 grams a day.

For a change, we actually want to increase some-thing in your body. You also want as high an HDL level as possible, and at least greater than 40. Increasing your HDL can be done in several ways:

★ consuming healthy fats like those in olive oil, fish, and walnuts (one tablespoon, four ounces, or twelve a day, respectively) or DHA omega-3 supplements (600 mg of DHA or 2 grams of fish oil)

★ walking or doing any physical activity for thirty minutes a day

★ taking niacin (check with your doctor on how to take a large dose of this in a way that doesn't cause flushing)

★ taking 300 milligrams of pantothenic acid (vitamin B_5) a day

★ having a drink of alcohol every night (seven on Saturday night doesn't count, and avoid drinking if you have a family member who becomes angry when he/she drinks)

Alcohol is a double-edged sword. It decreases inflammation, for reasons not fully understood. But too much of it can cause aging of the immune system, perhaps by inactivating the cells that defend you. Anything over about two and a half drinks daily for men and one and a half drinks for women is a net increase in risk.

Homocysteine A by-product of the body's digestion of protein, homocysteine causes nicks and inflammation in arterial walls, possibly by the simple physical fact that it is made of little crystals that directly bombard and gouge the walls.

High homocysteine levels are easily reduced to normal by taking the vitamin folate (400 micrograms a day is what we take). You should aim for a homocysteine level of 9 mg/dl or less.

C-Reactive Protein

HsCRP (hs stands for high sensitivity) measures the level of inflammation in your body, including anything from a chronic sinus infection to urinary-tract infections or gum inflammation. If it is high, your risk of heart disease is higher, because any significant inflammation in your body increases inflammation in your blood vessels. The Women's Health Initiative study of more than twenty-eight thousand women showed that those with elevated hsCRP had a cardiovascular death rate that was 3.1 times higher than that of people with the lowest hsCRP levels. There are ways to reduce your hsCRP (which will make your RealAge younger by four to seven years if you do), including a course of antibiotics, as well as exercise, aspirin, and non-steroidal anti-inflammatory drugs like ibuprofen (do not take aspirin and ibuprofen in the same twenty-four hours—stick with just one; more on that in Chapter 10), and statins.

Blood Sugar

Keep it lower than 100 mg/dl. The excess sugar in the blood that's caused by diabetes damages the arteries by inactivating a specific phosphokinase, a substance that makes it possible for your arteries to dilate smoothly and contract. Without that phosphokinase, the risk of holes or cracks appearing at junctions in the arterial walls increases dramatically. So all of us, not just diabetics, really want to avoid foods that are high in simple sugars and saturated and trans fats, like jelly doughnuts.

THE PHYSICAL TESTS Two simple physical tests can tell you a lot about the health of your heart. Both of them involve how your heart deals with vigorous exercise—how hard you can work out and how quickly you recover. Each of these tests independently can predict your risk of death or disability in the next ten years, from all causes, not just heart disease or arterial aging. Here's how to carry out your own personal exercise stress test (do these only to the maximum exercise level you normally do or if your doctor says you can do them). You will need to have a method of measuring your heart rate, such as a device that is built into the handles of an exercise machine or a heart rate monitor that straps on your wrist and chest.

Maximum Heart Rate	After exercising as hard as you can for three minutes, check your heart rate: How close does it come to 80 or 90 percent of the maximum for your age? (Calculate the maximum by subtracting your calendar age from 220: If you're forty years old, your maximum heart rate should be about 180 beats per minute; 90 percent would be 162, 80 percent would be 144.)
Recovery Time	Right at the end of the most strenuous workout you do, note your heart rate. Then stop all exercise (just this once, don't cool down) and check your heart rate two minutes later.

If you achieved at least 80 percent or greater of your maximum heart rate, or if your heart rate declined by 66 or more beats in the two minutes after you stopped, your RealAge is at least five years younger than your calendar age.

Action 3: Get Mental and Develop Lifelong Friends

As you know from your first love (whether it was Sammy in seventh grade or Cheryl Tiegs in a bathing suit), there is a strong mind-body connection. You *feel* different when you're happy. In fact, you're healthier when you're happy. So it shouldn't be a surprise that your emotions—specifically, how you handle some of the nonscientific things in your life—can have an enormous impact on the way your body works.

FIGHT ANGER AND HOSTILITY   Powerful negative emotional states are bad for your heart and are important enough to make your RealAge effect eight years older, so this is not just touchy-feely stuff. These emotions can cause high blood pressure, as well as disrupt your body's normal repair mechanism and also constrict your blood vessels, making it even harder for enough blood to work its way through. Various kinds of therapies—including learning relaxation techniques and meditation, and having friends you'd never think of getting angry with—can help you handle these damaging feelings in a healthier way (see below).

STAND UP TO DEPRESSION   When we say depression, we're not talking about how you feel after losing twenty bucks in the office Super Bowl pool. A more passive negative emotional state over the long term is strongly associated with heart disease. In fact, people with depression are statistically four times more likely to have a heart attack than people who are not depressed. A feeling of helplessness appears to weaken the immune system. Beyond that, there's a lot we need to learn about how the depressed state of mind affects the body—what we know now is that it does affect it profoundly. For instance, one study has shown that depression increases platelet aggregation, which means that being depressed may make you more prone to arterial clotting and arterial aging. Seeking professional help and managing depression require recognizing it in yourself or friends; getting help or helping your friends get help results in a more than 90 percent reduction in symptoms and consequences in just three months. Seeking help, whether through therapy or medication, is a needed first step to help you and your heart.

DESTRESS Stress is the greatest ager of your body in general, especially the nagging, unfinished-tasks kinds of stress that hang over you day after day or the stress of things that are out of your control (as opposed to the acute stresses—like having a flat tire or adjusting to a traffic jam when you are in a hurry—that eventually get fixed). We don't fully understand the mechanism of how emotional stress produces physical stress, but we know it is a powerful connection: In the United States for the thirty days after September 11, 2001 (compared to the thirty days before), heart attacks increased about threefold in Washington and New York, and threefold even in Missouri, Chicago, Kansas City, and Alabama. Even implanted defibrillators, which help manage dangerous heartbeats, discharged more than twice as much as usual in those thirty days following September 11. Three major life events or sets of unfinished tasks can make your RealAge more than thirty-two years older.

Just as chronic stress can damage your heart, actively working at reducing stress will keep your heart healthier. Therapies like meditation and relaxation techniques can teach you how to tolerate the stressful elements in your life—the tough boss, the rebellious teenage daughter, the dog hair on your suit—and how to tone down your body's physical response to stress (the racing heart, the stress hormones). Some people also find great stress relief in social contact, religious devotion or involvement, even playing with a pet. Find whatever refocuses your attention and give time to it. The most consistent stress reducers that also help with depression and anger: exercising, meditating, and nurturing friendships. We teach you how to do the first for maximum health benefit in Chapter 4.

Action 4: Eat Your Heart Out

It's becoming clearer every day that food is one of your most powerful tools for keeping your body (and especially your heart) in optimum condition. Now, we'll be the first to admit that sometimes the evidence has been confusing, even contradictory (we remember as well as you do how we were all told to eat margarine instead of butter—until it turned out that the trans-fatty acids in margarine were at least as bad as the saturated fat in butter). But there are some nutritional recommendations that are as clear as a Caribbean lagoon.

GO NUTS Eat at least one handful of nuts a day. Nuts are an excellent source of both healthful fats and healthful protein; they also can be concentrated sources of flavonoids, an antioxidant (see below). In the Iowa Nurses Study and three other studies, one ounce of nuts a day decreased the incidence of heart disease between 20 and 60 percent. The best nuts (those highest in omega-3 fatty acids) are walnuts, but all nuts—even legume peanuts—are good for you.

OIL YOUR BODY Olive oil contains large quantities of monounsaturated and polyunsaturated fats, which help raise your HDL cholesterol—the "healthy" cholesterol that is carried through your body by high-density lipoproteins. It actually helps clean out your arteries as it moves through. While it may seem repetitive, we think it's important enough to do it. When it comes to HDL, higher is better—so an HDL level of 60 versus one of 39 will make the average fifty-five-year-old woman four years younger. In fact, you should make sure that healthy fat makes up about 25 percent of your daily calories. Vegetables and flavonoids, in addition to the tricks we told you above, have also been shown to raise HDL.

GO FISH   You should eat three portions of fish per week. Fish, especially fatty fish like salmon and whitefish like cod or bass, is high in those omega-3 fatty acids, which have several powerful benefits. They appear to reduce triglyceride levels in the blood (high levels cause plaque buildup in the arteries), stabilize the heartbeat (reducing irregular rhythms), make platelets less sticky (reducing clotting), and may bring down blood pressure as well. (If you do not like fish or fish oils, DHA supplements [600 milligrams a day] or echium oil may do the same thing.) Some studies have suggested that eating fish once a week cuts your risk of heart attack in half. The best fish (those with the least mercury and PCBs [polychlorinated biphenyl]) are wild, line-caught salmon (almost all canned salmon is wild, healthful salmon), mahi mahi, catfish, flounder (sole), and whitefish.

PICK YOUR FAVORITE FLAVO   Get 31 milligrams of flavonoids a day. Flavonoids are powerful antioxidants and anti-inflammatory substances that occur in certain plant foods, including nuts; any tea, including green tea; red wine; grapes; cranberries; 100 percent natural orange juice; onions; and tomatoes and tomato juice. You can take in this amount by drinking two and a half glasses of cranberry juice or several cups or glasses of tea.

KNOW YOUR ENEMIES   As mentioned above, limit your saturated and trans fats (a mostly artificial form of aging fat) to less than 20 grams a day. No food element has been more closely linked to arterial aging than these kinds of fats, found mostly in meats, luncheon meats, full-fat dairy products, baked goods, fried fast foods, and palm and coconut oils. They increase arterial inflammation, which promotes plaque buildup, and they also turn on the mechanism that increases LDL cholesterol in the bloodstream—yet another way to slap more plaque onto your arteries. They're truly the four-letter words of heart disease. In the same way, you should also avoid simple sugars, including syrup (corn, malt, rice, maple—that's just another name for sugar) and most white processed foods, which have a very direct effect on your arteries. When your blood is high (over 106 mg/dl) in sugar, it disrupts the cells lining your blood vessels, allowing nicks and tears to occur in the inner arterial lining that lead to inflammation and plaque buildup. Simple sugars can also contribute to obesity or lead to insulin resistance and ultimately diabetes, which is also very damaging to your arteries.

Action 5: Don't Ignore the Relatives

Go around a Thanksgiving table, and every family can pick out one or two relatives they'd rather have dine at another table—preferably in someone else's house. But we shouldn't just hide from those relatives; we should learn from them (*then* hide from them). If a parent or other close family member developed heart disease or hardening of the arteries relatively early in life, your chances are significantly higher than the average person of developing it also. Abnormalities in lipid production can be inherited—that is, a tendency to have higher LDL or lower HDL levels. Other risk factors like high blood pressure or high homocysteine levels can be inherited as well. But, as we said earlier, behaviors can be inherited, too. Whatever the mechanism, anyone with a family history of heart disease should be extra vigilant about heart-risky behaviors, and should also begin routine tests at an earlier age than the general population. If you're doing all that, you may beat the genetic odds.

Action 6: Go on Da Pills

As you'll learn throughout this book, we're proponents of the power of certain nutrients, supplements, and occasional medications that can work preventive wonders in your body. For your heart, these are our top picks:

ASPIRIN   Who would ever have thought that one little white pill could have such a powerful effect on the heart? But the evidence that aspirin helps prevent cardiovascular disease just keeps growing: one well-controlled study, for instance, showed that taking aspirin regularly reduced the incidence of heart attack by 44 percent. It is thought to achieve this in several ways, including making platelets less sticky and decreasing inflammation in the arteries. One primary downside is aspirin's effect on the stomach lining—it is acidic, so it can irritate or disrupt the protective lining. And because it inhibits clotting it can cause more bleeding in those who have stomach ulcers. You can reduce those side effects by drinking a half glass of warm water before and after taking a pill. But it is so beneficial against heart disease that men over thirty-five and women over age forty should consider taking half a regular aspirin (or 162 milligrams) a day for life (it takes at least three years to establish the full benefit). An aspirin a day makes the average fifty-five-year-old 2.3 years younger in RealAge.

A MULTIVITAMIN   Your multivitamin is a fountain of micronutrients, some of which are particularly key to your heart's health: Magnesium (400 milligrams daily) helps keep the heart rhythm stable and with calcium (600 milligrams twice daily) lowers blood pressure; to absorb calcium well you need vitamin D (1,000 IU daily for those under age sixty; 1,200 IU for those over sixty), which also may decrease in-

---

FACTOID

About 25 percent of us have a gene that interferes with the action of drugs called beta-blockers, commonly used to treat high blood pressure. People who take those drugs potentially get only the side effects, without the benefits. While 75 percent of us get a longer, more vibrant life, the other 25 percent will age more quickly. How do you know if you're in the affected group? Ask your doc for a simple (though expensive) blood test.

flammation in blood vessels. Vitamins C (600 milligrams twice daily) and E (400 IU daily) work as an antioxidant combination—they are much more powerful together than they are separately. (By the way, if you are taking a statin like Zocor or Prevachol, or Lipitor or Crestor, reduce the amount of vitamins C and E you take in supplements or pills to no more than 100 milligrams twice a day and 100 IU a day, respectively. C and E inhibit the anti-inflammatory effects of statins—the cholesterol effects are not altered, just the anti-inflammatory effects, but those account for 40 percent or more of the benefit of statins.)

Potassium promotes arterial health (get it from dietary sources: four fruits per day, especially bananas, avocados, and melon). And avoid more than 2,500 IU of vitamin A a day (minimum is 1,500 IU). The correct multivitamin taken twice a day can make your RealAge more than six years younger.

FOLATE   This B vitamin has proven to be essential to human health in various ways, but for your heart, it has a crucial role: a daily dose of 400 micrograms (half from food is normal) lowers homocysteine to healthy levels, and makes the person whose homocysteine level is 26 mg/dl (the level you should shoot for is less than 9 mg/dl) about six years younger. The folate in food is only partially absorbed by your body, so it's easiest to ensure you are getting enough by taking a 400-microgram supplement—but you must also take B_6 and B_{12}, as folate sometimes unmasks a deficiency in them.

Action 7: Schedule Sleep

We don't know why, but if you get less sleep than you need, you increase your arterial aging and your risk of heart attack. Studies have shown that the optimal amount is seven to eight hours per night for men and six to seven hours for women. And those need to be solid hours: You have to be snoozing about two hours in a row before your sleep becomes truly restorative. Inadequate sleep causes you to release less of the pleasure hormone serotonin in your brain. To compensate, you try to increase those levels with foods like sugar or harmful substances like tobacco. So ignoring sleep is like ignoring a leak in the roof—if you do, things will only get worse. See the plan in Chapter 5 for getting a good night's sleep, and make your heart and arteries younger still.

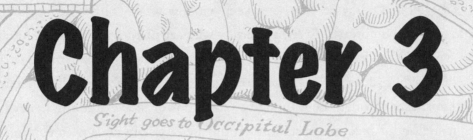

Chapter 3

Do You Mind: Your Brain and Nervous System

Major Myths About the Brain

Brain Myth #1	Memory loss is a natural, inevitable part of aging.
Brain Myth #2	The best way to determine brain power is with intelligence tests.
Brain Myth #3	Unless you get knocked out, brain trauma is negligible.
Brain Myth #4	You can will away depression.

We live in a world of wires. In computers, they connect the central processing unit to the monitor. In braces, they help shift the position of teeth. On skyscrapers, they keep window washers from falling. In bras, they do the same for breasts. Even in a society with cell phones and wireless Internet access, we still rely on wires for so many things—especially in our house. Strip a house of its siding, drywall, and insulation, and you'll see a labyrinth-like system of wires that snakes through the framing to supply power to every room. Everything flows in and out of one central station—your fuse box—but ends with you turning something on, whether it be a light, a TV, or your Jessica Simpson CD. Without a strong power source, your house would merely be a three-bedroom, two-and-a-half-bath turtle shell.

Your anatomical fuse box—your brain—has the same kind of responsibility. It has the power to control *everything* your body does. Your brain flips all of your body's switches. Most important, though, your brain is what makes you human, because it gives you the power to dream, imagine, reason, understand square roots, fall in love, fall in lust, invent flying cars, feel sorry about calling the boss a four-letter word, feel even sorrier for doing it to his face, joke, pray, and do the billions of things that so many other species can't.

Just like a house built in the 1950s has a different wiring capacity from one built during this decade, your brain has different power capacities as it ages. See, an older home could function fine with its original electrical system when all it had to handle was a refrigerator, a coffeepot, and a little Ed Sullivan. But if you were to try to pump up an old house with computers, surround sound, and your eight-year-old's video game setup, the strain would shock and overload the electrical system, blow a fuse, start a fire, and burn down your whole house. On the other hand, a young house is equipped to withstand all of the demands of modern society, so it can supply power to everything.

Your brain works the same way. In fact, most brains don't age very well under normal circumstances. Younger brains are equipped to handle overloads with only an accidental glitch here and there, but older brains need upgrading to avoid neurological blown fuses and major power outages. Luckily, cognitive upgrading doesn't require a subcontractor. It's a do-it-yourself project that has many wonderful outcomes: It will keep your brain function high throughout your life; it will minimize the deterioration that takes place as part of the normal aging process; and it will help regrow brain cells to keep your mind as sharp as a coral reef.

Don't believe us? Take a look at one of our favorite studies. The test measured the IQ of Harvard physicians as they aged. Though IQ tests are an oversimplified way to measure intelligence, for the purpose of this study, they provide a rough gauge for what's going on in our brains. The study, which started in the 1950s (and is still going), showed that the IQs of these doctors decreased on average by about 5 percent

Myth Buster #1

every ten years. But the key phrase is *on average*. Yes, many doctors lost IQ points quickly, but some doctors actually increased their IQs as they aged. That *shows* that you can become the exception to the rule. A decrease in brain function isn't inevitable and involuntary; you have the ability to influence what part of the roller coaster your brain function rides—steadily moving up, or going downhill fast. What's best is that you don't need to be a Rhodes scholar to stay mentally strong. Simple changes can do the trick. Take another study—one that measured the brain function of retirees who frequented a Starbucks in Illinois. The half who just sat and drank their coffee got no smarter, while the half who drank their coffee while walking for forty-five minutes at least three days a week actually improved their IQs (no word on how many bathroom breaks they needed). The explanation? Physical activity improves arterial function, and better arterial function improves brain function.

Weighing just three pounds, your brain is the most complex and least understood part of your body. It's only been over the last few decades that we've been able to break through and understand the maze underneath our skulls. Certainly, we're aware of the amazing things our brains do—in science, technology, art, music . . . in everything. Because we see its remarkable power, maybe that's why it's so disturbing when we see people affected by neurological problems. While understanding the anatomy of your brain can seem as complex as learning a foreign language, the fact is that you can take charge of preventing your brain function from declining as you age. Luckily, if you're reading this book, you care enough about your intellectual power source to add some fuses to your box.

Your Brain: The Anatomy

Many people equate brains with computers. They process a lot of information, and in older models they freeze a lot. Of course, there are many differences between brains and computers, but perhaps the most important difference is that your brain doesn't automatically come with any kind of maintenance policy—especially the lifetime variety. It's up to you to provide the technical support that'll keep your hardware and software running as smoothly as possible. We'll be your help desk, but it's up to you to learn what can make your system crash—and how you can prevent it from happening. Before we look at some of the most common age-related neurological problems, let's explore the inside of your mind to get a sense of how the wiring works.

About 80 percent of your brain is actually water, but the rest of it is taken up by both physical and biochemical structures. While it's not an extraordinary organ in terms of size, it is in terms of power. Making up about 2 percent of a 150-pound person weight-wise, your brain uses about 25 percent of the oxygen and sugar that your body circulates for nutrition. In general, a brain's anatomical structures are divided into two kinds of functions—executive (intellectual-type functions) and reptilian (based in movement and raw emo-

tion). Let's take a quick look into the different parts of your body's power source; you can see the big picture of brain function in Figure 3.1.

SKULL Because the brain has the consistency of a hard-boiled egg, it has to be protected by a skull, even at birth (at birth, the skull consists of folded plates to help get the head through the birth canal; then the plates connect and calcify after birth).

BRAIN STEM Connected to your spinal cord, it's responsible for controlling many involuntary functions, such as breathing, digestion, and heart rate.

CEREBELLUM It's responsible for muscle coordination, reflexes, and balance.

FIGURE 3.1 **Something on Your Mind** The cortex of the brain is separated into the major lobes: frontal (decision making), parietal (sensing pain and understanding speech), temporal (memory), occipital (eyesight), the cerebellum (balance), and the thalamus (relay station connecting them all together). If we flattened the folds and stretched out the cortex, it would be the size of a large pizza and have the thickness of an orange rind.

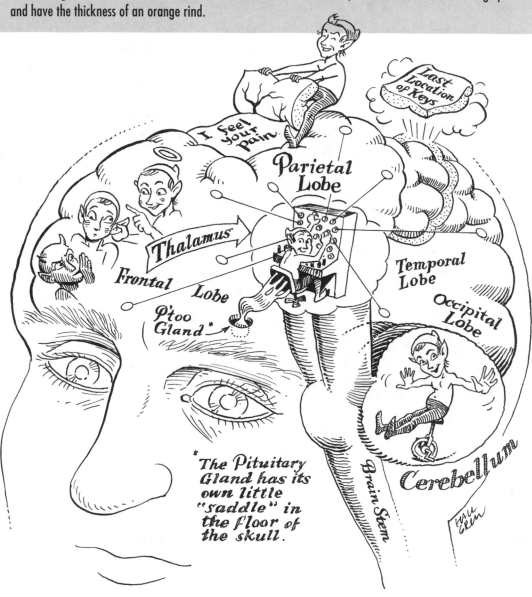

CEREBRUM   Much of your brain function takes place in the cerebral cortex, or outer layer of the cerebrum. It's the assembly line of human thought, where all the heavy work gets done.

LEFT HEMISPHERE   The left controls your concrete side: speech, writing, language, and calculation.

RIGHT HEMISPHERE   The right controls your imaginative side: spatial ability, music, and intuition.

THE FRONTAL LOBES   Control such things as planning, personality, behavior, and emotion. The area allows us to tell right from wrong and to help us think abstractly.

THE PARIETAL LOBE   Most associated with touching and moving our limbs, their junction with the occipital lobe is where speech and understanding speech is located.

THE OCCIPITAL LOBES   Control vision.

THE TEMPORAL LOBES   Located on both sides of your brain at about ear level, these lobes process sound and are also responsible for short-term memory.

NEURONS   You have 100 billion neurons in your brain, which, if stretched out in length, would reach thirty thousand miles. Each of these nerve cells contains pieces of information that need to be transmitted to another neuron so that your body can properly function. Neurons hold the information, but unless it's communicated to another neuron, it's virtually useless. That's where the edges of neurons come into play. They're called dendrites and they're like baseball catchers.

FIGURE 3.2 Instant Messaging Neurons communicate with one another using chemical messages. In one model of depression, serotonin is passed from the cell sending a message (presynaptic) to a cell that can "catch" the chemical and propagate the information (postsynaptic). If something bats the serotonin away, you feel more depressed. If something increases the serotonin that is released and received, then more postsynaptic cells are excited and the less depressed you feel. Many medications work in this way.

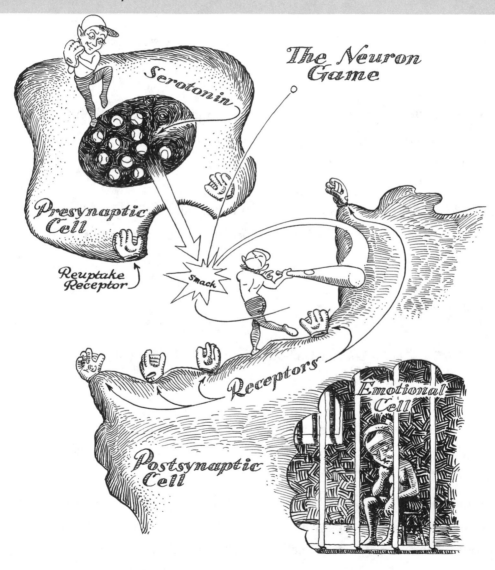

As shown in Figure 3.2, they receive the pitch sent to them from other neurons. Even more important, they act like catchers by communicating to the other players on the field. Specifically, the dendrite can influence how the signal is sent, received, and transmitted to other neurons.

NEUROTRANSMITTERS   These are the chemical messengers in your brain—like baseballs being tossed back and forth. When you turn a neuron on, the neurotransmitters ring or blare out to help send or receive information between neurons. When you experience neurological disorders, the cause often stems from a flaw in the neurotransmitter—if it can't transport one piece of information to another neuron, then you can't know how to complete a specific task. Also, a natural decline in the function of certain neurotransmitters is believed to make you more vulnerable to such conditions as dementia and depression.

THALAMUS   Think of the thalamus—pictured in Figure 3.1—as a train station in a major city that acts as a hub for many other smaller locations. That's because many different parts of the brain run through it; the thalamus takes sensory information from the spine and then fine-tunes what movements you make before they even start. It's really responsible for making actions smooth (problems with the thalamus can result in tremors, or nonsmooth motor movements).

LIMBIC SYSTEM   The limbic system isn't a structure but a series of pathways incorporating various structures deep inside the brain, such as the hippocampus and the amygdala (Figure 3.3). Why should you care? Information gained by vision and hearing passes from the eyes and ears directly to the cortex, so we recognize the sensation and can consciously consider its meaning. On the other hand, smell sensations bypass the cortex and influence the amygdala directly, so our body responds before we can consciously process the information. The amygdala is responsible for emotions, moods, and other functions related to depression and

FIGURE 3.3 **For Your Information** We usually process outside information by passing it directly from the sensory organ to the cortex, where we process what we have learned. The eyes send images to the occipital lobe, and the ears send sound and balance information to the parietal lobe. But smell is unique. An odor passes through the cribiform plate at the top of the nose and stimulates the olfactory nerve. This nerve bypasses the cortex, which filters information, and sends the information to the most ancient part of our brain (amygdala), where emotional responses occur almost subconsciously.

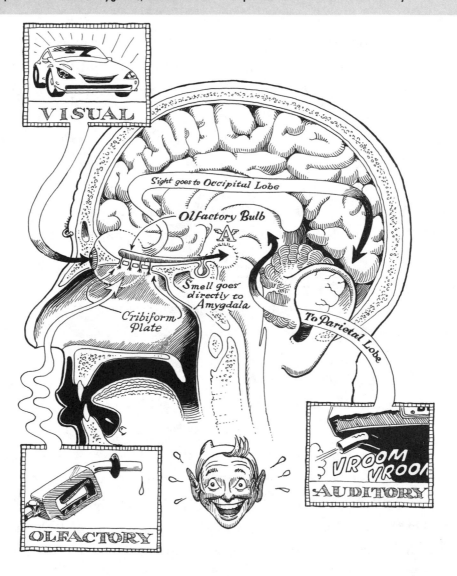

anxiety, and the nearby hippocampus is responsible for the processing and storage of short-term memory. See why the perfume manufacturers do so well?

The brain has many more parts and specific functions, and we could spend the rest of the book trying to dissect all of the anatomy. (But we can't, so we just gave you the most important.) Before we go on, it's worth touching on how we develop our brains to understand why we think the way we do. When we're infants, we have all of this brain material compacted in a small space. Like tree branches, they overlap one another. That garbled anatomy makes it difficult to do some things, like make decisions, because the jumbled structures crossing one another render it nearly impossible for our brains to focus on just one thing. As we get older—three, four, and five years old—our brain starts deciding which branch points get developed and which sort of fall off. So the more we use certain parts of our brain as toddlers, the more we develop those kinds of neurons, while the opposite holds true for those neurons we don't use. The way we train our brains at an early age actually has an effect on which of those neuron systems will become good and strong and which won't. (In autistic children, as the current best theory goes, those underused links don't fall off, meaning the jumbled mass makes it hard for autistic children to focus because there's too much going on.) This is different from attention deficit disorder (ADD)—a disorder affecting the ability to concentrate. Many of us actually had it as kids (but it was rarely diagnosed years ago), and difficulty concentrating on only one subject can be something we carry even into adulthood.

That explanation of neurological development can partly explain why our brains function in certain ways as we age. If we didn't listen to music as a child, or learn how to ski, or learn to speak French, then learning those things as an adult is more difficult because those neuron connections aren't developed for processing the necessary information.

But perhaps the most important distinction to make is this one: Traditionally, brain malfunctions have been broken up into two kinds. In one, the brain dysfunction has an obvious physiological, neurological, and medical explanation: things like strokes, memory loss, and Parkinson's disease. In the other kind, the neural dysfunction has no clear neurological explanation: things like depression, anxiety, and personality disorders. For years, these types of problems were as murky as floodwaters because their diagnoses were unclear and imprecise. More and more medical evidence will suggest what neurological malfunctions are taking place to cause some of these disorders. In the rest of the chapter, we'll distinguish between the two camps of brain problems, but, as we do throughout the book, we'll focus primarily on the most preventable diseases and conditions associated with aging.

Your Aging Brain: What Can Go Wrong

When you run over a nail with your bike, it's an easy diagnosis (flat tire) and an easy fix (seal the puncture and pump up the tube). But unless you're a tech expert, a computer malfunction is especially frustrating because you don't know what caused your computer to lock up or to erase your hard drive. When you don't know the problem, you don't know the fix. Because the brain is a mysterious and complex structure, the average person doesn't know whether to attribute a brain-related problem ("Now, where did I leave my belly button ring?") as merely a neurological hiccup or the signal of a serious disorder.

While there are many different kinds of brain disorders, we won't cover them all. For example, Parkinson's disease, a progressive disease characterized by rigid muscles, tremors, and difficulty walking, is one of the most common diseases of movement in people over fifty-five, but currently, there are no known substantial methods of prevention besides avoiding situations that cause traumatic injury. (We will briefly discuss two promising alternative therapies, coenzyme Q10 and deep brain stimulation, later in the chapter.) And we're also not going to discuss brain trauma, which can affect any age—except to say that the leading way to live younger, brain-wise, is to wear a helmet whenever you ride a bike or go in-line skating, and you might add DHA to your daily supplement routine. It's really common sense, isn't it? If you're hardheaded enough to ride a bike softheaded, it's sort of like throwing your computer against a wall and destroying everything inside—except your brain contents are a lot more valuable and a lot less replaceable than whatever is stored on your C drive.

Before we start, it's also important to make a distinction between brain function and intelligence. Brain function, as it relates to aging, really encompasses things like memory and concentration—not intelligence. In fact, intelligence isn't necessarily a factor in keeping your brain function young. Maybe that's because of all the different ranges and definitions of intelligence. For one, there are gender differences in intelligence. Men use their brains faster to act and solve a problem (it stems back from the days when

Myth Buster #2

men had to spear the wooly mammoth), while women have better lateralization—that is, the ability to analyze a complex topic. Here's a good way to think about it: When men go shopping, they know they need shaving cream, so they walk into the store, find it, pay for it, and leave. When women shop, they browse. They assess options, they make decisions based on numerous outside factors, and they could come out of the store with a large bottle of ibuprofen, the latest issue of *People,* and a birthday card for Mom (even though her birthday isn't for six months)—none of which was on the list to begin with. It doesn't mean one's smarter or more efficient than the other; it just means we assess and process information differently.

While the standard test of brain strength is the IQ test, which measures things like math, logic, and verbal skills, there's also such a thing as emotional intelligence. More and more people believe your emotional intelligence—that is, your ability to relate and interact with others—is just as important for your overall brain health. As we talk about things you can do to improve your brain, you should realize we all have unique brains that shouldn't be judged by one set of standards. Even folks who are mentally retarded as judged by IQ can have (or cause others to have) remarkable insights. That said, there are some things we do know about how the brain works—and how malfunctions cause serious problems. Here are several examples:

Artery-Related Disorders

A hurricane hits, the wind blows down power lines, and your electricity shuts off. That's a stroke. It's a major event that occurs in your brain to shut power down—but in your body's case, the power lines knock out the ability of your arteries to supply blood to your brain. Though there are several different kinds of strokes and several places where they can occur, the traditional stroke happens when a blood vessel leading to the brain becomes blocked or bursts, essentially causing the collapse of the major power line leading to your house. The parts of the brain deprived of blood die and can no longer function properly, which is why people with strokes may not be able to speak or move certain parts of their bodies. The risk factors are the same as other arterial diseases—high blood pressure, diabetes, arterial inflammation, gobbling aging (saturated and trans) fats, not enjoying enough healthful fat (olive oil, nuts, fish and fish oils, DHA, avocados, etc.), low healthy (HDL) cholesterol, high lousy (LDL) cholesterol, high homocysteine levels, too much couch time, cigarette smoking, and obesity (see Chapter 2 for more details).

Just like a storm can knock out power for a few minutes or indefinitely, a stroke can do the same—and have varying degrees of damage. A transient ischemic attack (TIA), for example, is a ministroke in which the arteries are blocked only a short time. A TIA is actually a precursor to a full stroke (though it's more easily treated). Multiple small strokes can have long-term consequences, like dementia. But recovery always depends on how much brain injury occurred from the lack of blood supply to the brain, so act quickly. While everyone knows it's important to get to the hospital as fast as Mario Andretti if you have chest pain, the same applies to the inability to move or express yourself from a stroke. But the biggest difference between a power line failure and a stroke is that you get to control Mother Nature—and prevent storms from wreaking havoc on your system.

Memory-Related Disorders

As we get older, everyone has bouts of forgetfulness. You might even forget things important to you and seemingly simple to remember, like names of friends, the date of your anniversary, the name of your favorite band (*You know, the four guys, c'mon, bad haircuts . . .*). Anyway, age-related memory loss is normal. But, as we'll outline later in the chapter (*the Beatles!*), we don't have to accept normal aging and we can take steps to prevent age-related memory loss. Memory loss can start as early as age thirty, but part of the complication of memory loss associated with aging is that there are several things that cause memory loss:

★ Vascular problems: When insufficient blood gets to the brain, the lack of blood flow can cause mini-strokes and impair memory.

★ Alzheimer's: Here, neurons tangle with other neurons, causing them to stop working properly.

★ Neuron loss: Many age-related problems are caused by the loss of neurons or the loss of the function of those neurons; literally, you're losing part of your mind.

★ Trauma: Memory loss can also come from trauma sustained during accidents or from participating in sports, like boxing, with repetitive injury to the brain. Forceful impact to the skull will bounce the brain around, resulting in bruises that cause concussions and more permanent damage. Memory at the time of impact is often lost as the brain is short-circuited, though surrounding tissue can make up for damaged areas.

And appearances can be deceiving. What might seem to be minor head trauma can actually play a major role in long-term memory loss. Though we usually associate brain trauma with the 1.1 million people who suffer concussions or worse, even seeing stars after a minor head injury can lead to later memory loss. See, your brain floats in a sea of liquid; when your head stops suddenly (such as from the impact of hitting it against another object), you can damage the sheath that protects your neurons as your brain gets jolted from the sea to the skull. And those damaged neurons are what could make you occasionally forget your spouse's middle name or the lyrics to "Hound Dog"; repeated minor traumas—no matter how inconsequential they seem at the time—can accumulate so that you suf-

Myth Buster #3

What Nerve

For a long time, the scientific community thought that memory problems all stemmed from chemical connections and processes, but today we're seeing that your body's nerves also play a role in the way you process and store information. The vagus nerve—the largest cranial nerve in your body (*cranial* means it comes from the brain but goes elsewhere)—carries a cargo ship's worth of information from your gut to your brain. The system is designed to help you (one of the signals that you're full after eating comes from the vagus nerve), but sometimes it can hurt you by overwhelming your brain—think lightning bolt hitting the grid. One way to slow memory loss is to temporarily cut off the nerve impulses from the vagus to the brain through meditation.

fer from neuron damage and memory loss even twenty to forty years later.

Though science hasn't pinpointed why and how memory loss happens, we do know that there are chemical changes in the structure of the brain that hinder the ability to process, store, and retrieve information. Many of us may think that memory loss comes at about the same time as our AARP membership cards, but the decline actually starts much earlier—in your mid-twenties. It's not uncommon to see some effects in your thirties and many more in your forties. What happens is that the speed with which you process information slows down naturally as you age (it's been proven to happen in mice, rats, and primates, as well as humans). Specifically, that comes out in an inability to store information in our short-term memory (say, not remembering a word that you recently heard). One theory for why this occurs is that a toxin eats away at that sheet of healthy fat that protects neurons; some believe that cholesterol is what creates these toxins. But other factors—including stress, thyroid disorders, diabetes, anxiety, depression, and

Myth or Fact? Treatments of forgetfulness are ineffective.

You may think forgetfulness is like a frayed wire—there's no repairing it unless you replace the whole thing. But you can strengthen your wiring in another way. Besides the steps in the Live Younger Action Plan, some research suggests that drugs, including the amphetamine Adderall, can improve your focus and decrease your forgetfulness. Imagine the wires in your electrical system are frayed, but once you have turned off the other appliances, you can focus all your energy capacity on a specific need, even though the underlying mechanism remains broken. So follow our lead to prevent fraying of your brain's wires—wearing a helmet during potentially dangerous sports is looking cooler all the time.

trauma—could all play a role in starting and accelerating memory loss. Fortunately, you can take steps to slow the process (see the Live Younger Action Plan on page 87).

But Alzheimer's is different. For example, symptoms of Alzheimer's start out with forgetfulness (usually spotted when a person cannot remember the way home when in the neighborhood). A person then loses short-term memory—often telling you a story from her past multiple times within fifteen minutes. It then progresses to the point where the person forgets major recent events or recent things about herself, and then to the point where she becomes more disoriented and confused. Often, a person with Alzheimer's can still remember remote events because long-term memory is the last to disappear. In reality, most memory loss is a little like vegetable soup. Your brain is really a pot of several cognitive ailments at once—some neuron loss, some neuron tangling, some vascular problems—that all contribute to losing some ability to recall information. In fact, almost all of us have some of these characteristics as we age. Whatever the official diagnosis, there are several points to remember. One, some memory loss is associated with the loss of nonfunctioning brain cells, so regrowing functional neurons is important to retain memory skills (we're not sure yet how regrowth can affect those with Alzheimer's). And memory loss is also related to blockages of the small blood vessels, so one of the keys to helping prevent memory loss is to keep your arteries young.

Conditions as complicated as memory loss don't have silver-bullet solutions, so you need to think about the problem in this way: There are a lot of factors that could be causing you to forget the name of your cockatiel, and a lot of things can help you remember it. Some are driven by medical technology; some are driven by you.

Chemical-Associated Disorders

One of the more serious brain-related disorders that's attributed to chemical malfunctions in the brain is addiction. We become addicted to substances that increase or release certain chemicals in our brain. Certain substances like nicotine release dopamine, the pleasure chemical, and your body craves more of it—which leads to a habitual behavior to keep pumping dopamine into your system. Not all addictions are caused by dopamine, but it may give some insight into the theory that such things like carbohydrates can be addictive. The feel-good chemical released after eating them is what drives the cravings for more. Lack of adequate sleep decreases the release of this feel-good chemical (and hormones as well). Not getting enough sleep may be one of the reasons you can get addicted to many of those simple carbohydrates and sugars, as well as the aging fats that are impostors of real food.

Nicotine is a leader in toxicity—especially because of its physiological effect on the rest of the body. The addiction itself is manifested not only in an emotional need for the drug but also in a physical need; your brain tells your body it needs nicotine to prevent the symptoms of withdrawal. One of the ways it works is by creating pleasure in the brain, causing a feeling of relaxation. Over time, nicotine keeps your brain from supplying these chemicals that create these good feelings, and you end up craving more nicotine and the feeling it produces. An alcohol addiction works in the same way, but with added disadvantages. Excessive alcohol can lead to other mental disorders, such as anxiety, depression, and liver failure—that is, failure of the liver to clear toxins that are damaging to your memory (see Chapter 7).

All of these chemical messengers control different rooms in your brain. Some make you happy. Some make you depressed. Some make you feel the urge to keep your snacks in alphabetical order in the pantry. You should remember that even though these chemical reactions do take place, you also have the power to make changes to your system—through things you eat, ways you think, and actions you take.

Myth Buster #4

That holds true for another chemical-related problem: depression. Here's a simple medical truth: When you have a broken leg, you can't run. No matter how hard you try, you're just not going to be able to do it. That's how your body works sometimes; it shuts down so you physically can't perform certain tasks. Surprising to a lot of people, depression works in a similar way. Depressed people also have broken parts—most likely a chemical reaction in their brain—that makes them unable to perform daily activities. And no matter how hard they try or how hard someone tries to convince them to be happy, they can't just get up and run.

Today, depression has become much more widely recognized for the physiological and psychological disease that it is. More than 11 million people take medication for depression, and the World Health Organization (WHO) lists depression as the second leading cause of disabilities related to illness. Of course, there are many different kinds of depression—ranging from seasonal affective disorder (SAD), caused by lack of exposure to sunlight, to reactive depression, associated with having an illness or suffering a tragedy. No matter the type, depression is generally defined by a feeling of sadness and disinterest in everyday life, and it can range anywhere from mild to severe. To be classified as clinical depression, the feeling of sadness must go on for more than two weeks. Physiologically, we believe depression stems from chemical imbalances in the brain—meaning that you may have abnormal levels of the chemicals that your nervous system uses to send signals to and from the brain. People with depression generally have low levels of serotonin, a feel-good hormone, in their brains—specifically, their neurons have trouble loading serotonin. While some drugs are prescribed to elevate serotonin levels by blocking degradation or inactivation of this neurotransmitter (see Figure 3.2), there are also natural ways to achieve the same effect, such as through relaxation techniques and so-called happy foods, like chocolate. (Chocolate also causes the release of dopamine, another feel-good hormone. Because of that release, people crave the

In the Mood

One way to think about the depressed mind is by looking at a mood circle. We tend to think of depression and anxiety as being on opposite sides of the emotional spectrum — one makes us jumpy, the other makes us slower than a 103-year-old driver on an interstate. But the reality is that they're a lot closer to being linked than they are to being apart. If perfect neural functioning is at the twelve o'clock position of a circle, then mild, introspective depression would be at about eight and agitation would be at four, with both extreme forms at six o'clock. The way antidepressant medications work is by getting your mind closer to those milder levels and toward that twelve o'clock spot.

good feeling and can become addicted, much like people can become addicted to caffeine or nicotine.)

Of course, depression is associated with any age, but it can make you feel, act, and look older fast. For one, depression is tied to cardiovascular aging. In one study, men and women who had heart disease and depression had a 69 percent higher rate of death from heart disease than those who simply had heart disease and no depression. And in another study, depressed women were found to have lower bone density than those who weren't, presumably from high levels of the stress hormone cortisol, found to be increased in the blood of depressed people. But perhaps the biggest reason is the indirect effect it has on aging. Depressed people are less likely to eat well, exercise, or take other actions to improve their health.

Mental illness is both chemical and environmental—as much as it is a chemical problem, there's also an emotional basis of depression. In fact, brain scans show that depression is localized to the parts of the brain that deal with emotion. We're often asked how much of mental illness comes from psychological factors and how much comes from brain chemistry. Many doctors answer, "One hundred percent of both." That is, depression is an interrelated illness that affects many different parts of the mind.

Personality-Related Disorders

One look at Joan Rivers and Eminem gives us a pretty good clue into the beauty of human personalities. We're all a little bit weird. There are all kinds of eccentric personalities in the world—the laid-back surfer, the cerebral artist, the nagging mother-in-law, the driven business executive, the self-deprecating comic. And you know what? You're included on this list, too, and that's good. The world would be pretty boring if we didn't have such diverse personalities.

While we applaud the weirdness of the world, we have to differentiate between healthy weird and unhealthy weird. When these personality traits start adversely affecting your life—in your daily activities and the way you interact with people—that's when you might have a problem. Keeping your house clean is good. Scrubbing your sink so often that your kids have to make a reservation to use the bathroom isn't. Being cautious about driving is good. But being so worried about the possibility of having an accident that you won't leave the house isn't. That's the line in diagnosing emotional disorders. Is your personality trait simply idiosyncratic and somewhat endearing? Or is it so destructive that it changes the way you and others around you live?

Sometimes it can be tough to distinguish between a personality trait and a personality defect. The telltale sign: whether you (or your wacky neighbor) can't adapt to social situations, or whether you (or your quirky cousin) are significantly impaired in social situations. Typically, in the case of people with these disorders, how you'd label the person might change from "quirky, unique, artistic" to "maybe a little crazy."

It used to be that people thought you could turn personality traits off and on, that all it took to change is the will to change. But now we know that brains are like college freshmen—sometimes they're going to do whatever they want to do no matter what you tell them. Anxiety, for example, which is characterized by a feeling of uneasiness, apprehension, or tension in response to stressful situations, can be mild or intense enough to trigger panic. Brought on by alcohol, caffeine, and certain drugs, as well as things like a heart problem or a lack of vitamins, some anxiety disorders manifest themselves in such conditions as obsessive-compulsive disorder, in which tasks like washing your hands become so habitual that you have to do them forty times a day: good for containing germs; bad for time management. Narcissistic personality disorder (*narcissism* comes from the Greek mythological character Narcissus, who thought no female suitors were worthy of him) happens in individuals who need constant attention, have a sense of superiority, and exploit others for their own gain. Sound like anyone you know? These people tend to have a higher incidence of depression later in life (not to mention a higher incidence of talking about themselves in the third person). The great news is that knowing about these disorders lets you get in control, so such a disorder will be an annoyance that you can manage (like peeling paint) and not a major life disruption (like a fire that destroys most of your house).

Your Brain: The Live Younger Action Plan

When you exercise, you can see your gut shrink. When you stop eating fried calamari, you can see your lousy LDL cholesterol levels drop. When you quit smoking, you can finally stop hacking phlegm out of your throat. As you change habits, you easily see changes in your body. But with your brain, it's a lot harder to gauge how well you're doing. It's not like you can walk around the gym, take off your hat, and flex for everyone. *(Man, your hippocampus is ripped, dude!)* But that's no reason to ignore the very organ that gives you the power to do so. Consider this your plan for building a better brain—for now and later.

Myth or Fact? You can work out your brain with weights.

Try this self-test: Stand on one leg and close your eyes. The longer you can stand without falling, the younger your brain (fifteen seconds is very good if you are forty-five or older). That balancing act is just one sign of your brain strength. To develop better balance, you should use free weights—that is, dumbbells and barbells—because exercising with them works your proprioception (your ability to balance). Weight machines don't have the same effect because the weights are attached to a fixed surface, so you don't develop your balancing abilities as you lift them.

Action 1: Keep All Lanes Open

To avoid the power-line accidents—the ones that lead to strokes—take two baby aspirin a day if you're over 40 because aspirin has been shown to help keep your arteries from being inflamed and your blood from clotting, as well as helping blood and oxygen flowing to the brain. Aspirin may also help the body build more blood vessels, so that if clots do form, there are alternate routes through which blood can flow around the clogged vessel. Recent studies on aspirin show a decrease in strokes, and the sustained use of aspirin (and other non-steroidal anti-inflammatory medications, like ibuprofen) also reduces the incidence of dementia and Alzheimer's disease, presumably because it keeps the arteries young. But don't take both ibuprofen and aspirin on the same day. In essence, the nonsteroidal anti-inflammatory occupies the site in the blood vessels and doesn't let aspirin do its work. They cancel out each other's effects on decreasing the aging of your arteries. Taking 162 milligrams of aspirin a day with a half glass of warm water before and after can have the long-term effect of making you 2.3 years younger when you're fifty-five, and as much as 2.9 years younger when you reach seventy.

Action 2: Exercise Your Brain

It doesn't matter what part of the body we're talking about, most everything follows the same mantra: Use it or lose it. If you don't work your muscles, they'll turn to mashed potatoes. If you don't exercise your heart, your arteries will become more clogged than Chewbacca's shower drain. And even urologists give men the same advice when it comes to erectile potency: If you want to keep on writing, you'd better sharpen the pencil. It's no different with your brain; in fact, you should approach exercising your brain with the same regularity as you do any other exercise. Keeping your brain emotionally and mentally active helps prevent memory loss.

The first thing you should do is avoid living on autopilot—that is, doing the same routine day after day. If you can find ways to stretch yourself mentally, you'll actually avoid brain shrinkage. The classic way to do this is to learn something new—whether it's learning how to speak Spanish, play Sousa tunes on the harmonica, or rebuild a car engine. The point is for you to use parts of your brain that you normally don't use. Like muscles, your brain grows when it's working outside of its normal routine.

Another way to build your brain is by, as researchers call it, "testing at your threshold." One large-scale project measured to see whether testing at your threshold was able to reverse and cause new growth of neurons and dendrites (the part of the neurons that catch information from neurotransmitters). In the project, computers were programmed so that an individual computer essentially understood a subject's ability in math, and then that computer programmed a test for its corresponding subject that stayed in line with the person's ability. Once the computer pushed the limit of each person's ability— testing them at his threshold—the researchers were able to see growth of neurons and dendrites (as judged by imaging scans taken of people's brains). But the best part is that the people didn't need to get the answers right in order to reap the benefits. Simply testing themselves just slightly beyond their capability (80 percent correct and 20 percent wrong answers) was enough to cause the regrowth. So for you, let's say you can always do Wednesday's crossword puzzle, but you get barely half of Sunday's answers. So while the best thing for your ego may be for you to continue to master Wednesday's puzzle, the best thing for your *brain* would be to continue taking a whack at Sunday's (as long as it's not so frustrating that there's no fun in doing it). Just as an athlete becomes

Myth or Fact? You can't get any smarter than you already are.

To show you the power you have to exercise your brain, look at a study measuring the brain size of London cabbies. Why cabbies? Despite the impression you've gotten from the profanities they've hurled at jaywalkers, cabbies have a very neurologically taxing job. They have to memorize the complex layout of a city and be able to figure the fastest routes between thousands of different starting and finishing points. The results of the research: the cabbies with the most experience—and therefore the ones who kept innovating to get more rides—continually challenged their brains to survive in the competitive industry and actually had larger right temporal lobes. They built bigger brains because they used them so often—and in different ways every day.

faster or stronger by training to attain goals that are just out of reach, you can train your brain to stay smarter and sharper.

An additional element, of course, is education. The more you know, the more you stretch your brain's capacity for learning. A study of nuns in a monastery is a great example. The researchers analyzed the sentence structure of essays the nuns wrote before entering the convent, then looked into their cognitive function some sixty-five years later. Those who used the most complex sentence structure when they entered the convent had the highest cognitive function as they got older. (Here's another important finding: Those who were most optimistic in their entries also had higher cognitive function.)

Bottom line: Everybody has such diverse interests that you're the only one who can choose the activities that will stretch your mind beyond its normal capabilities. You have to choose something you like; it should feel like recess, not study hall. But we can also offer some other suggestions for ways to improve your brain function in everyday life. At work, many people follow the same routine every day: Get coffee, sit down, check eBay, get more coffee, return e-mails, take bathroom break, do paperwork, call client, grab lunch, get yelled at by boss, and so on. Of course, only your boss can tell you how to do your job, but we'd like to suggest that you switch up the order every once in a while. Following the same routine every day will not stimulate your hippocampus—the part of the brain most responsible for memory. To keep your mind active, simply try to vary your routine at work or at home. Start with calls to your client, or write your report first instead of last. Whatever your normal routine is, change the order.

Here's one of our favorite ways to stretch your mind: vacations. Sure, vacations are great for both your stress levels and your sex life. But they can also help improve your cognitive skills. How? Maps. When you're driving, walking, or studying the subway system of a new city, you're using many different parts of your brain at once. You're using visual-spatial skills to read a map, and then you need to translate it into verbal code to whoever's driving. *(Honey, turn left! Now!)* When you're driving, you need to make quick decisions about where to go, which involves processing infor- mation quickly. And then you store things in your long-term memory to remember where you just visited. Get lost? Even better. Figuring out how to get back is actually contributing to the brain-building process. Of course, that kind of all-brain training can serve different purposes. For the vacationer, taking a wrong turn may lead you to a quaint antique shop you'd never have known about; but for a soldier in war, tak- ing a wrong turn can have serious consequences.

Really, everything just points to the same main advice: Keep learning. It even helps if it's in a formal system. People with higher levels of education and those who continue to be involved in activities that stimulate the mind undergo less mental aging. A college graduate who also continues to learn in formal educational settings is 2.5 years younger than a high school dropout. But informal activity helps, too. Keeping your mind active keeps arterial aging, immune aging, and even accidents in check, and has a RealAge benefit of making you 1.3 years younger. At the end of the chapter, you'll find a few ways to test and tax your brain.

Myth or Fact?
Coffee is good for your brain.

There have been enough studies performed that we can say that drinking twenty-four ounces of coffee a day decreases your risk of Parkinson's disease by 40 percent and your risk of Alzheimer's disease by about 20 percent. Why? We're not quite sure, except to say that it appears that caffeine has a beneficial impact on neurotransmitters. The effect of caffeine is substantial (whether it's in coffee or tea). It can help you live three to six months younger. Warning: For some people, too much caffeine causes irregular heartbeats, stomach upset, anxiety, or migraines; in men who suffer from an enlarged prostate condition called benign prostatic hypertrophy, caffeine can make it worse by causing spasms in the urethra.

Action 3: Some Food for Thought

Generally, what's harmful to your heart is also harmful to your brain. Make no mistake—while fried potato skins are busting your buttons, there's also a portion that gets shuttled up through your arteries to your brain. Saturated fats, for example, clog arteries that lead to your brain, putting you at increased risk of stroke, while omega-3 fatty acids—those fats found in fish—are helpful for your brain because they help keep your arteries clear. They also alter your neurotransmitters and reduce depression. The best foods for your brain are on page 93.

Action 4: Reduce Stress

In a lot of ways, stress is good. It's the physiological mechanism that helps us function. It helps us meet deadlines and run away from lions. Faced with a situation that requires action, we either decide to fight it (hustle to meet the deadline) or run away from it (aforementioned lion)—it's the process that defines "fight or flight." When those stressors reach extremely high levels, stress becomes dangerous. That's because of the effect of the stress hormone called cortisol. When you're constantly under stress, your cortisol is elevated too high. When your glands become exhausted, you end up with low levels. That's when stress is most damaging—when it exhausts your ability to increase your cortisol.

In fact, what we usually think of as stress—the daily hassles like deadlines and

Food	Why	Recommended Amount	RealAge Difference
Nuts	They contain monounsaturated and polyunsaturated fats to keep your arteries clear, as well as levels of precursors of serotonin to boost mood.	1 ounce a day is just right; more is fine, but remember to be careful of calorie overload—an ounce is about twelve walnuts or twenty-four almonds	Men: 3.3 years younger Women: 4.4 years younger
Fish (especially wild salmon, whitefish, tilapia, catfish, flounder, mahi mahi)	They contain artery-clearing omega-3 fatty acids.	13.5 ounces a week (or three servings about the size of your fist)	2.8 years younger
Soybeans	They contain heart- and artery-healthy protein and fiber.	1 cup a day	0.4 years younger
Tomato juice and spaghetti sauce	They contain folate, lycopene, and other nutrients to keep arteries young.	8 ounces a day of juice; 2 tablespoons of spaghetti sauce a day	at least 1 year younger
Olive oil, nut oils, fish oils, flaxseed, avocados	They contain heart-healthy monounsaturated omega-3 and omega-9 fats.	25 percent of daily calories should be healthy fats	3.4 years younger
Real (cocoa-based) chocolate	It increases dopamine release and provides flavonoids, which keep arteries young.	1 ounce a day (to replace milk chocolate)	1.2 years younger

getting the kids out the door—do not age our brain. It's the major stresses and nagging little stresses that age us. For years, researchers believed that having a type A, high-wired personality resulted in stress-induced illness, but your brain doesn't age from the stresses you bring onto yourself—like working hard and trying to achieve your goals. And your brain also doesn't age from the one-time, intermediate stressors, like the flat tire on your bike or the fender bender in the parking lot. These Important But Manageable events (we call them IBMs) do not cause us to age because they are problems we can solve. Instead, illness comes mainly from events that constantly stress you—even if they're minor to other people—and do so for a prolonged period. One category of these stressors is Nagging Unfinished Tasks (NUTs). For example, the nagging stress of sitting on a wobbly toilet seat and never fixing it will age you, if it is one of those things that just gnaws at you every time you use it. The other, as you'd expect, is from major life events—like moving, dealing with financial burdens, or coping with the death of a family member. Nagging stress wears you out, while persistent stressors are true killers.

You can have a major impact on your youth by reducing stress in your life with friendships, exercise, meditation, and group affiliation. In fact, doing so will give back thirty of the thirty-two years that major life events can take away. Two of our favorite stress reducers are laughing and meditating. Laughing, which reduces anxiety, tension, and stress, can make you between 1.7 and 8 years younger. With meditation, there's a multiple payoff. Meditation helps maintain your brain cells and preserve memory-related functions, and the stress-reduction component of meditation helps prevent such conditions as depression and anxiety disorder. To meditate, all you need is a quiet room. With your eyes partially closed, focus on your breathing and repeat the same word or phrase over and over again—like "um" or "one." Cardiologist Dean Ornish even starts the process with a small piece of dark chocolate. That process of repeating the same word is what helps clear and relax your mind, and it's what has the overall positive effect on your health, unless you use the phrase "I want nachos."

Action 5: Go Natural

These are the leading vitamins and supplements that can help elevate your brain function by improving mood, memory, or other aspects of your mind, and keeping it young.

FOLATE, B_6, AND B_{12}   As we covered in the heart chapter, elevated homocysteine levels are dangerous. They double the risk of stroke. We believe that homocysteine causes small openings between the endothelial cells that make up the inner lining of your arteries, leading to deterioration of the arterial wall, buildup of plaque, and inflammation. Taking 400 micrograms of folate a day in supplements, and 400 micrograms through your diet (the typical diet), can reduce homocysteine levels dramatically, essentially removing any excess homocysteine from your bloodstream and stopping its aging effects. It's important because as you age, you tend to take in less folate from food, and the concentration of folate in your body drops; in fact, lack of folate is one of the most common vitamin deficiencies among older people. Foods like asparagus, artichokes, Brussels sprouts, black-eyed peas, and sunflower seeds contain folate. Most of us also don't have high enough levels of B_6 and B_{12} (B_6 foods include chicken, bananas, and tomato paste, while B_{12} foods include salmon, tuna, hamburger, lamb, bran, and wheat flakes). By consistently taking 400 micrograms of folate a day, 6 milligrams of B_6, and 800 micrograms of B_{12} in food or 25 micrograms as a supplement (supplemental B_{12} is easier to absorb), you can make your RealAge 1.2 years younger in just three months, and probably 3.7 years younger in three years.

COENZYME Q10   Coenzyme Q10 has gained more attention than a celebrity wedding because of its alleged ability to prevent cardiovascular aging (as well as for helping critically ill patients awaiting heart transplants). We believe that it does help your heart and that it may also help prevent your brain from aging. Found naturally in the body's organs, coenzyme Q10 helps stimulate energy pathways at a cellular level, notably in muscle tissue and in all brain and nervous tissue cells. Our bodies naturally produce Q10—but only when we're not lacking vitamin C or any of the B-complex vitamins, such as B_{12}, B_6, and folate. In studies of Parkinson's disease and hypertension, high doses of coenzyme Q10 ranging up to 1,200 milligrams a day seem to decrease symptoms of Parkinson's disease, as well as decrease high blood pressure. According to these studies, this large group of potential patients would receive a benefit from taking coenzyme Q10: those who use statins (for example, Zocor, Pravachol, Lipitor, or Crestor)—that's more than 20 million people in the United States alone—will benefit; those with severe and life-threatening heart failure, Parkinson's symptoms, diabetes, and hypertension would also benefit from Q10.

ALPHA LIPOIC ACID AND L-CARNITINE   These two substances have been shown to improve cognitive function in mice. When old mice are injected with the substances, they find food at the end of the maze as fast as young mice—and faster than old mice that have not had them. L-carnitine is an amino acid that helps transfer en-

Go Deep

One extremely promising therapy for at least the movement disorders in Parkinson's disease is deep brain stimulation. One minute you can't stop multiple tremors. You turn on the deep brain stimulator, and the next minute, you can thread a sewing needle. So while coenzyme Q10 helps, and while we are waiting for stem cells to show more than promise, we are seeing miraculous changes caused by deep brain stimulation.

ergy between our cells; and in animal studies, it's been shown to decrease arterial aging and improve memory. For people over sixty, we recommend 1,500 milligrams daily of L-carnitine. Alpha lipoic acid (ALA), which also helps our bodies produce energy, is thought to help reduce the aging of our DNA caused by glucose and oxygen and to facilitate the movement of these materials to our body's power sources. Though enough data haven't been released yet, we will make recommendations on www.RealAge.com when more data become available. Stay tuned.

RESVERATROL This is a flavonoid found in red wine that seems to decrease the aging of the DNA in mitochondria—the cell's energy plant. Those flavonoids act as an antioxidant, which helps reduce aging of the arteries and the immune system. Red wine especially has this benefit because it's the grape's skin that contains resveratrol, and red wine has been in contact with the skin of the grape for a longer time than has white wine (which is why it's red). To get the maximum RealAge benefits (up to 1.9 years younger), drink alcohol in moderate amounts—one to two glasses a day if you're a man, one half to one glass a day if you're a woman.

SAME A natural amino acid, S-adenosylmethionine (SAMe), treats depression by altering the chemical reaction of neurotransmitters associated with depression. Some authorities worry that antidepressants with serious side effects are overprescribed. This one seems to have fewer side effects. If you feel you need an anti-depressant, get help. Usual dose for SAMe: 800 to 1,200 milligrams daily (on an empty stomach). While many studies have focused on St. John's wort as an antidepressant, it has interactions with many other medications. For example, it increases the metabolism of substances in birth control pills, essentially making them useless for 25 percent of the people who take both birth control pills and St. John's wort. SAMe is just as effective for mild depression, without the interactions with other medications.

Action 6: Think Hawaii

You're on a beach, with a cold drink in one hand and the latest Grisham in the other. The beach breeze kisses your face while the ocean tickles your toes. You hear gulls talking, waves crashing, and the steel-drum band jamming. You smell salt water and coconut sunscreen. Sound like paradise? Well, it's more than that. That quick mental picture just improved your brain function. See, daydreaming keeps your mind flexible. By stirring up the part of your brain that handles imagination, you keep your brain running outside of its normal thought process, which, as you now know, helps your cognitive function at the highest levels. Consider daydreaming an important part of your mental action plan. We just want your mind to stay active, so it's up to you what you daydream about, whether it involves Hawaii, Mount Everest, or a throng of sweaty Chippendale dancers.

Action 7: See the Pros

Just as there's no pill to teach Norwegian or instantly melt fat, there's also no cure-all medical treatment for personality disorders. Each person (and each disorder) is as unique as a zebra print, which is why a person suffering from a personality disorder actually needs to learn how to restructure his or her brain with the help of a professional. By the way, minor versions of personality disorders also help make us successful if we pick the right career.

Action 8: Don Your Helmet

It probably goes without saying, but we've seen enough bareheaded knuckleheads cycling the streets to know that it bears repeating: Wear a helmet when you're biking, blading, climbing, or jousting. Because your brain has the consistency of a hard-boiled egg, experiencing even minor trauma to your brain (*minor* being defined as a ding where you can't remember the event clearly) is akin to bruising that egg, which can cause outages in parts of your electrical circuitry that are related to long-term memory. Taking out a power plant with a head butt is never a good idea for the grid, and you often will not see the long-term effects on memory for decades.

Test Your Brain

How smart are you? Take this quick test to peek inside the power of your brain. *Test adapted from the Mensa test by Dr. Abbie Salny and America Mensa Ltd., copyright 1992 and 2004* Turn to page 102 for the results.

1. *While Bill was ironing his G-string, a person knocked on his door. It was his mother-in-law's only daughter's husband's son. What relation was this person to Bill?*

2. *What's the missing number in the series?*
    1 3 9 __ 81 243

3. *Which of the proverbs below best matches the meaning of "All that glitters is not gold"?*
    a.   A penny saved is a penny earned
    b.   You can't tell a book by its cover
    c.   A fool and his money are soon parted
    d.   Just because Boy George wears makeup doesn't mean he can sing

4. *Unscramble the letters to reveal this health term.*
    E E L L O C T O S H R

5. *If Britney is 10, Wolfgang Mozart is 20, and Prince and Sting are both 5, but Elvis is 10, how much is Madonna by the same system?*

6. *After paying for the Cabbage Patch Kid you bought on eBay, you have just $9.60 in your pocket. You have an equal number of quarters, dimes, and nickels, but no other coins. How many of each of the three coins do you have?*

7. Which of the following is least like the others?
    a. Lungs
    b. Ears
    c. Brain
    d. Legs
    e. Groin

8. How many 9s do you pass when you start at 1 and count up to 100?

9. One four-letter word will fit on all three lines below to make new words with the word preceding and the word following (example: IN [DOOR] STOP). The same word must be used for all three lines. What's the word?

    BACK _ _ _ _ SOME
    FREE _ _ _ _ MADE
    FORE _ _ _ _ BAG

10. What is the tree that contains all the vowels: A E I O U (though not in order)?

11. The following is a common proverb in disguise. Put it in its common form.
    A finely chosen pomegranate consumed at every eastwardly arrival of sunlight prevents the healer of all bodily malfunctions from knocking at the entrance of your abode.

12. The spy was captured easily, and his message proved to be so simple that the lieutenant saw its importance immediately. Here it is. What does it say?
    ALBERT: TOM TRICKS ARETHA'S CUDDLY KITTY, ANSWER TODAY: DO ANOTHER WIGGLE NOW. MARTHA'S OVARIES NOT DANCING. ARE YOU?

Answers, Brain Test

1. His son. Draw a box and label it Bill. Draw another box for his mother-in-law and connect them. Draw a third box for his mother-in-law's only daughter, who has to be Bill's wife. Then a fourth box, who also has to be Bill's son—and very disturbed at his father as well.

2. 27. Each number has three times the value of the number preceding it.

3. B, general knowledge question.

4. Cholesterol

5. Madonna is 15 in a system that awards 5 points for each syllable in the name

6. 24

7. Brain. All others have hair—legs and groin on the skin, while the ears and lungs have tiny hairs called cilia that serve a cleaning function.

8. 20

9. Hand

10. Sequoia

11. An apple a day keeps the doctor away.

12. Attack at dawn Monday. The lieutenant lifted the first letter out of each word and strung the letters together.

Score

11–12: Among the most intelligent people around

8–10: Very intelligent

5–7: Respectable score

4 or below: Chalk it up to a bad day

Chapter 4

Motion Control: Your Bones, Joints, and Muscles

Major Myths About Movement

Motion Myth #1	The more you exercise, the more you benefit.
Motion Myth #2	Your bones are solid structures that thin with aging at a predetermined rate.
Motion Myth #3	Men are safe from osteoporosis.

A house's wood beams define its shape, anchor heavy wall hangings, and shield the inside from the outside. Nailed together, these two-by-fours frame everything inside. If those beams weaken or those nails rust, the result would threaten not only that particular part of the house but the entire structure. Without a strong structure to hold up the drywall and siding, our valuables would be susceptible to damage by weather, looters, and hungry bears. In many ways, your 206 bones (as well as the joints that hold them together) serve the same purpose in your body. Your skeletal system gives you the shape that allows you to stand up straight, and it protects your internal organs from potentially destructive falls, accidents, and knife-throwing magicians.

Chances are, you've been brought up to believe that your bones are much like two-by-fours—solid and generally unchanging. They grow in size as we change from kids to adults, but besides that, they're static structures, right? Not exactly. The molecular elements in each of our bones right now are actually different from the ones composing the bones that held you up even a decade ago. The individual molecules in your bones rotate in response to what your bones need—and how well you nourish them. Just as you can take control of how efficient your heart pumps or how thick your waist becomes, you can take control of the way your bones age.

Together, bones, joints, and muscles make up the human machine of movement; they help you walk your dog, play golf, and outrun the paparazzi. Even if your bones feel more like steel girders than toothpicks, your musculoskeletal system does some surprising things as it develops. Maybe you're not terribly worried about your bones, joints, and muscles right now, but they're hugely important to the way we age, if for no other reason than this: Having Lance Armstrong's heart or Albert Einstein's brain doesn't mean a darn thing if you can't lift yourself off the toilet.

Of course, many things can put your skeletal system at risk—falling off a bike,

slipping on a patch of ice, being on the receiving end
of a machete. But what has the most potential for
damaging your skeletal system is a factor so important to your overall health: physical activity.
Though we can generally identify things good for
us in extraordinary amounts (vegetables, $100 bills) and

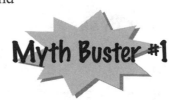

Myth Buster #1

the things that aren't (corn dogs, overdue bills), physical activity is one of those
things that's a little less clear. Certainly, physical activity helps our entire body—our
heart, brain, and bones—but the catch is that when it comes to your bones, joints,
and muscles, *excessive* physical activity can be just as destructive to your body as a
boxer's right hand.

We know it's a hard concept to imagine when today's athletes look as if
they're chiseled out of granite. But the reality is that excessive exercise is like a category 5 hurricane to your body. The more pounding you take—even if you aren't a
superathlete—the greater the chance that the foundation of your house is going to
be reduced to rubble.

Later in the chapter, we'll discuss how moderate exercise (done to the point at
which you push yourself toward your limits) and other choices can keep your bones,
joints, and muscles young. But first, let's spin through the amazing system of movement in your body.

Your Bones, Joints, and Muscles: The Anatomy

The trio of bones, joints, and muscles is a little like the Three Stooges. They're all different individually, but any one is virtually useless without the support of the others.
Here's how they work:

Your Bones

On the surface, bones seem easy: They're white and hard, and they're great for fetching and Halloween parties. But in reality, bones are more misunderstood than Bob Dylan's lyrics. The primary functions of bone are as follows:

★ To act as a suit of armor for our other vital organs
★ To store minerals like calcium and magnesium
★ To act as a series of lever arms needed for movement
★ To act as a factory for the production of blood cells and stem cells

Your bones also have some other unique characteristics. For one, they're living organs; they continually replenish themselves and regenerate to build new bone in place of old or damaged bone—making it one of the organs in the body able to do that (like the liver; see Chapter 7). In fact, it's the only material in your body that regenerates brand new; when you cut your skin, you don't grow new skin; you heal with a scar, which isn't really new because it doesn't grow hair, stretch, or secrete sweat. Bone is the opposite—it heals itself, and the new, repaired bone is eventually as strong as the original. The only downside—as anyone who's ever had to wear a cast knows—is that it can take four to six months to heal completely. While that process is going on, other parts of your system—like the muscles around those bones—can weaken.

The second intriguing thing about bone is its physical structure. Most people think that bones are bricklike—hard all the way through the entire mass. Yes, your bones are the second-hardest substance in your body (enamel is the hardest), but

Myth Buster #2

they're not solid like concrete. Their physical structure is more like a honeycomb—a solid mass dotted with tiny holes.

Normally, your body recycles old bone components to make new ones, and it also deposits new calcium and other minerals into your bones to make them hard and dense. But after you turn thirty-five, your bones stop growing and you gradually lose bone density, which means that those holes get larger while the hard substance gets thinner. So your bones become more porous, weaker, and more susceptible to injury and fractures if you don't do things to protect them from aging. To understand what the aging process does to your bones, think about what termites do to a house. They make holes all throughout the center of the wood beams. Left untreated, they'd create holes so big that the wood beams would eventually collapse. It's the same process with your bones, except that you have the ability to serve as your own exterminator.

OSTEOPOROSIS   If that decrease in bone density is significant enough, it can lead to osteoporosis—a condition in which the bones have thinned and weakened to the point where they can break very easily. In people with osteoporosis, those two processes of recycling old bone cells and depositing calcium are thrown out of whack, and the deterioration of old bone cells outpaces the formation of new bone cells.

When you think of osteoporosis, you probably think of bone breaks. Surely that's the danger of having thin bones. But it's not the break itself that makes osteoporosis so bad. It's what happens afterward. The fracture triggers a chain of aging-related events. When you're bedridden, you become weaker and more susceptible to infections. With less exercise, your arteries become less elastic and more prone to injury. And finally, your immune system becomes more vulnerable to dangerous diseases and infections.

More than 28 million Americans either have osteoporosis or are at risk for it, but the disease hits primarily people over the age of sixty-five. It's often considered a women's disease because of the current statistics: 25 percent of women over sixty-five have the disease, compared to 15 percent of men, and one-third of women will suffer a broken bone due to osteoporosis compared to one-sixth of men. But the disease, in fact, isn't gender specific. As the average life span of men increases, we're seeing the osteoporosis rate in men increase as well. When men reach the age of seventy-five, their rate of having the disease increases to 25 percent, too. Women just tend to get osteoporosis earlier because women's bone density and bone mass are naturally thinner. Women also lose bone density after menopause, since they lose some estrogen, which is paramount in helping deposit calcium. But men "catch up" later; as they reach seventy-five, they lack both the mass and sufficient estrogen and testosterone to help build bone.

Myth Buster #3

What makes osteoporosis different from so many other conditions is that you may have no idea you even have it. In most cases, there aren't any symptoms until you break a bone. Break an arm when you slip on the ice, and you think nothing of the way it happened—you know that the trauma was significant enough to cause a break. But break an arm when you bump into the doorway, and it's a tip-off that your bones are much weaker than normal and that you may have osteoporosis. (A doctor may also discover osteoporosis through an X ray taken for another problem. You can also have a test to measure your bone mineral density, such as a DEXA [dual-energy X-ray absorptiometry] scan.) That's one of the reasons why prevention is so important—you never see the injury coming until it's too late to do anything about it. The other reason is that treatment doesn't cure osteoporosis; it slows the thinning process and can help rebuild new bone. Because your bones grow when stimulated under the right circumstances, you can take steps now to prevent bone loss and osteoporosis.

We are optimistic about osteoporosis, especially because you can take control of your own body and keep yourself younger. If you are getting enough physical activity, controlling your blood pressure, and eliminating cigarettes, you're well on your way to keeping the disease at bay. Another item to celebrate: From 1988 to 2003, there was a sevenfold increase in the detection of osteoporosis *before* a fracture occurred. But don't feel comfortable just yet; over half the people who should have been screened for it in 2003 weren't, and over three-quarters of those diagnosed with it were not even prescribed appropriate calcium (let alone vitamin D). Soon we'll talk about the steps you can take to keep your internal bone-building factory right on schedule.

Your Joints

Take one look at the way a toddler can put her feet behind her head, and you'll see the full capability of our joints in action. Somehow evolution knew that we needed to reach the top shelf, make a quick cut away from the linebacker, and do the Electric Slide at our cousin's wedding. In response, evolution rewarded us with joints that can move in an infinite number of ways. As one of the more amazing parts of our bodies, all joints have the same overriding physiology, but they're also all unique because they're customized for their special function, depending on what part of the body they form.

The simple physiology of almost all of our joints is this: They link one bone to another to allow us to move at the point of connection—the way a hinge connects a door to a wall. Made up of ligaments and cartilage, joints are well lubed to keep your bones moving smoothly. They're also unique in that they don't all function like door

Myth or Fact? Football players have the highest risk of ACL tears.

Athletes get all the headlines when they get injured, but women are up to eight times more likely than men to tear their ACL. The looser construction of the female knee—and overall weaker skeleton—can compromise stability and predispose women to ligament tears. The injuries are also linked to hormonal changes around the time of menstruation, so female high school, collegiate, recreational, and professional athletes end up suffering many more tears than men do.

hinges—swinging back and forth in a two-dimensional motion. Also, they all must balance two opposing forces—stability versus mobility. Three joints—the knee, hip, and shoulder—are typically considered our body's most important joints, and they're all constructed differently to customize the relationship between mobility and stability. While the shoulder joint is the most mobile joint in the body (look how many ways you can turn and swing your arms), the hip joint is the most stable (for good reason, to carry you everywhere). Let's take a more detailed look.

KNEE Situated between the two longest bones in your body (the tibia and femur), the classic door-hinge joint bends in one plane of motion—backward, not forward or side to side (see Figure 4.1). It's at risk for strain and injury because of its limited range of motion, the heavy load your knees carry, and the torque (from twisting motions) generated by the two leverlike bones. While you may hear about knee injuries most commonly in the form of professional athletes who tear their anterior cruciate ligaments (ACLs), the more common knee injury for those of us who do and don't play with pigskin is actually a torn meniscus. Your meniscus, which is a piece of cartilage in the middle of your knee, not only acts as a shock absorber but also has several other functions. It helps lubricate the joint by increasing the surface

Why We Ice

You ice an injury for forty-eight hours after an injury because of the swelling. While swelling indicates an increase in fluid or blood deposits in the area, it slows down recovery from the injury. The presence of this additional fluid makes joints stiffer and more painful, which makes them weaker. Ice reduces the swelling—and the pain. After that forty-eight-hour period, you can use ice off and on, but you can also use heat alone on the injury to warm it up. The heat loosens up the joint or muscle, giving you more flexibility and allowing you to move more freely during rehabilitation.

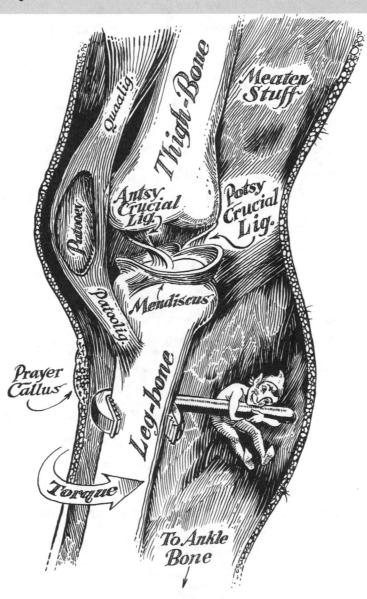

area of the cartilage. It adds stability to the joint in that it's shaped like a suction cup to keep the round femur on top of the flat tibia. And it also helps produce synovial fluid to feed the cells of the cartilage. It can tear from traumatic injury (when a football player gets a cleat wedged in the turf, his body may twist, but his knee won't be able to because his foot is stuck), but it can also tear from overuse and doing simple movements like squatting. Your meniscus acts as a shock absorber when you're walking, and when it tears, it leads to inflammation and a lot of pain. Doctors can detect a tear using an MRI; treatment involves anti-inflammatory medication, icing, aggressive rehabilitation (and, if all else fails, arthroscopic surgery).

SHOULDER From Figure 4.2, you can see that your two shoulder joints each consist of three bones (the clavicle, scapula, and humerus), and they're essentially what gives you the ability to rotate your arms in many different directions. The top of the humerus bone lies on a shallow shelf of bone within the shoulder, like a golf ball on a tee. Some shoulders dislocate easily because the top of the humerus falls off a damaged joint, just like a ball on a chipped tee. This anatomy allows a wide range of motion and allows you to swing clubs, play tennis, and do the backstroke. But that wide range of motion also makes it the most prone to dislocation. Those people who play sports with throwing motions are at most risk of suffering an injury to their shoulder joints; a rotator cuff injury is usually a strain or tear of the muscles or tendons around those shoulder bones. Diagnosis comes from a physical examination—no, the doc isn't just trying to see if you're tough—confirmed by an MRI, and the treatment is similar to that undertaken for a meniscus tear. You can most likely avoid shoulder problems by paying attention to your arm position during movement. Avoid any exercises that require you to put your hands outside of your line of vision. In those positions, you're more likely to pull the ball farther from the golf tee than it wants to go.

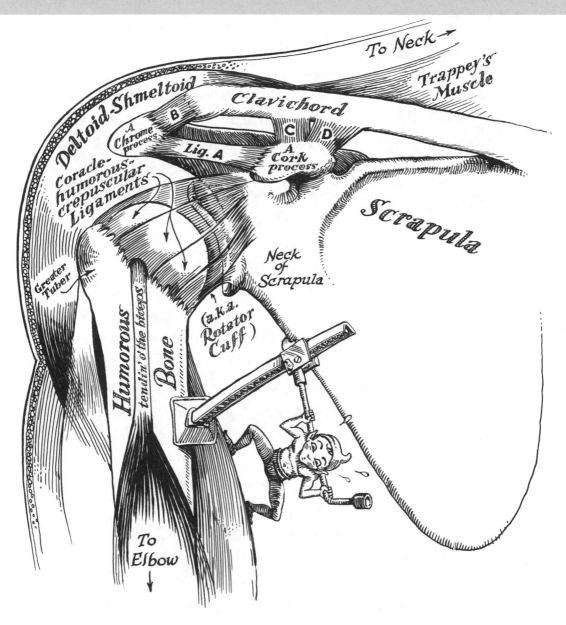

Myth or Fact?
Your hips hurt;
you're going to need
a replacement.

Belly dancing isn't the only thing hips are good for. Hip joints are the ones that provide the hinge for any kind of forward motion. While they're not as flexible as shoulder joints, they're large joints, and a lot of things can happen in there. Any chronic pain needs to be addressed by a doctor, but hip pain does not automatically mean you have arthritis. If the pain is coming from the front of the hips, in the groin area, it's probably a sign of some form of arthritis. But if you're experiencing some tenderness along the sides, your pain more likely stems from tendonitis or bursitis, which can be treated in a number of different ways, including anti-inflammatory medication and physical therapy.

HIP   The hip joint (Figure 4.3) gives you a lot of stability because it needs to carry your body weight, but the ball-and-socket anatomy also gives you the ability to rotate and to move forward but not back. One of the foundations of your body, the hip joint is a place where many different muscles and tendons attach; many of the injuries that happen to this ball-and-socket joint stem from overuse and the wear and tear of being in constant motion. But because it's more stable than mobile, it's more prone to fracture than dislocation (especially as you get older, when it's more likely that you'll lose balance on a rug or an uneven part of the pavement and land on your side).

No matter which one we're talking about, joints are vulnerable parts of your body. They're soft substances, so if there's some kind of trauma, the joint is the first thing to take the hit. But as you age, your concern shouldn't revolve around injury. It should revolve around degeneration and how you can keep your joints young and strong.

OSTEOARTHRITIS   As you age, the density of those slippery shock-absorber surfaces thins, and you gradually lose your cushioning. When that happens, the effect is similar to walking in shoes without socks. While socks provide cushioning (and contain odor), they also provide a buffer to absorb the friction that would occur if the shoe rubbed up against your skin. Without the sock, your exposed skin would rub against the shoe, get irritated, blister, and become inflamed. It's the same con-

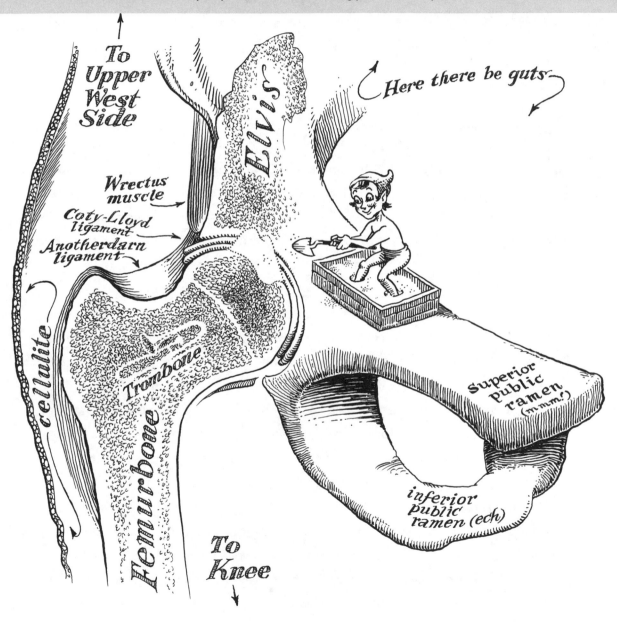

FIGURE 4.3 **Hip Hip Hooray** Our strongest joint, the hip, has a ball-and-socket construction that gives us stability, but at a price. The joint is difficult to stretch out and is prone to stiffening with arthritis. The effect is that your joint feels as if sand is being poured into the joint.

Myth or Fact?
Cracking your knuckles will give you arthritis.

Cracking your knuckles makes you sound like a bowl of Rice Krispies and never goes over well in church. While it's painful for *us* to hear, you're not doing any harm to your joints, bones, or muscles when you crack — unless you feel pain when you crack them. It's just caused by the high pressure suction of gas being expelled when your joints move apart. If it hurts when your knuckles or knees crack, you need to see your doctor to assess what kind of joint damage you may have.

cept with your joints. As you lose your internal sock, your bones lose their ability to slide, and they can rub directly against each other. When that happens, the effect is like stick on stick—and it hurts. In simple form, that's what osteoarthritis is. It's a condition in which the cartilage that covers the bones and forms the surface of the joints becomes thinner, rougher, and less protective of the bone, so the bones grind against each other, and the joint becomes inflamed. It's painful and makes walking— or any kind of movement—difficult (by the way, not all arthritis shows up on X rays, and not all painful arthritis means there's significant joint damage). Currently, osteoarthritis affects more than 20 million Americans, and that number is expected to grow to 40 million by 2020, making it one of the most common health problems in the country. Eighty-five percent of us who reach eighty-five will have knee osteoarthritis if we do not do something to prevent it. When it's detected by X ray alone, it's usually not a problem, but when there's pain associated with it, there is.

Joint deterioration really affects those super- and professional athletes who put an excessive amount of pressure on their joints throughout their careers. Since many of you are not training for the next Olympics, you can prevent damage to your joints while you're young—and even regenerate damaged cartilage.

Though osteoarthritis can occur in any of your joints, including your hands, hips, and spine, we're going to focus mainly on your knees, because they're the largest hinges in your body and because you need your knees an awful lot. On the surface, your knees seem very strong, because they're one of the most powerful joints in the body; you use the knee joints to both push off and absorb force. But they're also prone to wear and tear for one major reason. Your knee joints are the UPS men of your body. They carry your body no matter how heavy the package—and without the help of dollies. Just as it's easier for the UPS guy to carry a book than a refrigerator, it's easier for your knees to haul lighter freight. When you gain ten pounds of body weight, it feels more like a thirty-pound weight gain for your knees. (No matter how much you weigh, your knees are constantly under strain. When you walk up stairs, that ten pounds feels like seventy pounds of weight to your knee joint.) Unlike osteoporosis, osteoarthritis is a disease that you will feel—often—in the form of mild to severe pain, creaking, or swelling

and stiffness in your joints. And though MRIs will show that 85 percent of us will have osteoarthritis by the time we reach eighty-five, only about 50 percent of us will have the symptoms. Many things can make osteoarthritis more likely, including bad posture, overuse, heredity, obesity, the lack of vitamins C and D, and the lack of calcium. Since symptoms usually occur in middle age, osteoarthritis is like osteoporosis in one important way: You can prevent progression of the disease, and even reverse it, by following the right antiaging guidelines (see later in this chapter).

Your Muscles

You might not know it by our country's obesity epidemic, but we certainly do love our muscles. We see them on everything from magazine covers and CD cases to Brad Pitt movie posters and Times Square billboards. Despite our visual fascination with the lean mass of tissue that swiped the term "six-pack" from the beer industry, muscles are really important because of their physical function. The 650 muscles in our body give us the strength to do *everything*. While we all have varied levels of muscle mass, all of our muscles work the same way. Attached to ligaments, muscles are made up of tissues that contract and relax. To understand how they work, think of an extendable ladder that is extended—that's your muscle at rest. When you put tension on one end, the ladder ratchets together and consolidates the rungs—making the ladder shorter. When you release tension on your muscle, it relaxes and extends back to its rest length. A muscle works when you put it under a certain amount of tension, and the energy you consume (food) gives you the power to contract and relax. When a muscle is under full tension during a workout, it is actually damaged by that tension, but it grows when it recovers. When you put your muscles under just the right amount of tension (that at threshold), that's when you feel soreness—a soreness is caused by toxins in that damaged muscle. (Postworkout massage and stretching have been shown to reduce muscle soreness because they both help work those toxins away from the muscle, to be drained in the lymphatic system.) Too much tension, and a muscle rips—that's not soreness; that's pain.

BACK PAIN   Of course, while every one of those muscles serves a different purpose and each is susceptible to its own form of strain, tears, and other kinds of injuries, we want to focus on the most common and debilitating muscle problem in terms of aging: back pain. First, let's tour your back. Your spine is the snakelike curved structure made up of small bones called the vertebrae, which are stacked one on top of another to form a column. Between each two vertebrae, there's a disc that provides cushioning. Think of the spinal structure as a series of jelly doughnuts—with the vertebrae acting as the semihard casing and the discs as the squishy substances inside that casing. Tendons and ligaments hold the entire spine together, and an opening in each vertebra line up to form a long hollow canal that houses the spinal cord from the base of the brain down the spine. Small nerves from the spinal cord jet out the spine through the space between the vertebrae. (A bulging or herniated disc happens when too much torque is put on the spine and the disc bulges out, like pinching the doughnut so the jelly oozes out. If that occurs close to a nerve, that leads to inflammation of your nerves leading down to your legs and arms, which is why a pinched nerve hurts down the legs or arms more than directly in the neck or back.) Though we all have heard of the severity of injuries that can come from trauma to the spine, the more common forms of pain come from strained muscles in or surrounding the lower back.

The muscles in your lower back have a function similar to your knees'—they support a lot of your body weight. Yet they are just not as strong as they need to be to support you by themselves, and they are often abandoned by the stomach and pelvic

Myth or Fact?
Your spouse can accelerate your recovery from back pain.

If you've ever strained your back, you know that on the scale of 1 to 10, the pain ranks at a 692. It can be paralyzing—making it difficult to walk, to sit, to get up, to sleep, to do anything. All you want to do is to lie down, prop your head on some pillows, flick on *Ally McBeal* reruns, and remain still. And you can think of nothing better than having your spouse deliver ice packs, ibuprofen, and the latest issue of *Tattoo Today* directly to your bed. But your spouse shouldn't play nurse. Why? Statistically speaking, married people with back pain suffer two and a half times longer than single people. Attentive spouses may be doing the right thing emotionally, but by encouraging the suffering to stay in bed, they're doing the wrong thing physically. If you stay in bed for longer than forty-eight hours, your back muscles weaken—and can increase your risk for further injury. In order to recover from strain, your muscles need to grow stronger and stay active, and the only way they'll do that is by working, even if it's just a little bit. The best method: Walk around the house. Keep moving.

Myth or Fact? Weight belts will save your back.

Go to one of those mega-hardware stores, and the employees are all wearing weight belts — those large beltlike straps that provide extra support to their waists when they haul heavy boxes. But you know what? You have a natural weight belt — your abdominal muscles. And if your abdominal muscles are strong enough, they'll give you the support your lower back needs. In fact, some studies have shown that weight belts are actually detrimental, because wearing one means that the muscles in your abdominals will learn to rely on the belt, so they won't develop and grow stronger. That'll leave them more vulnerable when you call on them to protect your back during times you're not wearing a weight belt, such as when you slip on ice, twist in an unnatural way, or lift your child out of a grocery cart.

muscles, which work in harmony to support our upright structure. The people who are most at risk for back pain are those who go long periods sitting or standing, those who are in poor physical condition or who have a poor exercise regimen, and those who do heavy labor. They're less likely to recover quickly from lower back pain because their lifestyle exacerbates the pain—or their bodies aren't equipped to recover. They may also have overused or underdeveloped muscles in their lower back. In that case, doing anything from getting off the couch to stepping into a car may be enough to trigger excruciating tension in your lower-back muscles. That's the strain that causes the pain. (To test yourself, lie on the floor and raise one leg straight up. If there's pain in the back of your leg when you raise your foot about a foot off the ground, it's probably more of a nerve problem than a muscle problem.)

With about 65 million Americans suffering from back pain, it's the second most common reason for medical visits. The way the odds play out, you're likely to have about one serious episode of back pain for every fifteen years of your life (serious is defined by pain severe enough that you seek medical attention). For those who plan to live ninety-plus years, that means you're likely to have six severe episodes of back pain in your life. But in only 5 percent of cases does the pain keep you from all daily activities. The really interesting part of this is that, unlike your bones and joints, your back muscles seem to be under the most strain from the ages of thirty-five to fifty-five. Back pain is much less common in older people, presumably because older people carry less tension in their back. Luckily, nearly 95 percent of lower back pain can be treated without surgery. And even more can be prevented by doing exercises that center around the pelvis and abdomen.

Your Bones, Joints, and Muscles: The Live Younger Action Plan

Just like a car can't move without wheels, you can't move without a properly functioning set of bones, joints, and muscles. To make sure you can continue to do everything from walking to scoring a perfect 10 on the pommel horse, you need to build a system of movement that gives you not only the power to move but also the power to do so pain- and problem-free. As essential as it is to keep your tires inflated, it's as crucial that you do the few things that will keep your body comfortably set on cruise control on the interstate of life.

Myth or Fact? You can't have a herniated disc without pain.

The sciatic nerve passes from your lower spine to your feet; when a bulging disc compresses it, it causes leg pain, which helps indicate the cause and severity of back pain. Doctors do not like removing a disc and fusing the spine because the extra pressure on surrounding discs can cause premature damage. But be warned: Lots of folks have herniated discs without pain; many people have joint and back pain with normal X rays; others have abnormal X rays with no pain at all. Just because the MRI is irregular doesn't mean you found the culprit, which makes back pain one of the most difficult conditions to diagnose.

Action 1: Do the right amount—and all three kinds— of physical activity

Some people exercise to lose weight. Some exercise because it allows them to feel good, to reduce stress, to win races. And some people just love to sweat. But of all the reasons to be physically active, we think one trumps all the others: Do it to live younger. In fact, if you follow these steps, the result will be a RealAge royal flush—

Myth or Fact?
Doing sit-ups (crunches) will save your back

It is true. Not only will abdominal exercises strengthen your bones and the muscles of the back, but they'll also strengthen your entire midsection—which takes weight and pressure off your back. So add exercises like the ones in the "Owner's Manual Workout" (page 433). Your magazine cover contract awaits you.

men who exercise right live eight years younger, and women who do so live nine years younger.

Of course, an important reason to do physical activity is that it will help you lose weight and keep the weight off. If your body is a plastic grocery bag and you load it up with a loaf of bread, a box of rice, and a small bag of apples, everything's just fine. Now drop a can of beans in a bag. Then another can. And another. Keep going. Eventually, if you add enough cans, the bag will break under the weight and strain. Your body works the same way—it can take only so much extra weight before it starts to break down. Physical activity, even a little in small doses, removes cans from your plastic bag and even strengthens the bag. It has an effect not only on your appearance and on other areas of your health, as we've talked about in previous chapters, but also on how your joints feel. (In one study, women who lost just ten pounds had a 50 percent lower risk of osteoarthritis.)

That said, because we all have different goals and reasons for exercising, we also all have different programs. A boxer's training program is different from a marathoner's, whose program is different from your cousin Lenny's. We do know the value in extreme exercise—whether it's for the thrills, glory, or emotional satisfaction—but you won't be protecting your bones, joints, and muscles from the deterioration associated with aging; in fact, you'll be doing it at their expense. What follows is our recommendation for the best bone-building exercise plan you can have.

SHOW SOME RESISTANCE Go to the gym and you'll see two camps of exercisers. There are the ones who use the cardiovascular machines, and there are the ones who lift the weights. If you fall into the first camp, you may have little experience with weight training or you may fear that one day in the gym will somehow morph you into a Hulk-like creature. But if you fall into the latter camp, you need to know that weights aren't just made for twenty-year-old guys trying to impress the coeds. There are benefits to weight training—no matter your age or fitness level. For one, weight training adds to your body's lean muscle mass, which, over time, consumes more calories than fat and therefore helps keep your weight down. For another, it makes your muscles stronger and better equipped to go through the motions of life. In fact, increasing the strength of your lower back is the top way to avoid lower-back pain. And somehow it decreases the aging of your heart, arteries, and immune system. Most of all, weight training builds bones—it's one of the best things you can do to maintain and build bone density and prevent osteoporosis. How? Bone will form in response to stress, so when muscles pull on the bones during weight lifting, they stimulate the bone to increase its density—making resistance training a bone-stimulating activity.

Myth or Fact? Training for marathons is healthy.

Finishing a marathon will earn you many things: a medal, increased cardiovascular stamina, and blisters the size of Australia. While we respect marathoners and admire their passion, dedication, and athleticism, we can't endorse the training it takes to complete a 26.2-mile race. The constant pounding your joints take with every step increases the likelihood that you'll suffer from joint problems and osteoarthritis down the road. And once you exceed more than eighteen to twenty miles, you are likely to be consuming your own muscle proteins to provide energy. Sure, we'd love to see you cross the finish line, but we'd also like to see you live your whole life in the best — and youngest — shape possible. To live long and young, you need to be physically active. But too much activity can actually put the accelerator on aging, instead of the brakes.

Now, weight training doesn't have to come in the form of bench-pressing monster trucks. What's important is that you do some kind of weight-bearing, resistance exercise—that is, exercise in which your body pushes and pulls against some kind of resistance, whether it's by lifting dumbbells, using an exercise machine, pushing and pulling exercise tubes or bands, or even using your own body weight. (See the

"Owner's Manual Workout" on page 433.) In some way that we don't fully understand, the right amount of resistance training—that done "at threshold," where your muscles fatigue to the point of failure at eight to twelve repetitions—puts your bones under the stress they need to regrow, maintain, and build their density.

Your bones don't need much resistance to grow. In fact, they don't need much resistance at all. Just thirty minutes of weight-bearing exercise *a week* is all you need to maintain and build your bone density. What's better is that you not do it all at once; if you split it into three ten-minute sessions, you'll still gain the maximum benefit. And you'll be reaping the benefits exponentially. Doing just thirty minutes of

Myth or Fact?
You can spot-reduce by exercising a specific muscle or using an electrical stimulator.

Let's say you have a gut, or some love handles, or some cellulite on your hips. Do a thousand crunches a day or put an electrical stimulator over your hips, and you'll eventually fry away the fat, right? Sorry. That's not how your body works. One exercise—or any kind of electronic or exercise gadget—cannot burn fat from specific parts of your body. Think about when you see someone who has lost weight. Where's the first place you notice it? The face. Since we don't see too many people doing face crunches in the gym, it just goes to show that your body dictates where it burns fat. Very often, the place you most want to lose it is the last place it burns. While it's true that you can build muscle in different locations of your body based on what exercises you do, there's no way to "spot-reduce" fat. The only way to address target areas is through an overall program that includes both stamina training and resistance training, as well as using a calorie-controlled diet. If you want to build muscle in a particular area, you can make it look younger and firmer. But losing fat isn't a targeted process the way building muscle is—you have to lose it under the chin to lose it from your belly. With smaller-portioned meals and more physical activity, you'll reduce *everywhere* and make yourself feel, be, and look younger.

resistance training a week has a RealAge effect of making you nearly two years younger.

If you're a novice in the gym, some of the best bone-building resistance exercises don't have to involve any outside weights; rather, you can use your own body weight as resistance. Squats and lunges not only help build all the muscles in your leg and butt, they also help strengthen the muscles in your lower back to protect you from strains. You can also add upper-body exercises—and exercises that work your midsection—to help provide stabilization and increase strength in your entire body. Best of all, strength training helps you stay slim. If you don't do strength-building exercises, you lose 5 percent of your muscle mass every ten years (the average woman loses two pounds of muscle every ten years after age thirty-five, the average man three pounds). Adding muscle burns fat because muscle needs energy to survive: A pound of muscle uses between 50 and 150 calories a day (remember, it's working and using energy), while a pound of fat needs only 3 calories a day (fat, the ingrate, does nothing to help your body, so it doesn't need much energy to maintain itself). That muscle building takes only a few minutes—ten minutes, three times a week, to be exact—to maintain muscle mass.

Resistance training strengthens your muscles, but the benefits extend to your bones and joints as well by increasing the flexibility of your joints, remodeling your

Myth or Fact? You're too overweight to exercise.

Saying you're too overweight to exercise is like saying you're too skinny to eat. Your body needs exercise just the way your body needs food. No matter how overweight you are, you can do something to start the process of losing fat, strengthening your bones, and relieving your joints of the load that they're carrying. If you're overweight or have other medical conditions, you should consult your doctor before starting any exercise program. Start small: Walk five minutes a day, and increase by one or two minutes every few days. Soon you'll be fit enough to walk an hour a day. You can even start small with resistance training. Doing simple exercises with soup cans or books will stimulate your muscles in new ways—and will begin the process of kick-starting your metabolism so your body can burn fat. If you want to live longer, start today. Your family—and your younger body—will thank you.

bone structure, and building a skeletal support system with stronger muscles. When done together (see Chapter 14), these exercises form a total-body strength-building workout.

BE KIND TO YOUR BODY As doctors, we see all kinds of people and patients. We get to know not only their medical history but also their lifestyle passions—what makes their hearts tick, literally and figuratively. For instance, we've come across people who would choose open-heart surgery as a medical option rather than give up running; an athlete's passion is admirable and the dedication impressive. Certainly, many people simply get addicted to exercise—addicted because it makes them feel good. But we also see what happens to people whose knees, shoulders, and hips take constant pounding from running, throwing, skiing, and playing tennis or basketball. Let's take the example of Arnold Schwarzenegger. As brainy as he is brawny, Arnold knew what to do when his body started slowing down. He had to cut back, or else he'd develop more pain and chronic problems, especially in his joints. So he tapered off to a lighter workout regimen. By taking some of the pressure off the very structure that gave him the unworldly ability to squat buses, he's essentially ensuring that his bones and joints *vill be back*. So he incorporated a routine that decreased his weight training because he was doing way too much of it, and he increased his stamina training because he was doing way too little.

A quick note: Stamina training will not help your bones. Stamina training, as our plan in the cardiovascular chapter outlines, is all about strengthening your heart and keeping your arteries young. The problem with some cardiovascular training, like running and stair climbing, is that it whoops up on your bones and joints like a lion on raw meat (and usually does little for your muscles, depending on what kind of stamina training you're doing). To live longer and best protect your joints from the onslaught of impact, the best stamina workouts you can do are swimming, rowing, cycling, and exercising on an elliptical machine. These activities elevate your heart rate, and they work various muscles (with swimming working just about every part of your body), but your joints don't absorb the shock, trauma, and pounding of your body step after step. And that's a major advantage to those people suffering from joint pain and osteoarthritis—they're the best ways to maintain your cardiovascular health so your joints can recover. With swimming and cycling, you get the benefits of cardiovascular training without the stress. (Walking is also a super form of exercise, but most people don't walk quickly enough to elevate their heart rates high enough to be classified as stamina training, although we recommend frequent walking—at least thirty minutes a day, no excuses—for overall health.) The perfect workout program actually includes both weight-bearing and non-weight-bearing stamina activities, because cross training—that is, choosing different types of stamina exercises on different days—helps you use different muscles. And strength training builds muscles. Those

The Replacements

Live in a house long enough, and you know the inevitability of age. The roof will spring leaks, the carpet will get worn down, the appliances will sputter, and you'll end up spending most of your free time patching and plugging (and cursing every step of the way). In a lot of ways, your body works the same way. Exposed to so many external forces through everyday life, your joints carry much of the burden of getting you to the bus stop, up the stairs, and through the jungle of life. The price you pay for that wear and tear can come in the form of joint replacement surgery. The two most prevalent (and successful) procedures include knee and hip replacement—with osteoarthritis being the primary cause of them. While successful, most replacements last only about ten years—underscoring the fact that prevention is key. Getting a knee replaced at fifty certainly is a lot different from getting one replaced at seventy-five. While you may like seconds when it comes to mom's cooking, getting seconds in the OR isn't quite as appealing. So if you can take steps to delay the decline of your joints, you'll quite possibly save yourself from multiple surgeries throughout your life. Of course, as technology develops even further (soon we'll even have some serious bionic and ultratechie artificial limbs), a replacement might end up lasting longer than a decade. But why even try to find out?

Myth or Fact?
Swimming will save your joints.

Unless you're a mermaid or your last name is Spitz and you spend all day in the water, swimming won't unconditionally save you from getting joint pain, but it may help delay the onset. And it will certainly help you stay in shape while you're recovering from problems associated with your joints.

muscles will help support your joints without damaging them.

As with any issue concerning your health, you will have to make choices. You'll have to weigh your risk factors and make decisions. In some cases, you may be hurting your body in one way but helping it another. So running, which may be phenomenal for your heart, can hurt your joints. That's why we recommend a "best of both worlds" approach—by choosing an activity that pumps up your heart without sacrificing your knees.

GET LOOSE AND STRONG AT THE SAME TIME

In the weight room at any coed gym, there's only one thing that smells worse than the locker room—the machismo. Guys bang out three-hundred-pound bench presses, grunt like agitated bulls, and lift their shirts to see how closely their abs resemble tire treads. Not every gym is like that, but there's always a fair share of one-upsmanship when you mix together a bunch of testosterone-filled guys with barbells. That can be an intimidating setting for any novice, and frankly, it's not for everyone. But yoga is. The ancient method of exercise—which is based on the principles of stretching, breathing, and being in tune to all of the ways your body can move—has become popular in gyms and homes because of the major health benefits you can derive from it. Though there are many, we see yoga as having three major advantages in terms of longevity: One, it increases your flexibility. Your muscles aren't static tissues. They move, they expand, they contract. The more flexible they are, the better range of motion you have and the less stress you'll have on your joints doing normal activities.

Two, yoga increases your strength. No, you're not holding any weights in yoga, and yes, yoga looks more tranquil than a Pacific Ocean sunset. But some of these poses are as taxing as they are relaxing. They force your muscles to hold your body weight, which counts as resistance training—and that gives you the additional benefit of building bone density. Yoga also helps you focus on your breathing (see our chapter on lungs for proper breathing techniques). There's certainly a meditative component to holding one position for a minute or longer, and that helps you concentrate on proper breathing and posture—both of which have not only spiritual effects but physical effects as well. And we love that true yoga is not about ego. Yoga is all about how much *you* can do—knowing your body and its limits.

But perhaps the best part about yoga is that it really isn't some form of anatomical pretzel making. It's easy—so easy that a lot of the basic stretching moves you did in elementary school PE are just derivations of yoga. Combine the fact that you can gain benefits from as little as five minutes at a time with a simplified yoga plan. So c'mon. Are you willing to admit that your life is so out of control that you can't spare five minutes? Though there are hundreds of yoga poses to work all different parts of your body, you can incorporate these right away as you focus on your deep breathing. Do the Sun Salutation in the morning. (For a full explanation of the positions involved, see the following pages.) In addition, the Physical Activity Crib Sheet (page 135) can serve as a useful reference.

Myth or Fact? It's good to combine walking with resistance training by walking with light dumbbells.

People think that using three-pound dumbbells while walking a couple miles will get them both stronger and leaner at the same time. But using three-pound dumbbells while walking is like observing toddlers entering the terrible twos — their size makes them *look* harmless, but they can actually cause tornado-sized trouble. The seemingly harmless activity of carrying three-pound dumbbells actually turns out to be a leading cause of orthopedic surgery. Why? Most people don't pay attention to the way they swing the weights when they walk, so they get sloppy in their form. That causes trauma and wear and tear to your shoulder joints because the motion is throwing the joint out of its normal range of motion over long periods. In terms of joint health and exercise, proper form is essential.

Yoga Sun Salutation Crib Sheet

1. 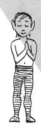 Stand with both feet touching. Bring your hands together, palm to palm, at the heart. Make sure your weight is evenly distributed. Exhale.

2. 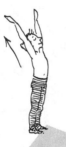 Raise your arms upward. Slowly bend backward, stretching arms above the head. Relax your neck. Inhale.

3. Exhale while you slowly bend forward until your hands are in line with your feet, touching your head to your knees, if possible. Press your palms down, fingertips in line with toes (bend your knees if you have to), and touch the floor.

4. 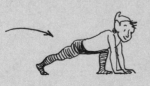 Move your right leg back away from your body in a wide backward lunge. As you inhale, keep your hands and feet on the ground, with your left foot between your hands, and raise your head.

5. 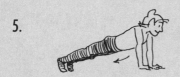 Bring your left foot together with your right.

6. 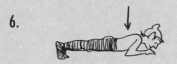 Lower your body as you exhale by putting your elbows on the ground.

7. 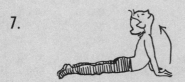 As you inhale, lower your pelvis to the ground and raise your head and bend backward as far as possible, while straightening your arms.

8. 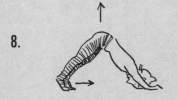 Putting your hands on the ground and keeping your arms straight, raise your hips and align your head with your arms. Exhale.

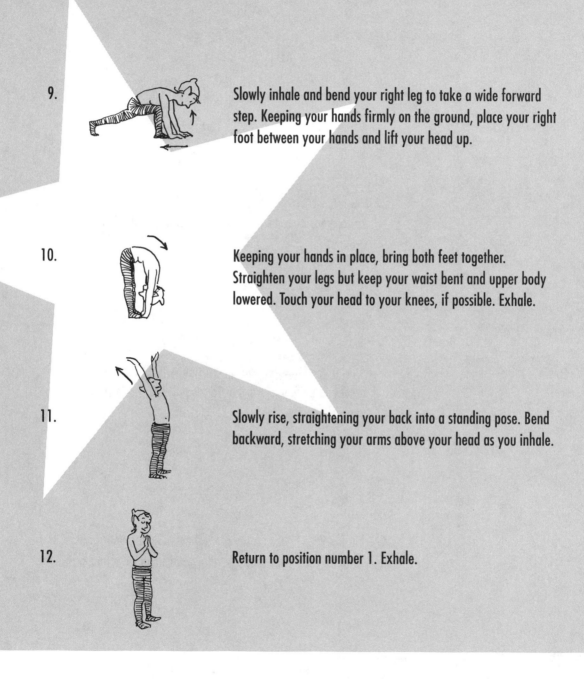

9. Slowly inhale and bend your right leg to take a wide forward step. Keeping your hands firmly on the ground, place your right foot between your hands and lift your head up.

10. Keeping your hands in place, bring both feet together. Straighten your legs but keep your waist bent and upper body lowered. Touch your head to your knees, if possible. Exhale.

11. Slowly rise, straightening your back into a standing pose. Bend backward, stretching your arms above your head as you inhale.

12. Return to position number 1. Exhale.

The Owner's Manual Physical Activity Crib Sheet

★ Thirty minutes of walking every day, no excuses (can be broken up throughout the day into shorter periods to add up to thirty minutes)

★ Thirty minutes a week of resistance training, broken into three ten-minute workouts

★ Sixty minutes a week of stamina training (swimming or cycling), broken into three twenty-minute workouts

★ Thirty minutes a week of yoga or stretching, broken into five five-minute stretching sessions

Sample Schedule

Thirty minutes of walking every day, plus:

Monday:	Twenty-minute stamina workout,	followed by five minutes of yoga or stretching
Tuesday:	Ten-minute resistance training,	followed by five minutes of yoga or stretching
Wednesday:	Twenty-minute stamina workout,	followed by five minutes of yoga or stretching
Thursday:	Ten-minute resistance training,	followed by five minutes of yoga or stretching
Friday:	Twenty-minute stamina workout,	followed by five minutes of yoga or stretching
Saturday:	Additional thirty minutes of walking (for a total of one hour) plus ten-minute resistance training,	followed by five minutes of yoga or stretching
Sunday:	Additional thirty minutes of walking (for a total of one hour)	

Action 2: Eat for Strength

When it comes to your bones, joints, and muscles, healthy eating comes in the form of just a few different foods and nutrients that do great things for structure of movement. Integrate them into your diet, and you'll be rewarding your body with longer living.

CALCIUM   Calcium is the Derek Jeter of nutrients. Derek earns a lot of his Yankee-pinstripe reputation for his great hitting, but he also runs and fields just as well. Like Derek, calcium gets top billing for one thing—what it does to your bones. But calcium is actually responsible for a lot of things in your body. Proper amounts of calcium help keep your joints free of inflammation and arthritis, as well as help your muscles contract. Calcium also helps your brain communicate with your nerves, keeps your blood pressure normal, and reduces the risk of colon cancer. Still, the reason calcium is your skeletal all-star is that it solidifies and strengthens your bones.

Your body stores excess calcium until you reach your early thirties—the time you reach your peak bone density. After that, your body stops storing calcium, and you must rely on getting all the calcium you need from your diet. If you don't, you'll deplete the calcium stores in your body. It's as simple as maintaining your pantry at home. When you remove a jar, you have to replace it, or eventually you'll be left with an empty pantry. As your body depletes the calcium stored in your bones, they become weaker and weaker until finally they're almost hollow—which makes them especially vulnerable to a break. Further, as you constantly remake and replace your bone, being short on calcium (or vitamins D or C) means that your body can't make bone perfectly. So as your tendons, cartilage, and nerves rub against the newly formed, yet imperfect, bone, the joints can become inflamed. That contributes to further inflammation, pain, and the development of arthritis.

The best plan is to fortify your diet with calcium supplements to ensure you get the minimum amounts. To keep your bones young, men should take 1,000 to 1,200 milligrams of calcium a day; women under sixty should take about 1,200 milligrams—best broken up twice a day in the form of 500 or 600 milligrams (that's because most of us cannot absorb more than 600 milligrams of calcium at a time). Over the age of sixty, women need 1,600 milligrams of calcium a day to keep their bones the youngest and strongest possible. (Those amounts refer to actual calcium, not calcium combined with citrate; if you choose supplements with citrate, check the label for that supplement's actual amount of calcium. We do not recommend calcium carbonate as your choice of supplement.)

You've surely seen enough milk-mustache ads to know that there's a lot of calcium in dairy foods such as milk, cheese, and yogurt. But the problem is that most American adults don't eat enough of these foods to get the minimum daily requirement. If you do hit the mark, make sure that you choose low-fat or fat-free versions of dairy foods, because the extra fat often leads to too much saturated fat a day (more than 20 grams a day ages you). That saturated fat causes inflammation in your arteries, increases your chance of immune dysfunctions and cancer, and causes weight gain—which, as you know, can have a negative effect on your bones and joints. While you're at it, you might as well choose milk fortified with DHA (the active omega-3). Other foods rich in calcium include green, leafy vegetables. You can eat these foods to complement your calcium intake, and if you do get a lot of calcium in your diet, you can adjust the amount you take through supplements. To make sure calcium is properly absorbed, add an additional 20 milligrams of calcium for every twelve-ounce caffeinated soft drink or four-ounce cup of coffee you drink. And for every thirty minutes of sweating exercise, add an additional 100 milligrams (calcium comes out in sweat). But in all situations, choose that 1,000 to 1,600 milligrams a day to build bones stronger than redwoods.

If you want to choose a great calcium supplement, don't do what desperate game-show contestants do—guess. Take charge—it is your body—and read the labels. You want one with 600 milligrams of calcium at a time, plus 200 milligrams of magnesium and 400 IU of vitamin D (see why below) and in a size and taste that you can swallow. If it takes four pills to get the dosage right and that works for you, great. If candy helps you, great (as long as the candy has real chocolate and no trans or milk fats). If you enjoy your doses in four glasses of low-fat milk, perfect. There are lots of ways to do it right; just avoid things that have iron in them (iron inhibits calcium's absorption, and you typically get enough iron from food; if you're anemic and take calcium, take the iron two hours apart from the calcium). Also, calcium needs an acidic environment for absorption, so calcium in an antacid that neutralizes acid may not be optimal.

VITAMIN D AND MAGNESIUM   If calcium is the ingredient that absolutely, positively has to get to your bones on time, then vitamin D_3 is FedEx. Essentially, vitamin D_3 increases the absorption of calcium, making it more efficient to deliver calcium to your bones so they can stay strong. Besides being essential for good bone health, it also may be effective for your joints. Vitamin D_3 also helps slow the progression of arthritis. Individuals with low levels of D_3 and calcium are three more times more likely to suffer from, and age from, arthritis.

You can get vitamin D_3 from three sources: the sun, food, and vitamin supplements. The sun actually triggers a chemical reaction that turns inactive vitamin D_3 into active vitamin D_3, but most people aren't exposed to enough sun to get the recommended amount of D_3 (and prolonged exposure can increase your risk of skin cancer; sunblock also blocks the vitamin D_3 conversion). Also, between October 1 and April 15, the sun does not have enough energy north of the line that stretches between Los Angeles and Atlanta to convert vitamin D_3 from inactive to active, so many of us cannot get active vitamin D_3 from the sun even if we sit out in it all day. So food and supplements make the most sense. Some foods, like fish and shellfish, have D_3 naturally, while other foods, like milk, 100 percent natural orange juice, and cereal often are or can be purchased fortified with it. Since most adults don't drink enough milk or orange juice or eat enough cereal to get the recommended dosages, supplementing your diet with D can give you the levels you need. We recommend that you take 1,000 IU of vitamin D in a supplement if you're under sixty and 1,200 IU if you're over sixty. That's how much is necessary for the optimal absorption of calcium and the optimal incorporation into the bone. We also recommend 400 to 500 milligrams of magnesium (a nutrient found in almonds), because magnesium helps balance the effects of calcium on nerve function.

OMEGA-3 FATTY ACIDS Omega-3 fatty acids—the good fats found in fish such as salmon and tuna and in walnuts, canola oil, flaxseeds, avocados, echium oil, foods fortified with DHA from algae (where fish get their DHA), and olive oil—are good for just about every part of your body. Think of omega-3s as a can of WD-40 for the body. Omega-3s are believed to help provide the lubrication that the joints need to function at an effective level. By keeping the joints lubed, you experience less friction, less grinding, and less pain as you age. Omega-3s have been shown in repeated studies to decrease inflammation in inflamed joints. Though there's no widely accepted data to support its use to prevent joint aging in people without inflammation, we advise our family and friends to consume omega-3s in the form of fish at least twice a week. Snacking on walnuts is another way to boost your omega-3s. Another bonus: Fish oil and fish protein have been shown to regenerate the membrane of the meniscus, which is important if you suffer a painful tear or have chronic meniscus discomfort. If you don't like fish, try fish oil capsules—about 2 grams a day is the equivalent of thirteen ounces of fish a week (and, because it is usually distilled, comes without the contaminants some fish have)—or foods supplemented with 600 milligrams of DHA a day.

VITAMIN C While most research in relation to osteoporosis is linked to vitamin D and calcium, more studies are focusing on the role of vitamin C. In earlier chapters, we outlined C's all-around abilities—from being a powerful antioxidant to boosting immunity—but more research is showing that C can help prevent bone loss associ-

Bone-Busting Foods

We're a country of crazes: hula hoops, parachute pants, Chia pets. They come, they go, some stick around. One that appears to be around for a while is the high-protein diet craze. Although as effective for pure weight loss as other diets, the ultra-high-protein diets can accelerate bone loss. Large amounts of protein eaten every day—in the amount of more than 140 grams a day (that's the equivalent of a pound of chicken, fish, beef, or pork, or two and a half pounds of nuts in a day)— are believed to be threatening to your bones because the extra protein can cause your body to excrete calcium rather than absorb it. Same goes for carbonated and caffeinated drinks; the caffeine may actually make you excrete the calcium before your body's been given a chance to use it. The phosphates may be even worse for your bones' calcium stores. Add 20 milligrams of calcium a day for each twelve-ounce carbonated soft drink, four-ounce cup of coffee, and four ounces of protein you consume.

ated with osteoporosis and cartilage inadequacies associated with aging. Specifically, when your joint has cartilage that needs to be repaired, vitamin C is needed for such repairs to keep your cartilage young. To do so, shoot for 1,200 milligrams of vitamin C a day—spread between your diet and supplements throughout the day. (Be careful, though, because some data suggest that too much C—over 2,500 milligrams a day—can do the opposite and increase osteoarthritis and DNA abnormalities.)

Action 3: Think of an Alternative

In a world where we can choose whether we want our cosmetic-surgery fix in the form of *The Swan* or *Extreme Makeover,* it's no surprise that you also have a lot of options when it comes to your health. As the sole decision maker regarding your health, you have the ability to try different methods—to see what works for you. We've outlined the basic principles for the strategies that have been proven to be effective—as well as the ones we believe to be, through our more than fifty years of collective medical experience. Though definitive studies might not have been done on some of the following recommendations, we want to give you the best advice possible for keeping your body young, and we believe these methods can play a major role in doing that.

INCREASE YOUR LUBRICATION   Put your windshield wipers on when it's not raining, and you can almost feel the friction of the rubber grinding against the glass. To glide smoothly, they need rain or wiper fluid. Your joints need lubrication, too, for smooth gliding. Two supplements can help keep them lubricated at optimum levels or may actually result in cartilage regeneration. Glucosamine sulfate—a chemical surrounding your joints—is also found in the hard outer shells of shrimps, crabs, and lobsters. Your body needs it to make cartilage, ligament, and joint fluid. By taking extracted glucosamine, you might be able to keep the cartilage pliable enough to help maintain adequate lubrication between your joints and to act as a shock absorber between bones.

Both glucosamine and the supplement chondroitin have also been shown to be effective in decreasing the symptoms of osteoarthritis for those who are already experiencing joint pain. The theory is that they work like aspirin and ibuprofen by decreasing inflammation at the joint that's causing the pain. Though no one is quite sure how or why they work, there are some excellent data in four randomized and controlled studies (the gold standard of science). These studies show that the supplements actually restore youth to your joints by modifying the basic disease process—they cause the regeneration of cartilage in the knee and hip joints and repair damaged cartilage. While there is some confllicting data, the majority favors the benefit of these supplemets. Take 1,500 milligrams a day of the two combined (many supplements have both in the same pill) to increase and maintain lubrication between joints. Only three current preparations of the supplement have more than 25 percent of the ingredient on the label in the pill, so we recommend you use these three brands, which have between 80 and 100 percent of the ingredient in each pill.

They are Triple Flex, Osteo Bi-Flex, and Cosamin DS. A plant-based version is also available (see www.drtheo.com).

SUPPORT HAWAII'S ECONOMY Bromelain—an ingredient found in pineapples—isn't really a nutrient for preventing bone and joint disease, but it can be used to help speed recovery. That's because bromelain has shown anti-inflammatory abilities. Take 100 milligrams once a day if your joints feel stiff.

LIVE ON PINS AND NEEDLES Western medicine has made great advances in the way we treat disease, the way we alleviate pain, and the way we can help people live longer, more productive lives. But some people also use methods from Eastern medicine as alternatives. Acupuncture—one of the oldest healing systems in the world—has been used for thousands of years to treat everything from insomnia to migraines. Since back pain is such a widespread problem in the United States, many people are trying acupuncture to help relieve the pain.

Here's the acupuncture theory in a nutshell: Energy meridians pass through all aspects of our bodies and reflect our health. Healers use the surface of the body to access these streams of energy and heal internal injuries. They believe that each energy channel represents an internal organ—and by stimulating that external part with a needle, you can redirect negative energy from the internal organ that's in pain or ill. So, for example, Chinese physicians see the ear as a microcosm of the human body, almost like an upside-down fetus. One of the long curves in your ear represents the spine. So healers treating people with lower-back pain will place small needles in the upper part of that curvature (remember, the ear is upside down, symbolically). Those needles stimulate energy flow from the lower back and help eliminate pain. Healers use needles ranging in length from one-half inch to five inches, and it's surprising how little the needle hurts when it's inserted (we've tried it and usually cannot feel the prick). The needles stay in for fifteen minutes, and some clinicians say they have up to a 90 percent success rate in alleviating pain.

While Eastern medicine attributes the success to the redirection of energy flow, Western medicine is also looking for reasons why acupuncture might be effective. Some possible theories: Acupuncture releases neurochemicals—endorphins—that relieve pain, and researchers have even theorized that it increases circulation to help the healing process. While it's certainly an alternative treatment to back pain, Eastern methodologies are not regulated in the United States the way Western medicine is. Before seeing an acupuncturist, make sure the practitioner has both a state license and national certification.

Action 4: Make Minor Changes

Sometimes the smallest changes in your life can lead to the biggest results. Besides eating right and exercising, you can also maintain proper bone and joint health by making a few adjustments to the way you live.

STAND UP STRAIGHT One of the easiest ways to strengthen your abdominal muscles—and support your back—is through good posture. You may feel like you're standing straight, but in reality, most of us stand like the Leaning Tower of Pisa. Practice good posture by bringing your head and neck back. The key element is breathing in to tighten your gut. That's the component that lifts your chest and will give you Marine-like posture. Sucking it in while you do crunches, or even when taking the elevator, helps your body look and stay younger.

WEAR WELL-CUSHIONED SHOES Your body is pretty good about providing its own natural shock absorbers—like the fluid between your joints and the cushioning between your vertebrae. But when we evolved from living on all fours to living on just two, we took advantage of it. We run marathons *just because;* we walk Wal-Mart Super Centers that are the size of entire counties; we spend summers hiking a trail that spans from Georgia to Maine. No matter where we're walking, our feet take more of a beating than a carton of eggs in a baker's kitchen. Sure, with twenty-six bones in our feet, we were designed to move. But our feet don't have the natural shock absorbers other parts of the body have. To protect them better, always wear well-cushioned walking or running shoes when you'll be on your feet for extended periods of time (even if you're just standing). Running shoes are usually a good option, because they're well cushioned in the back of the shoe—where your heel strikes the ground first and absorbs most of your body's weight.

GO SKIM   By now, you've heard us say it enough—being overweight or obese exponentially increases the risk factors associated with so many diseases and conditions. The slimmer you are, the less joint pain you'll have. Fat is a learned taste, so you can change your desire for it. Avoiding the bad fats—saturated and trans fats—will keep you thinner and slow the aging of your arteries and immune system substantially. And it will also help with joint pain. One of the first places you can cut fat is with dairy products. We know that if you're drinking whole milk now, you think skim milk tastes like lake water. So try this trick: Mix 2 percent milk with whole milk for one week, gradually changing the proportions until you're drinking a glass of entirely 2 percent milk. Do the same thing by mixing 1 percent milk with 2 percent milk, and then by mixing skim milk with 1 percent milk. Over the course of about eight weeks, skim milk will taste normal, and whole milk will eventually taste *too* fatty.

STOP SMOKING   You wouldn't blast your living room with smoke twenty times a day, so why do it to your body? In Chapter 5, we talk a lot about the damage smoking can do to your lungs, and it's even tougher on your arteries. It's safe to say that smoking is just as destructive to your bones. Smoking increases your risk of osteoporosis, making your bones weaker over time.

Chapter 5

To a Lung and Healthy Life: Your Lungs

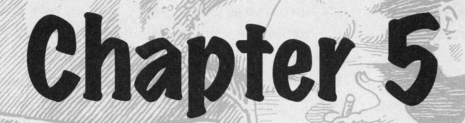

Major Myths About the Lungs

Lung Myth #1   If you're not a smoker, you have nothing to worry about.

Lung Myth #2   Being in good cardiovascular shape means you have healthy lungs.

Lung Myth #3   Snoring is a sign of a serious breathing problem.

Most people think about their breath at three points in their lives: when it stinks (garlic shrimp over linguini); when it's in imminent danger (boa constrictor); and when it's heavy (after a workout or on your wedding night). Besides those times, breathing gets about as much attention as Janet Jackson's backup dancers. As your body's main ventilation system, it's responsible for your overall airflow throughout your house. Like heating and air-conditioning, breathing is one of those things we take for granted when it's working. We live, so we breathe.

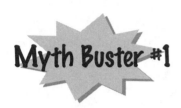

In our body's ventilation system, our lungs involuntarily pull air in and push air out of our body. Most people conclude that as long as you don't pollute your body with such duct-destroying toxins as nicotine or factory smoke, then your vents should function smoothly throughout your whole life.

Sounds good, but it's dead wrong. While smoking and other environmental toxins surely are potent attackers of your airways, many things can change the way your lungs bring oxygen in and push carbon dioxide out.

In fact, when it comes to your airways, the small things pose the greatest threat. A vent door keeps large pieces of debris out of your vents, and your nose acts almost like an air filter, too. But there's still room for dust and dander to make it through. When you take bacteria, viruses, and other particles into your lungs, your system is able to stop the larger particles, because they get trapped by the lung's natural defenses. They beat the particles out of your windpipes with little brushes called cilia and force them out of your body through coughing, sneezing, and blowing your nose. But even smaller particles—particles we can't actually see—can slip through the defense system much like a great running back breaks tackles. Undetected, these particles actually cause an inflammatory reaction that destroys part of your lung tissue—and puts you at greater risk for various lung disorders. (That's why nanotechnology manufacturing may be dangerous: the waste product is all small particles.)

You might remember when investment guru Warren Buffett quipped that trust is just like air—nobody appreciates it until there's a shortage. Even if you're in

Myth Buster #2

great cardiovascular shape, you can still have breathing issues.

And even if you don't have asthma or any other lung problem right now, you can learn more about your airways—and how to ensure that you are breathing as efficiently as possible. What's astounding is that, as easy as it seems, many of us actually don't have the slightest idea of how to breathe right. In Chinese medicine, lungs are the orchestra conductor of the entire body—they set the rhythm from which everything else follows. And that's why yoga incorporates so much time teaching proper ways to breathe—to put your whole body in balance. In this chapter, we'll take you through the steps of proper breathing, but we also want you to start thinking that your lungs are just as much of a headliner act in your body as your heart is. In fact, if all the organs are separate parts of the house, your lungs and heart are like adjoining rooms. They work so closely together that if there's a problem in one, there's almost sure to be a problem in the other.

As with almost every part of your body, you can make changes to your system that ensure smooth airflow throughout your life. In fact, your breathing can actually be somewhat of a voluntary process—one in which you control the thermostat for keeping your lungs young and healthy.

Your Lungs: The Anatomy

Quick quiz: Name the person who normally consumes six quarts per minute.

    a.   Frat guy on his twenty-first birthday

    b.   Owner of car with three hundred thousand miles on it

    c.   A Starbucks addict

    d.   You

The correct answer is D, but it has nothing to do with lager or lattes. It has to do with how much air you take in with each breath—that's enough air to fill 10 million balloons in a lifetime (you gotta feel for the poor graduate student who had to prove that theory). As you can imagine, there's a lot of stuff going on in your lungs every few seconds; grab your flashlight so we can crawl up into your ducts and see what's inside.

You probably have a good image of the way your lungs look on the outside. While you may think they function a little like balloons in that they expand when air is consumed, it's probably better to think of your two lungs as large sponges. They're light and fluffy when filled with air, but they get bogged down when they get wet (as they do in some diseases) and don't exchange air very well in those cases.

To start, think of your respiratory system as an upside-down tree (see Figure 5.1). If we follow a breath of air, we'll start with your mouth and nose. When air enters your body, it goes down your trachea. That's your trunk—the one airway at the beginning of the process. Then it quickly divides into two airways to feed into two lungs; those are your bronchial tubes. Then, like tree branches, those airways break off into four, then eight, then hundreds of thousands of little airways in each lung. Those airways are your bronchi. At the end of each airway are tiny sacs called alveoli. Think of them like leaves at the ends of the branches. Healthy lungs have hundreds of millions of alveoli. Each alveolus is covered with a thin layer of fluid that helps you breathe by keeping the alveoli open so oxygen is absorbed and carbon dioxide is excreted.

Of course, your lungs also have other parts that are integral to the breathing process. Your bronchial tubes are responsible for cleaning out your lungs. Typically, they're like a four-year-old's birthday cake—covered with mucus, which dirt and germs stick to. Your lungs also have millions of tiny hairs called cilia. Cilia act like little brooms that sweep away all the stuff that's caught in your mucus. They're fast-action sweepers, like high-speed windshield wipers—constantly moving back and forth to clear your lungs of nasty stuff that makes its way in with every breath (that's why where you live can have a sizable effect on your aging process, because of the

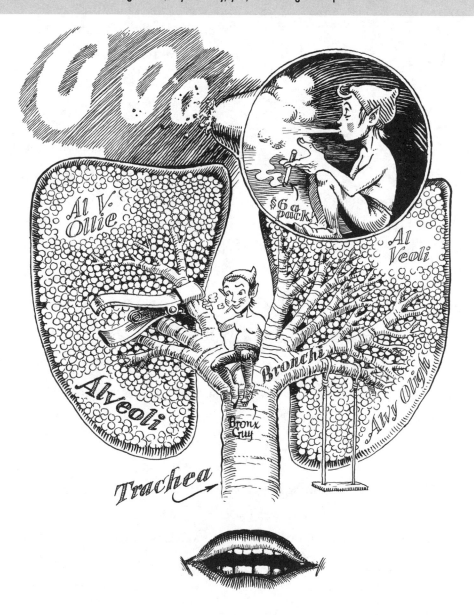

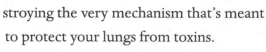

toxins and pollutants more prevalent in larger cities). What's important to know here is that cigarette smoke kills cilia, essentially destroying the very mechanism that's meant to protect your lungs from toxins.

The last part of your lungs that influences healthy breathing is the musculature around them. Your diaphragm (see Figure 5.2) is a large muscle at the bottom of your chest cavity that pulls air down into your lungs. We'll talk about proper breathing in a moment, but it's important to know that the movements of breathing are like other movements in your body. They're controlled by a muscle; imagine fireplace bellows that are sucked open and then passively eject air. By using the diaphragm, you can develop techniques to help you breathe deeper.

The Diseases:
Common Respiratory Distresses

The lifesaver of your body, your lungs need air to keep you afloat. With restricted airflow, they don't have enough fuel to support the rest of your body. At best, labored breathing is uncomfortable. At worst, it's life-threatening. No one wants to be at sea without a fully inflated life ring, and no one wants to live without fully inflated airways. These are the important aging-related conditions that can deflate—or destroy—the structures that help keep you alive. Sleep apnea and asthma are the most common lung abnormalities, so we discuss these two at length in this chapter.

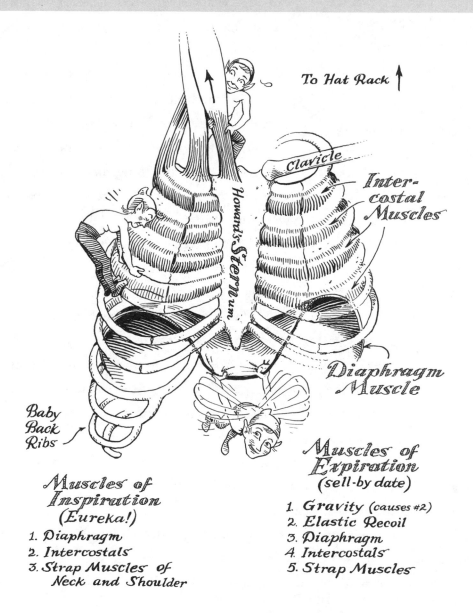

To Hat Rack ↑

Clavicle

Inter-costal Muscles

Howard's Sternum

Diaphragm Muscle

Baby Back Ribs

Muscles of Inspiration (Eureka!)
1. Diaphragm
2. Intercostals
3. Strap Muscles of Neck and Shoulder

Muscles of Expiration (sell-by date)
1. Gravity (causes #2)
2. Elastic Recoil
3. Diaphragm
4. Intercostals
5. Strap Muscles

Myth or Fact?
Raspy voices are a sign of sexiness.

Well, in Demi Moore's case, it may be true. But hoarseness can signify actual changes of your vocal cords, especially in people who often speak loudly, like schoolteachers and football coaches. When you smoke or strain your voice (which professional singers—even those who lip-synch—are taught not to do), you irritate the vocal cords and form scars and subsequent overgrowths that are called polyps.

Sleep Apnea

We put this problem first it because it is caused by changes right at the start of your breathing passage and is the most rapidly increasing airway problem. If you sleep—or try to sleep, shall we say—next to a snorer, you might compare the sound to a garbage disposal, maybe? Jet engine? The amplifiers from your teenager's band? Without question, snoring is second only to karaoke as the most annoying thing that can come out of your mouth, and most of us know the roar all too well. Almost 50 percent of adults snore occasionally, while 25 percent snore regularly. Anatomically speaking, snoring occurs when there's obstruction of the free flow of air through the passages in the back of your mouth. That obstruction forces air through a tiny hole and out your mouth; the air rubbing against the lining of your throat is what makes that sound (see Figure 5.3). If the jackhammer-like vibrations firing from your partner's face aren't enough to scare the sheets off you, this fact will: Snoring can reach up to 85 decibels—the sound level of a New York City subway (that's actually enough to cause hearing damage over time).

While snoring can damage your ears (and your relationship), it isn't necessarily a health problem by itself. The important thing is whether snoring can be a sign of sleep apnea—a condition that affects 20 million Americans. Almost 10 percent of people who snore have sleep apnea.

Sleep apnea is defined as any period during your sleep in which you stop breathing for more than ten seconds at a time. This isn't snoring. This is actually a stoppage in snoring that, like a beautiful painting or person, takes your breath away. Here's

FIGURE 5.3 **Clear Your Throat** Fat accumulates in the back of the throat and causes snoring and sleep apnea when the surrounding muscles relax during sleep. At the back of the tongue, the epiglottis protects the trachea (windpipe) from food and prevents choking. The thyroid gland, which is nestled just in front of the trachea in your neck, can be seen in some folks.

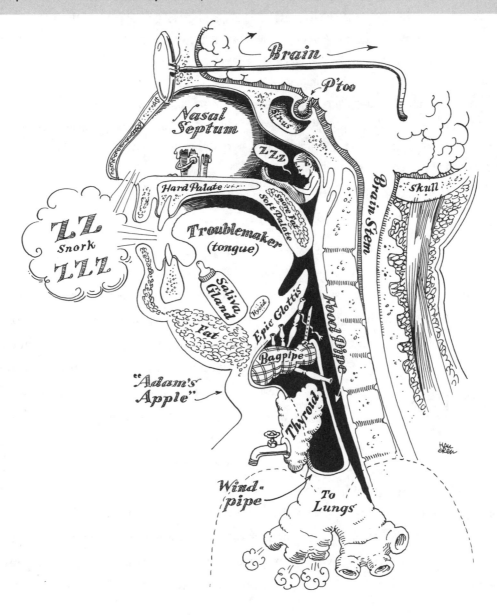

Little Lumps

Sarcoidosis may sound as if it's an arcade game from the 1970s, but it's actually something that can slow down the function of your organs—primarily your lungs and respiratory system. Affecting mostly people from twenty to forty, sarcoidosis causes little lumps of granular white blood cells (called granulomas) to form and changes how organ function—namely by giving you such symptoms as fatigue, general muscle aches, swollen glands, and difficulty breathing. Though docs don't know the cause, they think that it may happen when your immune system overreacts to a threat (like a toxin or drug) and inflammation causes the formation of those granules. When it happens in your lungs and the disease progresses, the tissue between your air sacs can scar. That can stiffen your lungs and decrease the amount of air your lungs can hold. Steroids and other classes of drugs have been used to help treat the disease and reduce the size of granulomas.

what happens. Remember that blockage that causes snoring? Well, when that blockage gets complete, it can stop all airflow and cause sleep apnea. Here's how. As you get older, the tissue in your throat softens, and the area around your tonsils is one of the primary places that fat pulls up a seat and stays awhile (see Figure 5.3). That swollen tissue and fat constrict your airway. When you're asleep and your muscles fully relax, the tissue collapses, so that there's no room in the back of your throat. That fatty tissue essentially acts as a lid over a manhole, and no air can get into and out of your throat. That's obstructive sleep apnea (there's also a form that's caused by neurological problems, as well as kinds that are caused by both obstruction and neurological problems).

Myth Buster #3

Though it would seem that the lack of breathing would be the problem, it's actually not the only danger with sleep apnea. When you stop breathing, your body actually wakes itself up—without your consciously knowing it. The effect is that you

Sleeping Duty

People who suffer from sleep apnea can choose a number of treatment options, the most popular being a CPAP mask that's worn at night. The mask—which looks like a traditional oxygen mask that's hooked up to a machine with tubes—gauges levels of the swollenness of tissue and pushes air past the swollen tissue so that you can breathe easier. Though it has a 90 to 95 percent success rate, its downside is inadequate patient compliance because many wearers don't like looking and sounding like Darth Vader when they go to bed. There are also surgical treatments, which are about 50 percent successful. Surgery removes some of the obstructing tissue, which helps you breathe better and cure the apnea, and procedures that help you lose weight (that is, gastric bypass surgery) are also effective and can help some people who have severe sleep apnea. But the biggest change can come from you. Losing just ten pounds can decrease your episodes of sleep apnea by 30 percent, while gaining ten pounds does the reverse—making weight loss even more effective than surgery.

can never get into a deep sleep, so your body never gets the rejuvenating effect of deep sleep. Your body needs two things during the night (three, if you count back massages). It needs REM (rapid eye movement) sleep, and it needs slow-wave sleep. To get into REM sleep, you need about ninety minutes of consistent sleep. So if you're waking up ten times an hour, which is typical for people with sleep apnea, you're never getting into REM and won't wake up refreshed.

In the early stages of sleep apnea, there's no real damage to your body, except for occasional low periods of oxygen, which can kill some brain cells. But as the condition progresses, it leads to more serious issues, including hypertension. The breathing stoppages cause your lungs to hold on to some carbon dioxide, which is what leads to the high blood pressure. You'll also be faced with excessive fatigue throughout the day, memory loss, and morning headaches. Over time, it can also increase the risk of stroke, and in some cases, sleep apnea can even trigger abnormal heartbeats and other cardiovascular events that can cause death.

Owner's Manual Crib Sheet for Sleep

With some major exceptions, sleep is a lot like sex. It's something you really look forward to, and it makes you feel great when you're done. Most important, though, sleep is more like your boss—it's much more agreeable when it goes uninterrupted. Getting a good night's sleep is one of the most crucial things you can do for your body. Getting about 7 hours of sleep a night can make a profound difference on your brain and your heart and make you up to three years younger. Lack of sleep makes you less mentally aware and more fatigued, causes you to eat more, and places you at a higher risk of accidents. Plus, being fatigued puts you at greater risk for making choices that age you (when you're tired, it's easier to order the bacon double-fat burgers than the grilled salmon). But if you have sleep apnea, it means you're simply not getting enough of the rejuvenating REM and slow-wave sleep. While sleeping pills may seem like a good idea—because they do work in the short term by shutting off the Leno-watching neurons—they have harmful effects over the long term because of their addictive qualities. Instead, you can try these ways to help yourself sleep like a teenager during summer break.

Get on a schedule. Your body clock runs best as it did when you were a baby. It gets up at the same time every day—whether you have a full day of work or a full day of cartoons. On the weekends, try to rise within one hour of the time you get up during the week.

Change your temperature. The ideal setting is a cool, dark room. If you're having trouble sleeping, try removing a layer of clothing (like socks) or lowering the thermostat.

Eat small portions before bed. Eat foods that contain melatonin—a substance that helps regulate your body clock. That means oats, sweet corn, or rice. Or try a complex carbohydrate that has serotonin, like vegetables or whole-grain pasta. You can also go with the classic remedy: skim milk. Of course, you know to avoid stimulants like caffeine and exercise near bedtime.

Use your bedroom for only sleep and sex. It is best to take work materials, computers, and televisions out of the sleeping environment.

While your partner's snoring might make you want to stuff socks down his throat, you should look for risk factors. The most critical is that pause in breathing for more than ten seconds. But be careful. Breathing can be an illusion. Remember your diaphragm? It's a muscle that pulls the air down your lungs. So you may look over at Mr. Lawn Mower Mouth and see his belly moving up and down. You assume he (or she) is breathing, but he actually might not be. That's just his diaphragm trying to pull air down. His gut can be moving even if he's not breathing air in. What you want to do is listen for changes in breath. Snoring is actually a good thing (never thought you'd hear that, huh?). It signals that some air is actually moving in and out. No snoring after a period of snoring can be a warning sign that no air is moving in and out. If there's no sound for ten or more seconds, and there isn't a whoosh of air out of the nose or mouth, it's an indication he isn't breathing.

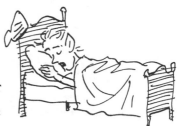

How Do You Sleep?

It's likely that you already know whether you're getting enough sleep (a head on your desk is one sure sign). But if you're unsure, ask yourself these questions. If you answer yes to one (yup, just one) or more, then you need to revaluate your sleep hygiene.

★   Are you often tired or sleepy during the day? Do you fall asleep in meetings, while operating heavy machinery, or while performing other mundane chores?

★   Has your partner told you that your snoring sounds like a construction site?

★   Have you kicked or thrashed like a fish out of water while you're sleeping?

★   Is the time it takes to go to sleep your own personal purgatory?

★   Do you have a family history of sleep problems?

★   Do you have an unusual sensation in your legs that interferes with your ability to fall asleep?

★   Do you talk, laugh, juggle, or conduct orchestras during your sleep?

★   Do your sleeping or waking times change more often than the CNN Web site?

★   Have you had sleep problems for more than three months?

You can also check yourself if you live alone. For example, if you can fall asleep anywhere during the day (and you do not work or play all night long), it's probably a sign of excessive fatigue that could indicate apnea. Another clue is neck size. If it's over seventeen inches, you have more than a 50 percent chance of developing sleep apnea or a better than 30 percent chance of making it as an NFL offensive lineman.

Asthma

Take a look at the picture of lungs affected by asthma (see Figure 5.1) and imagine what happens if you take a deep breath and then clamp a vise on the bronchus that drains air from the lung. The air stays bottled up at the point of obstruction. You hear a whistling sound and the noise intensifies when the airflow has trouble making it through the ventilation system. That's asthma. In patients with asthma, the trouble isn't with getting air into the lungs; it's with getting air out, and as Figure 5.1 shows, it feels like a vise is squeezing the bronchus. The clamps come in different sizes and strengths, so you can have different degrees of airway obstruction, some of which are dangerous. You can make many choices to prevent and control asthma. Once the obstruction is cleared—often through medication—air is released and you can breathe smoothly.

More than 15 million Americans have asthma, and one-third of them are under eighteen. It can start anytime in your life. While asthma is not a disease that seems primarily associated with aging, its implications for aging are important. In some ways, the final pathway for many diseases is in the lungs (if you live long enough, eventually, it's the lungs that will get you). Historically, in fact, pneumonia was called an old man's best friend, because it would allow you to slip into a coma and die peacefully when lack of oxygen would cause an abnormal and lethal heart rhythm.

Asthma is a complex disease and can be caused by a mix of factors, including

What's an Allergy?

If you or your doctor can hear wheezing, that means something's constricting your bronchi (the smaller breathing tubes). One of the causes—asthma—can be triggered by an irritant like smoke, nervous impulses like stress, or an allergy. Allergies are exaggerated reactions of the immune system to substances that don't cause symptoms in most people. Those reactions can come in the form of:

★ skin rashes (typically from chemicals)
★ runny and stuffy noses (from dust, pollen, etc.)
★ itchy eyes (from dust, pollen, mascara, etc.)
★ upset stomach or intestines (from food allergies)
★ coughing, shortness of breath, wheezing, or any distress to the respiratory system (from any kind of allergen)

More than one-third of Americans have allergies, but most don't have their symptoms under control. While the worst a rash or red eye will do is crimp your enjoyment of the 1980s flashback party, allergies that affect your lungs can be life threatening. This is called an anaphylactic reaction. If you're allergic to a wasp sting, for instance, your blood vessels develop holes that leak fluid (you need blood inside the vessels, not outside) and you may get so short of breath that no air can move (the fluid constricts the bronchi so much no air can pass, and you cannot even hear your wheezing). And you'd need immediate help to open your airways.

The three basic ways to treat allergies are medication, allergy shots (also called immunotherapy), and avoidance. We recommend avoidance for allergens you know, but if you have an allergy that triggers a respiratory reaction, you might need to carry an EpiPen to inject yourself with epinephrine to help you open your airways enough to get to a hospital for further treatment.

environment (like dust mites, house dander), lifestyle (where you live dictates toxin levels), and genetics (kids have at least a 25 percent of developing asthma if their parents have allergies). Even if you have a genetic disposition for asthma, you can control the symptoms and the disabling effects that come from the chronic inflammation caused by frequent acute attacks.

It all starts when pollen or another allergen works its way down your airway. As it moves past the cilia, the pollen sticks to your lungs. In response to the foreign matter, your body sends immune cells to the area. When they attach to the pollen, they explode like a grenade and call in more white blood cells to investigate. That migration of white blood cells to the area causes the area to inflame and move mucus into the lung and chemicals into the immediate area, including near the muscles. When that happens, the muscles in the area become red, swollen, and more likely to go into spasm—which constricts the bronchi to trap air in the alveoli, which causes the plastic kazoo sound of trying to force air through the small opening.

Of course, the scariest part of asthma is an attack. While asthma may be mild, an attack—a period of time when it's extremely difficult to breathe—may last for several minutes or even up to a few days. Severe attacks can be fatal, but that doesn't mean you need to live in fear of attacks. In fact, many treatments can help asthma patients enjoy life performing their normal activities. First, you'll want to try to avoid the things that are triggering the attacks. But you might also benefit from medications to open your airways during an attack. One of the more common categories of medications is bronchodilators, which are inhaled medications that relax the muscles in your airway so the airways become larger, making room for more air to pass through—it's kind of like a new filter or cleaner for your exhaust line. Another common prescription is the category of inhaled steroids. Steroids are the librarians of the respiratory system; they prevent symptoms from occurring by telling your airways to be quiet by reducing the inflammation in the area, and that can prevent the aging that inflammation causes (that's why you should take your medication as prescribed—you may feel well without drugs, but if you

What's That Coming Out of Your Mouth?

Coughing   Begins with a deep inspiration, then forced expiration against a closed airway trapdoor. The explosion of airflow travels at six hundred miles per hour. Sneezing is similar, and both work to expel irritants and keep your airways clear.

Hiccups   A spasmodic contraction of the diaphragm and other muscles that produces an inspiration when the glottis suddenly closes. The closure is what causes the sensation and sound. Hiccups also occur in the fetus in utero.

Yawning   Why we yawn is unclear. One theory is that when underventilated alveoli collapse, the deep inspiration of a yawn stretches them open. It's also been suggested that yawning is a nonverbal signal used for communication between monkeys in a group (and perhaps humans as well).

avoid the chronic inflammation, you avoid the aging of lung tissue associated with the inflammation as well).

Your Lungs:
The Live Younger Action Plan

There's a reason why the swoosh-happy shoe company branded the word "air" on a whole line of shoes. Air is everything. It gives you power. It blows out birthday candles. It tickles a lover's ear. It gives you life. Nike may have the Air Max and the Air Jordan, but you have an even more important air—yours. You have the opportunity to make your respiratory system as efficient and clog-free as possible. By making a few simple changes—and at least one life-altering change, if you're a smoker—you have the ability to make your pipes powerful. So let's take a look at the ways you can clear the air.

Action 1: Go Deep

Most people breathe the way they dance—they think they know what they're doing, but they really don't have a clue about how to do it right. Stop right now for a second and focus on your breathing. Now look down. See anything moving? Probably not. That's because most people typically take very short, shallow breaths—the kind that come simply from your chest. For you to really improve your lung function, you need to practice taking deep, whole breaths.

Remember what makes the lungs move? Your diaphragm. That's the muscle that pulls your lungs down, so your lungs expand and you can really circulate oxygen down throughout the whole lung (see Figure 5.2). To learn proper breathing technique, take yoga lessons—where people focus as much on their breathing as they do on their ability to scratch their heads with their toes. Lie flat on the floor, with one hand on your belly and one hand on your chest. Take a deep breath in—slowly. Lying

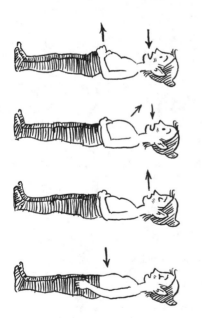

on the floor at first when you practice is important, because if you stand up, you're more likely to fake a deep breath by doing an exaggerated chest extension, rather than letting it fill up naturally. Imagine your lungs filling up with air; it should take about five seconds to inhale. As your diaphragm pulls your chest cavity down, your belly button should be moving away from your spine as you fill your lungs. Your chest will also widen—and maybe rise ever so slightly—as you inhale. When your lungs feel fuller than a sumo wrestler's lunch box, exhale slowly—taking about seven seconds to let all the air out. You can pull your belly button toward your spine to force all the air out of your lungs.

Okay, so now you know how to breathe deep, but what's the benefit? What will deep breathing get you, besides stares on the subway? A lot, actually. For one, it helps transport nitric oxide—a very potent lung and blood vessel dilator that resides in your nasal passages—to your lungs. So it makes your lungs and blood vessels function better. Taking deep breaths helps your lungs go from 98 percent saturation of oxygen to 100 percent saturation of oxygen. Another benefit is that it helps improve the drainage of your lymphatic system, which removes toxins from your body. Of course, it also helps in stress relief. The deep breaths act as a mini-meditation and, from a longevity standpoint, are an important stress reliever. Shifting to slower breathing in times of tension can help calm you and allow you to perform, whether mentally or physically, at higher levels.

Our recommendation: Take ten deep breaths in the morning, ten at night, and as many as you need when shooting free throws or after chasing your toddler down the cereal aisle.

Action 2: Take a Test

We know tests are about as appealing as catheter insertion, but this one's easy. You can do it in just a minute, you can grade yourself, and you'll get the results immediately. The test? Briskly run up two flights of stairs or walk six blocks. That's it. If you can do either of those without pausing to rest, your lungs are probably in pretty good shape. (This is actually a test to determine whether someone is fit for surgery. For those who pass the test, it indicates a decrease in your risk of dying

---

Myth or Fact? You yawn because you're tired.

Actually, that's part of it. But the technical reason you yawn is because your body senses a dip in the oxygen level in the blood, so your body wants to yawn to take in more oxygen and get it back into the bloodstream. What we don't understand is why yawning is contagious.

Myth or Fact? Shortness of breath always means there's a problem with your lungs.

Sure, a lack of air means something's not working in your respiratory system, but the problem doesn't always start and stop with your lungs. If your heart isn't working properly, it can't pump blood forward, meaning that blood can back up into your lungs—making the dry, fluffy substance soggy. And that means they can no longer exchange air. So in many cases when you feel shortness of breath, the solution is in finding out and addressing what's wrong with the heart to help move blood out of the lungs so they can work properly.

or being disabled in surgery to that of someone who is about ten years younger. It indicates your lung's ability to provide oxygen and exhale carbon dioxide.)

It's a simple grading system: pass/fail. Make it up the two flights without spewing out more air than an industrial-size fan, and you pass. But if you experience extreme shortness of breath or have to stop, it's a sign your lungs are suffering at least some distress, even if it's the heart's fault. We recommend that you do this test every month, as a way of periodically checking your lung function, plus you will gain insights into your overall fitness level. That's important, because one of the major warning signs of decreased lung function is seeing a severe change in your ability to complete the test—from being able to run the flights easily to suddenly having a lot of trouble with it. The reason? When you exercise over this compact period of time, shortness of breath means all your organs are feeling deprived of oxygen and that some of them might not be getting enough.

Action 3: Be Your Own Air Traffic Controller

In chili recipes and golf swings, little changes can make a big difference. The same holds true for managing your air quality. Since you can control what goes into and out of your mouth and nose, you have some say about the traffic pattern of air waiting to enter your system. Here are a few additional things you can do to go with the flow.

GO TO THE NURSERY Quite simply, plants improve air quality because they produce oxygen, increase the oxygen in the room, and remove pollutants from the air. One NASA study showed that philodendrons, spider plants, and golden pothos were the most effective.

TAKE SUPPLEMENTS Magnesium is a mineral that relaxes the bronchial tubes and can help with asthma. Take 400 milligrams a day. If you routinely cough up mucus from your lungs (rather than mucus coming out only when you blow your nose, which is usually from sinus conditions), consider N-acetylcysteine. It's a substance that loosens mucus and boosts production of a substance called glutathione, which helps prevent damage in lung tissue. We recommend 600 milligrams twice daily. (By the way, we actually use a related compound with intensive care patients.) Even caffeine can help people with asthma. Caffeine seems to stabilize and shrink the lining of the airways to help make breathing easier.

TRY NETI A Neti pot device can clean out your nasal cavity (via water running through the pot into nostrils). These pots are sold over the counter.

AVOID TOXINS It's just part of today's society that we'll be exposed to such toxic substances as pollution, carbon monoxide, and some morning-drive DJs. But

Myth or Fact? Air filters rock.

On the surface, air filters sound as if they'd be the best things for your lungs since snorkeling tubes. Air filters are supposed to work by taking allergens out of the air so you can have cleaner breathing. But many of them don't work that well, and the primary reason isn't a mechanical malfunction but an owner malfunction. Most people don't change air filters or clean humidifiers with enough regularity, so they're not that effective. Unless humidifiers are cleaned regularly, they'll form a cesspool of water, which grows mold and fungi, and then you end up breathing it. If you stick to regular maintenance, however, they can be useful for taking allergens out of the air.

you can take steps to avoid being exposed to many indoor pollutants like radon, asbestos, and mold. Test for radon before buying a house, for instance. And did you know that one hour of driving on a Los Angeles freeway gives off the same carbon monoxide as the average tunnel that's not well ventilated? Keep your windows closed when on the freeways in large cities (or take the side streets). While you might not pick up and move from the city to the country to avoid pollutants, it is worth noting that if you can avoid jobs where you are exposed to pollutants and toxins, it can have a RealAge effect of up to 2.8 years younger. That's because avoiding pollution at work decreases arterial hardening and decreases all diseases related to arterial aging, like infections of the lung, asthma, heart disease, stroke, and memory loss. And if you can choose to live in a city on the Environmental Protection Agency's (EPA's) list of cities with low pollution, you can make yourself 2.2 years younger. It's especially important because the EPA rates cities based on the size of the pollutant particles. The smallest pollutants get the farthest into your lungs, which can have a detrimental effect on your immune system, as well as increase the rate of inflammation in your lungs, arteries, and entire cardiovascular system. (See the EPA Web site for the ratings of individual cities. It changes the Web site on which it posts this information more frequently than most people change their house air filters.) By the way, the better sealed a house is, the more you lock in toxins emitted by newer construction materials. So keeping your windows open at times to let in fresh air can make you and your family younger.

Action 4: Take Cover

Here's a tip about good bedroom behavior that has nothing to do with lingerie, orgasms, or pretzel-like sex positions. The average pillow infested with mites builds up two pounds of mite excrement within two years. It seems that a high incidence of asthma isn't necessarily linked to pollution but to mites in pillows and mattresses. Mites in your mattress and pillows digest the skin you shed and produce feces in the 2.5 to 10 micron range, the most dangerous for your lungs. The increases in mite feces from pillows and mattresses are thought responsible for the large increase in asthma. Get new pillows frequently and wrap the ones you have in vinyl casings (less comfortable) or with small-micron-protected cloth that's impermeable. You can find the vinyl ones at virtually any store and the 1 micron ones at CleanRest.

Action 5: Shake Your Butt

Smoke may be great for grilling and haunted houses, but you don't have to be the Marlboro man to know what kind of damage smoking can do to your lungs. In fact, pumping smoke down your airways makes you eight years older—and puts you at risk for lung diseases like cancer, emphysema, and bronchitis. While we'll talk more about cancer in Chapter 12, one of the greatest things you can do

Myth or Fact? Vitamin A and beta-carotene are good for your lungs.

Supplementing your diet with vitamin A and beta-carotene can lead to megadosing—that is, taking in more than 2,500 IU of vitamin A or the vitamin A equivalent in beta-carotene. When you get more than that amount from supplements or vitamins, it doesn't serve its purpose as an antioxidant. In fact, it does the opposite and oxidizes tissue, which causes DNA damage. One study from Finland showed that people taking vitamin A had a higher risk of lung cancer, atherosclerosis, and, for smokers, stroke. So keep your vitamin supplement dose to 1,500 to 2,500 IU a day.

for yourself is clear your life of smoke—whether you or someone in your family is the one smoking. Unlike a White House press secretary, a good damage-control plan won't bail you out. Your only option is to stop. The positive side is that just two months of being smoke-free can make you one year younger. After five years of smoke-free living, a former smoker can regain seven of the eight years lost to smoking.

IF YOU'RE A SMOKER . . .   We're a society that doesn't like quitters—not in sports, not in school, not in wing-eating contests. So it's against our human nature to give up something that we've started—even cigarettes. One of the toughest parts about quitting smoking is that they're both physiologically and psychologically addictive. From the physiological end, it seems that the release of dopamine—a naturally occurring substance in your body that dulls pain and causes pleasure—is triggered when you're smoking. When you smoke, you get used to the elevated dopamine levels, so when you don't smoke, you crave the cigarette with no explanation as to why, almost like the way a pregnant woman craves chocolate-chip relish. Luckily, those dopamine levels don't stay elevated all the time, and if you can quit, you can switch your dopamine level back to normal.

Psychologically, smoking becomes a behavioral addiction—you have a cigarette with a beer, after dinner, after sex. And you get used to the feeling of picking something up and putting it in your mouth. The hardest part of quitting comes in the first week. You feel cravings, you're sluggish, and you start producing and expelling a lot of gunk from the lining of your lungs. But all that subsides after a few weeks, if you can push through. Luckily, there is an effective way you can stop smoking. Here's the plan:

Days 1 through 27 (don't try to stop yet; establish another behavior in its place): Walk thirty minutes a day, every day. When you're done, report to another person that you've completed it (use the same person every day). Walking thirty minutes a day will help prevent the weight gain for when you do stop, but it also proves to you that you have the discipline to stick with a plan. Only one rule: You can't act like an eleventh-grader who blew off doing his chemistry homework. No excuses. Tired? You walk. Hurricane swirling outside? You walk for thirty minutes, taking laps around the dining room table. Want to watch *Seinfeld* reruns? You buy a treadmill and walk while you watch. You walk *every day*.

Days 28 and 29: Start taking 100 milligrams of Wellbutrin (bupropion) once a day in the morning. An anticraving drug (it's also an antidepressant, if you take much more of it) can help you make the transition from being a smoker to being a quitter. (Check with your doctor if you have high blood pressure or seizure disorders, because bupropion can have side effects when taken with other medications.)

Keep walking thirty minutes (or more) every day, no excuses, and keep checking in with your support person.

Day 30: Quit. Throw away all your cigarettes, cigars, tobacco, ashtrays, lighters, pipes, and Kool boxer shorts. Put on a nicotine patch as prescribed by your doctor (usually about 7 to 10 milligrams if you smoke less than half a pack a day, 14 milligrams if you smoke between a half and one pack, and 21 or 22 milligrams if you smoke more than one pack a day). Also, increase your Wellbutrin to two a day—100 milligrams in the morning and the same dose in the evening. Keep walking. The toughest days will be three to five days after you quit, but if you can make it to Day 33—seven days after you quit—you'll have crossed the desert and made it past the most difficult part of the quitting cycle. You'll decrease the size of the nicotine patch after two months and again after four months, and you'll also gradually come off the pills so that you won't be taking any after six months. Walking? You do that as long as Elvis keeps selling albums. In other words, forever. After thirty days (or earlier) off cigarettes (Day 60 or so), you begin lifting weights ten minutes a day (see Chapter 14).

One of the biggest concerns with quitting smoking is the potential weight gain. On average (and without the walking), men gain ten pounds after quitting and women about eight. Six months later, the typical woman is just two pounds heavier than when she was smoking, but those men and women who use the plan above and do the walking and weight lifting average six pounds *lighter* than the day they quit. Though the dangers of smoking far outweigh the dangers of this additional weight, you can prevent weight gain during the quitting process. Walking will help. Chewing sugarless gum will ease oral cravings. Put a rubber band around your wrist so you have something to do with your fingers besides pick up baby back ribs. Concentrate on low-fat snacks, like fruits, vegetables, and unbuttered popcorn, with a few healthy-fat snacks like six walnuts with the fruit.

If you can make any change that will improve your health and make you live younger, it's this one. For once in your life, be a quitter—and be proud of it. Think of the rewards: No matter how much or how long you've smoked, you can reverse seven-eighths, usually, of the bad effects of smoking within five years.

IF YOU'RE AROUND A LOT OF SMOKE... Secondhand smoke is one of the few actions that another person can do that can actually contribute to your aging process. Spending an hour in someone else's smoke is like your smoking four cigarettes yourself. In other words, for every cigarette that a smoker smokes, you're inhaling about a third of it yourself. Just look at the consequences: Spending four hours a day in a smoky environment can make your RealAge up to 6.9 years older.

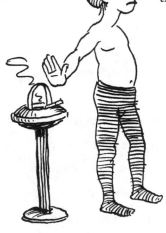

That's all the more reason that if you live with a smoker, then you have to encourage that smoker to follow the steps to quitting. It'll help your partner—not to mention you.

Smoking Cessation Plan

1. Start walking thirty minutes every day, no excuses, every day. Start this on Day 1, one month before quitting. Call a support person.

2. Fill prescription. Ask your doctor for prescriptions for 100 milligram Wellbutrin tablets and nicotine patches dosed according to the amount you smoke, as indicated below:
    *   ★ for ½ pack a day, take 7–10 milligrams
    *   ★ for ½–1 pack a day, take 14 milligrams
    *   ★ for 1–2 packs a day, take 21 or 22 milligrams
    *   ★ for more than 2 packs a day, ask your doctor

3. On Day 28: two days before you plan to stop smoking, take 1 Wellbutrin (bupropion).

4. On Day 29: take 1 Wellbutrin.

5. Apply your nicotine transdermal patch system on Day 30 (this is your stop smoking day). Place one patch on your arm, chest, or thigh (replace daily).

6. On day 30 and subsequent days, take Wellbutrin each morning *and* each evening. Most folks wean off Wellbutrin between days 90 and 180.

7. Continue walking thirty (to forty-five) minutes each day and call your support person. Feel free to drink as much coffee or water as you wish.

8. Phone or e-mail your support person daily to discuss your progress.

9. Begin weight lifting on Day 60 (_____ , or earlier). Do not increase your physical activities by more than 10 percent a week.

10. Decrease patch size by one-third every two months.

11. Decrease to one Wellbutrin in the evening after six months, and eliminate that one at twelve months.

12. Carry one Wellbutrin tablet with you at all times to take if you feel a craving.

Chapter 6

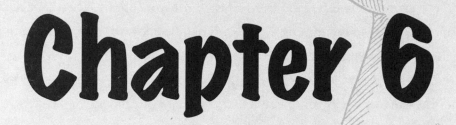

Gut Feelings:
Your Digestive System

Major Myths About Digestion

Gut Myth #1	Stress causes ulcers.
Gut Myth #2	Bad breath comes from your mouth.
Gut Myth #3	Blood in your stool usually indicates cancer.

When you think about it, it's amazing how many things go down your drains—razor stubble, toilet paper, soap scum, onion skin, dinner crumbs, spiders, sand from a beach trip, toothpaste, an occasional wedding ring . . . A house's plumbing system can handle a lot (thank goodness, or we'd all be living in hazmat suits). It takes away what we don't want, shuttles it to some processing facility, and we never have to think about it again—unless some kink prevents our waste from being drained. Whatever plugs your pipes, you know you have to clear a clog with Drano or some piece of heavy artillery. Without clean pipes, life stinks.

That's why you take steps to keep all your pipes clear. Before winter, you may shut off the outside water supply to keep pipes from freezing, and though your toddler may have a different agenda, House Rule Number 26 is: No Tonka trucks down the toilet. Really, it's much easier to keep your pipes working than to call a belt-phobic plumber to fix them.

It's the same thing with your body's pipes—your digestive system. We all put an extraordinary variety (and amount) of things down our anatomical drains, and we expect our plumbing system to shuttle everything away. Because our pipes don't always appreciate the jalapeño-laden burritos or fraternity-prank goldfish we slide down them, we can experience digestive problems like clogs, spills, leaks, breaks, and spouse-scaring explosions. A key element in this factory of consumption and elimination is your intestinal tract. Most people don't realize that your intestines are living things; they're organs just like your heart's an organ. They're not inert tubes; instead, they actively absorb, secrete, send signals, and metabolize. In some ways, your intestines are the democratic government of your body. They give us the freedom to eat whatever we want, which means our intestines allow us to be omnivores instead of carnivores or herbivores. Depending on what we crave, we have the intestinal freedom to eat plants, animals, or a dozen Krispy Kremes at one sitting. That's because our intestines let us micromanage what we allow within the borders of our body. But with that freedom comes responsibility. As young people, we think that our bodies are like machines, that they'll convert whatever we want to eat into something our cells can convert to energy. That's not entirely true, especially as we get older or don't exercise as much. That's because your body—as you can attest from your gastrointestinal reaction to your mom's eight-bean casserole—responds differently to various types of food.

For a lot of people, talking about digestive sewage sounds as appealing as playing in it. It's just not something that we talk about much (*"How about that rain today? Did you see Shaq's dunk last night? Your bowels chugging along regularly these days, Frank?"*). Maybe so, but foul shouldn't mean taboo. And that's an important point: Colon cancer is silent because there aren't many outward symptoms, but also because people would rather talk about the kind of colon that appears earlier in this sentence rather than the anatomical pipe that launches your enchilada submarine into the great porcelain ocean.

Of course, we all know that your digestive system is as dirty as George Carlin's jokes, especially when you start throwing around words like colon, rectum, and feces. But it's crucial to talk openly about these things, because a well-lubed digestive system helps you live younger and better. When you consider how many different kinds of foods are out there and how differently all of our bodies respond to them, you'll want to understand how your pipes work and what can cause them to break. Look, we're not trying to be a pain in the butt (but more on hemorrhoids later); we just want your sewer system to get your food from one end of your body to the other as efficiently as it can.

Your Digestion: The Anatomy

Like a house, the inside of your body contains a series of overlapping pipes and cables. You've read so far that your veins and arteries pick up and transport blood, oxygen, and other nutrients all over your body. Your neurons send messages throughout your brain and body to other neurons and muscles. And then you have the largest pipe (at least in terms of mass) in your body—the digestive tract. Like your house's piping system, this digestive pipeline has primarily one way in and one way out—though it also has many, many other smaller entrances and exits that help deliver nutrients throughout your body. The typical travel pattern flows from top to bottom, except at times when gravity or illness force food and liquid back up, as in the cases of heartburn, roller coasters, or a tequila-induced hangover. Of course, high school biology class taught us the basics of digestion: Food passes through the esophagus into the stomach, then through twenty-six feet of small intestines, to rest finally in the colon, until you are ready to pass it out of your body. But the devil is in the details of this process, especially since this system has the complexity of a brain part and micromanages how you interact with the outside world of food and water. So let's follow a piece of food along the digestive tract to see how things start—and how they end.

Mouth

The food-consumption process starts right here—in your body's food processor. Though opera singers, politicians, and courtside fans are known mostly for what comes out of their mouths, what makes our mouths so special is how we handle what goes into them. For starters, consider your mouth to be like the guy who buckles you in on a Ferris wheel—it's there simply to prepare the food for the journey. We're different from most other animals in the way we chew. A crocodile, for instance, has nail-like teeth so it can grab its food and rip it apart. While intimidating, it's actually not energy-efficient, because it cannot start extracting energy until the food is halfway through its intestinal system. Elephants have grinding teeth; they're flat teeth made to chew in a grinding motion, which allows them to eat all kinds of food but at a slow pace. Neither way is very efficient (in fact, elephants have to make

Chomp Chomp

Everybody knows the two primary things teeth are used for—eating and stopping hockey pucks. But what may surprise you is that your teeth can provide clues into your health like virtually no other outward part of your body. Why? The biggest concern when it comes to aging and your teeth isn't the presence of cavities; it's the presence of periodontal disease, which can make you up to 3.7 years older. Gum disease (gingivitis) has been linked to many other health problems, presumably because the same bacteria that cause periodontal disease can also trigger an immune response that causes inflammation and hardening of the arteries. That same plaque that causes tooth decay—that sticky coating of bacteria, saliva, and three-day-old cauliflower—can also contribute to the plaque in your arteries. And that has a profound effect on all kinds of vascular problems, from heart attacks to erectile dysfunction. Here's a telling fact: Many people in Great Britain don't have regular dental care because it's not provided free by the National Health Service. But when people in Great Britain go to the hospital with chest pain, they're given an aspirin, a beta-blocker, and an antibiotic for gum disease—because doctors know there's a strong link between the inflammation of gum disease and an aging and unstable cardiovascular system.

new teeth to replace the worn-out ones throughout their lives; when they lose their last tooth, they die of starvation.)

Humans actually get the most energy possible from food because we don't waste a lot of energy as we eat. We can thank our opposing molars for starting us off right. For chewing efficiency, the grooves of our upper teeth are supposed to fit perfectly together with the grooves in our lowers. If one tooth falls out, the opposing tooth actually grows longer to try to make up the space (ever hear of someone who's "long in the tooth"?). The other advantage we have is through our jawbones, which allow us to crush food efficiently. As the only joint in the body that purposely dislocates itself during a motion, the jawbone has two points of attachment—a lever point in the back of the jaw and another two inches in front (see Figure 6.1). Every time you chew, your jaw dislocates and relocates, which allows you to crush the food like a foot crushes an aluminum can and starts the process of getting all the energy out of what you're eating. We also pay a price for that efficiency. If you chew too much, it can stress the joint and cause the joint to come slightly out of alignment. That leads to TMJ (temporomandibular joint) disorders, which are signified by intense jaw, neck, or eye pain. And, much to the dismay of sex-starved men, it's one of the leading causes of headaches in young women.

As you're chewing, your tongue takes its turn, too. You already know about the four major taste receptors—sweet, sour, bitter, salty. But there's another one—one that delivers deliciousness—called umami. It's why we crave foods; it's why some foods literally make you salivate more than a Gucci half-off sale. And it's partly what creates a dietary tug-of-war in your body. Your tongue wants to eat certain foods—foods that have lots of taste and energy—even though your body may not have a place for all that energy to go. Sweet, sour, bitter, and salty are inherited tastes—so you either like them or don't like them, depending on what your genes tell you. But fat is a *learned* taste. That means you can also learn how *not* to like fat. (For example, if you drink whole-fat milk, you can train yourself to prefer skim milk by gradually diluting whole milk. The phenomenon takes only eight weeks). Taste buds can also play tricks on you—making you think you have a problem when you really

Figure 6.1 **Jaws of Life** Our remarkably efficient digestive system extracts the most calories possible. The process starts in the mouth with a temporomandibular jaw (TMJ) joint that purposely dislocates during chewing in order to allow the masseter muscle to compress food more forcefully. The teeth fit together like puzzle pieces to ensure that no morsel is left unchewed and underdigested. Clenching teeth and having a tight jaw often cause TMJ pain and headaches.

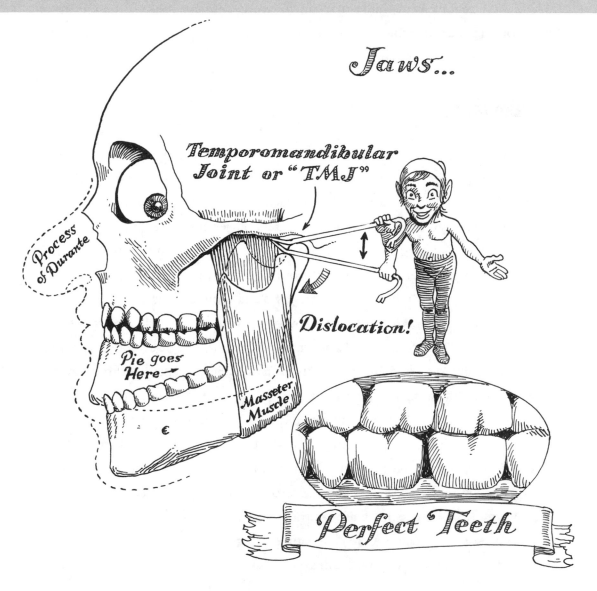

don't. Part of the way taste buds work is through expectation. When you eat something that's salty and you weren't expecting it, it surprises you. And that can happen with all kinds of food—if you're not expecting them to taste the way that they do. This is really a matter of taste expectation rather than something destructive going on in your digestive system. Your mouth acts as the doorway to your internal plumbing, so there're only a few things that can go wrong here in your mouth in terms of digestion: trouble with the enzymes in your saliva, with your teeth, or with your gums (see Chomp Chomp on page 177).

Esophagus

Once you're done chewing your food, it passes into the esophagus and through the gastroesophageal junction. Let's look at the anatomy of the esophagus. In Figure 6.2, do you see where it enters the stomach?

It doesn't enter from straight down; it enters like Jennifer Aniston trying to sneak into a restaurant—through a side door. As your stomach curls around your esophagus, that side entrance actually helps prevent stomach fluid from regurgitating back up to or at least toward your mouth. When you get older, though, your stomach becomes more sensitive to the foods you eat, and you wind up with more acid than that found backstage at a 1970s rock concert. Regurgitation is actually one of evolution's greatest gifts. That ability to regurgitate protects us. Horses, for instance, can't vomit, so when they eat poisonous stuff, they can't get it out of their system. That promotes a condition called colic—or severe abdominal pain caused by trauma in the digestive tract—and that's the leading cause of equine deaths. So the stars of MTV's *Jackass* aren't the only ones who should be thankful humans can vomit, spit up, and vent air with Richter-registering burps. This poison-control system helps us clear harmful substances out of our bodies, but it also contributes to acid reflux.

Your esophagus enters at an acute angle, which kinks off after the food passes to prevent the stomach contents from going back into your esophagus. If the acute

FIGURE 6.2 ## You've Got a Lot of Guts

We are born to eat, and our stomachs can digest nearly anything, but in order to be able to experiment with new and sometimes poisonous foods, humans must have the ability to vomit food or burp gas. The esophagus makes a sharp angle as it enters the stomach to reduce this regurgitation, but if the junction is opened (the angle is reduced), we get burning and indigestion from GERD (gastroesophageal reflux disorder). The gallbladder stores bile, which can be secreted into the small bowel once the food bolus has passed through the stomach. The stored bile can harden and form painful gallstones.

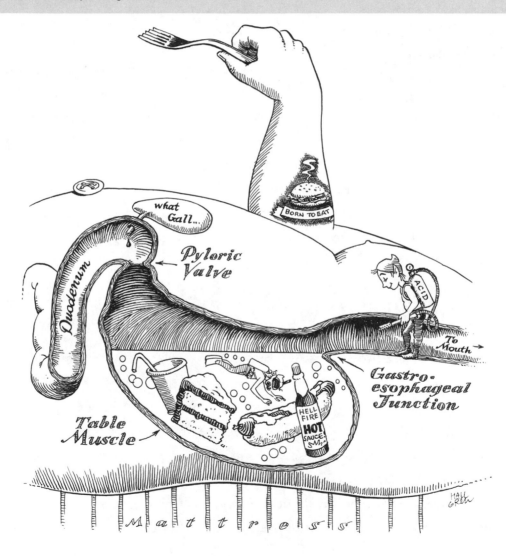

angle is distorted, for example by a hiatal hernia (an abnormal hole where muscle should be to keep the angle acute), the acid can flow backward into the esophagus. When you produce a lot of stomach acid—or overeat late at night—you risk becoming bloated and having that fluid top off in your esophagus. Think of it as being like when you overfill your gas tank—all that fuel runs out of the opening through which it entered.

Because your esophagus has less protective lining than your stomach does, it's much more sensitive. And that's what causes the pain in your throat that feels as if somebody's running a lit match up and down it. When that kind of heartburn recurs, that's GERD—or gastroesophageal reflux disease. Besides being more uncomfortable than high heels that are two sizes too small, GERD can also be dangerous because it leads to chronic inflammation in your esophagus, which has been linked to cancer.

Stomach

You know it. You love it. You rub it. Your kids bounce on it. You stretch shirts with it. It's your stomach—the storage bin of food. Once your food drops down your esophagus, it lingers there. The longer it stays, the fuller you feel and the less you eat. A lot of things happen in your stomach because of the accumulation of all that food. When you feel that burning sensation in your gut, you assume it's a mild case of GERD or heartburn. But that's not always the case. In your stomach, you have a very protective layer of mucus that lines the gut and helps keep it from being injured by acid and digestive fluids. But if the mucus erodes (from such things as inflammation, infection, alcohol, or spicy foods) and the protective layer is injured, you can develop a stomach ulcer—which is a raw or open sore in that stomach lining. Sometimes that crater—the ulcer—erodes multiple layers of your stomach tissue and gets deep enough to hit the blood vessels and to cause bleeding within the digestive tract.

Now, we all know the stereotypical pictures of people with ulcers. One's the hard-driving, type A personality who works too much and is so stressed that he freaks out if his coffee shop runs out of lids. And then there's the type B—the one who holds everything in and lets stress eat him or her away slowly, like a baby vulture on a zebra carcass. Well, the answer usually isn't type A or type B; it's Type H—as in a bacteria called *H. pylori (Helicobacter pylori)*, which is the most common cause of ulcers. The easiest way to distinguish the difference between GERD and a stomach ulcer is to locate the pain. Pain associated with ulcers tends to be in the abdominal area, especially just above the umbilicus (belly button); with GERD, you'll often feel pain in your chest or throat. Eating often makes stomach ulcers feel better because food neutralizes some of that stomach acid; in GERD, eating often makes symptoms worse. If the ulcer is caused by a bacterial infection, you can pass the bacteria to other people you're living with. Through kissing, you can ping-pong the bacteria forth between you and your partner, and you'll never get rid of it until you're both treated. Though ulcers caused by *H. pylori* can be treated successfully with antibiotics, the worry is that ulcers can also be harbingers of gastric cancer.

Myth Buster #1

The next stomach condition is the one most associated with failed first dates: bad breath. Sometimes bad breath originates from your mouth, and it's easy to check your teeth and gums for culprits. But often your mouth is only the porthole for bad stomach odors. Think of it as a sewer main breaking. You may smell it aboveground, but the actual problem comes from underground. It's the same with bad breath. Severe bad breath—called halitosis—usually comes from your stomach and digestive

Myth Buster #2

Myth or Fact? The best cure for diarrhea is waiting it out.

Diarrhea is usually caused by an infection releasing a toxin that paralyzes the small intestine wall and allows water to leak wherever it wants, which is why you feel like a water pistol while sitting on the toilet. The best solution isn't making camp on the toilet and waiting for the infection to run its course. It's chicken soup with rice. The combination of the rice and broth seems to protect the lining cells of your intestines by providing critical sugars so you can minimize the onset of Ole Faithful. Or even calcium tablets work. We're not sure why, but they do slow all muscular movements, which may help keep sewage from propelling through your intestinal pipes.

problems. As the bacteria in your stomach breaks down foods, it releases odors back up into and out of your mouth. Understand, though, that we're not criticizing your hummus breath. Let's just say that we really do think people are a lot like jade stones. What makes a jade stone beautiful is its imperfection, not its purity. We all have imperfections, and we all have varying levels of odorous breath. You're not striving for so-called perfect breath; you just don't want your breath to have the same effect as a serious headwind the minute you meet someone. When it comes to your breath, you should approach the problem the way you look at your favorite 1973 neon-green polyester three-piece suit. You're so close to it that you don't realize how really bad it is. In this case, you're unable to detect your own imperfections. So you need someone else to give you an honest opinion—and to tell you if you should be arrested for assault with a deadly weapon. A tongue scraper or change in diet can clear up mild cases.

Gallbladder

After the stomach, food moves into the small intestine and mixes with green bile—the liquid material made by the liver that surrounds and emulsifies the fat you gobbled down at last night's movie. Bile works the way soap dissolves grease; this green fluid makes fat soluble in water so you can digest food more efficiently. The gallbladder stores your body's bile so it can be squirted as a bolus when food comes

The Stone Age

Gallstones and the Rolling Stones aren't the only stones that can change your life. The other is the one that'll make you keel over like a rugby player who's been kneed in the groin. Kidney stones form when urine becomes so concentrated that small crystals and then stones are formed—creating intense pain in your lower back and side and when you urinate. The main method of prevention is to treat your body like an empty swimming pool and flood it with water to flush it out, which inhibits the formation of the crystals by diluting them with water.

gushing around the corner from the stomach. But in between meals, your bile is stored in the gallbladder, and with the wrong combination of fatty meals, some of the particles may fall out of the liquid solution and become solid crystals. When those particles congregate together, they form gallstones. As stones, they try to pass through your gallbladder ducts, and if they're small enough, they can. But if they're too big, they clog the orifice, which can cause the gallbladder to swell like a bursting balloon and cause abdominal discomfort beneath the right rib cage. In fact, gallstones are the leading cause of belly pain. Overweight women in their forties who haven't reached menopause are most at risk (fat, female, forty, fertile is an easy—albeit politically incorrect—way to remember).

Fatty meals, which cause your gallbladder to contract, can increase the pain from your existing stones. So there's a way that you can actually test yourself to see if your belly pain is caused by gallstones. Go out and eat a small amount of a highly fatty fast-food meal, like a piece or two of original Kentucky Fried Chicken (yes, this is the only time you'll hear us recommend *that*). If you can eat it without pain, you likely don't have gallbladder disease. If you have pain when you're eating it, that's a probable sign of gallbladder disease, and you'll need to see a gallbladder surgeon before another trip to the fried-food store (which you should be avoiding anyway).

Intestines

If you were to stretch your intestines vertically out in front of you (which we highly discourage), they'd reach from the ground in your front yard up past the second floor and all the way to your attic window. That's twenty-six feet of tubing—and this is where the serious plumbing takes place. The small intestine comes after the stomach and is the tubing where most of foods' nutrients are absorbed; the large intestine, or colon, is wider and shorter than the small intestine and absorbs water to form feces.

Chemically, your intestines are the organ most similar to your brain, in that the neurotransmitters and hormones are remarkably alike. Your intestines are loaded with neurons that keep the muscles that line your intestinal pipe working to move food down. When your intestines shuttle food into and out of your system, they act

What GALT You Have

The intestines' defense against aggressions from the external environment works through gut-associated lymphoid tissue (GALT) and is based on three constituents that are in permanent contact and dialogue with one another: the microflora, mucosal barrier, and local immune system. The bacteria colonizing our gut block new bacteria from moving into the neighborhood. The intestinal mucosa is a cellular barrier and the main site of interaction with foreign substances and exogenous microorganisms. It defends us by using a slimy layer that provides both a physical and chemical boundary. The intestine is the primary immune organ of the body represented by the gut-associated lymphoid tissue through innate (you're born with it) and acquired immunity. This immune system can tolerate dietary antigens and the gut-colonizing bacteria, and it recognizes and rejects dangerous microorganisms that may challenge the body's defenses. In cooperation with these native barriers, some in-transit bacteria, such as probiotics, can strengthen the defense system of the intestine.

almost like a celebrity's personal assistant who goes through fan mail. They decide what stays and what gets tossed. Foods have such a huge effect on so many things that affect our life—lethargy, depression, pants size—and most people don't even realize how closely related the chemical compounds in our brains and intestines are. Much the way we all respond differently to outside stimuli (some of us enjoy a rousing game of beach volleyball, while others prefer spelunking around a damp, dark cave), our intestines respond to elements from the outside world differently too. Kielbasa, for instance, may give your buddies enough energy to hoist trees out of the ground, but it may dull and bloat you. Either way, it's your small intestine that's screaming clues to you. The delicate lining is armed with unique immune cells that guard your borders and recognize foods

FACTOID

Grapefruit juice can add to the potency (and side effects) of cholesterol-lowering statin drugs. The good side: If you drink eight ounces of grapefruit juice a day, you may need to take only a quarter of your statin dosage. The bad side: Grapefruit juice increases the effective dose and the side effects of other drugs like calcium channel blockers, benzodiazepines, amiodarone, and Zoloft. So if you like grapefruit juice, work with your doctor to determine the right amount of each of your pills to take.

that you—or your ancestors—could not tolerate. When dissed, this finicky organ sends SOS signals to wake you up in the form of gas and spasms. And it rebels by squeezing you. Often, the small intestine is a kind organ—holding its temper unless there's truly a nutritional emergency (*"Yo, slow down on the chili dogs, will ya?"*). It's the intestine's way of asking you to be more attentive in the future.

Throughout, you have vascular systems that transport nutrients from the food and deliver it to your body's major organs (which scientifically proves that a way to a man's heart is through his stomach). After the small intestine decides what to keep, it shuttles the waste along into the cecum, a reservoir at the beginning of the large intestine that holds fluid from the small bowel.

That watery remnant of your past meals goes from the cecum (which is where the appendix lives, by the way) through the colon, whose major goal is to suck fluid

FIGURE 6.3 **End of the Line** Adequate fiber in the diet cleans the colon as the stool is stored in the curving rectum. Too little fiber or water can increase the risk of diverticuli forming. At defecation, the "caca"—an important diagnostic for measuring your digestive health—is expelled and should retain its banana shape in the toilet bowl unless you are constipated. Hard stools may injure the hemorrhoid veins, which can bleed and hurt.

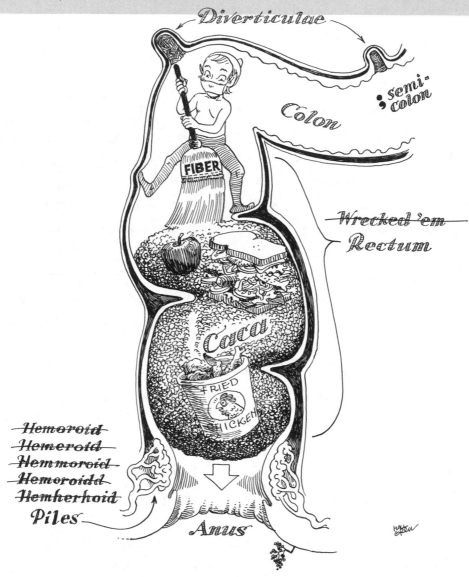

back into your body. Typically, as the liquid gets drained out, a solid mass of waste remains—your feces (or caca, if you're trying to be polite or potty-train your child). As feces gets harder and harder, it moves down to the muscular rectum at the bottom of your digestive system, as you can see in Figure 6.3. And when bacteria from an unsanitary cheese dog in Mexico City hinders its function . . . that's right, you get diarrhea.

There are three layers in the walls of your intestines. Where there's a little break between muscles, feces can squeeze into the gap and become as hard as clay. When that happens, the small out-pouches (they look a little like small thumbs poking out of the side of the colon) can get inflamed and cause diverticulitis. It usually occurs when the colon wall has to squeeze too hard to move the feces along—which is an indication of too little fiber in the diet.

While your waste exits your body through the rectum when you relax your sphincter muscles, preparing waste for the toilet bowl is really a function of your intestines—and the end product of it all proves a good glimpse into your intestinal health.

Let's look down into the toilet and do a self-test (c'mon, you're alone anyway). Your feces should be S-shaped (the shape of your rectum as it nears your anus), as opposed to gumball-size pellets. If it's not the proper shape, it's a sign that your intestines are temporarily not working as well as they could be. You can also do the sound test. The optimum feces enters the water like Greg Louganis—no splash. You want to hear a basketball through the net sounding (*Swish!*) rather than machine-gun rounds (*PopPopPopPopPopPopPop!*). Ideally, it should still be attached to you when it hits the water.

Hold the Syrup

Your digestive system has two main hormones that control hunger and appetite. Ghrelin is secreted by the stomach and increases your appetite. When your stomach's empty, it sends ghrelin out requesting food. Leptin tells your brain that you're full. When you eat, your fat cells secrete it so that you stop eating. One of the biggest evil influences on our diet is the presence of high-fructose corn syrup (HFCS), a sugar substitute that is found in soft drinks and many other sweet, processed foods. The problem is that HFCS inhibits leptin secretion, so you never get the message that you're full. And it never shuts off ghrelin, so, even though you have food in your stomach, you constantly get the message that you're hungry. The double whammy on our hormones has contributed enormously to our collective enormity. When you consider that many American women often obtain as much of 50 percent of their daily calories from salad dressing (which contains HFCS), you can see the problem. While food manufacturers may eliminate fat, they make up for its taste with sugar and HFCS—which are simply empty calories that serve no nutritional purpose.

Through sleep, your brain also plays a role in gut functions. If you want to eat less, get more sleep. When you don't sleep enough, more ghrelin is secreted and less leptin is released. So lack of sleep can have the same effect as HFCS by causing you to eat more often.

Fiber and liquids, which we'll discuss later, will help keep systems moving. And, of course, you'll want to check to make sure there's no blood in your stool. A small amount of bright red blood is usually nothing to be alarmed about. It most likely indicates hemorrhoids, and just a single drop of blood can turn the whole bowl red. But you can detect microscopic levels of blood with an at-home Hemoccult test, which is available at pharmacies and should be done every year after age forty. Don't worry—it's actually not as gross as it sounds; just follow the directions on the label. But this test, as many at-home tests do, can produce a false positive, so you'll need to follow up with your physician (this week,

Myth Buster #3

not next year) if you do have a positive reading. Blood can be a sign of many things, but it's important to look for it so that a colonoscopy—recommended every ten years for people over fifty or every five years for people over forty who have a family history of early onset colon cancer—can catch the precancerous polyps before they lead to colon cancer. Considering that you produce more than a thousand pounds of feces every year—that's the approximate weight of a concert grand piano—it's one of the best self-diagnostic tools you can use to measure your intestinal health.

Just like aspiring football players, your intestines need bulk—namely, in the form of your feces. With a bulky stool, your intestines can easily squeeze on it and push it toward the anus. But if your stool's consistency is more like that of toothpaste, then it travels through your intestines like traffic on the day before Thanksgiving—slowly and painfully. As the fluid is sucked out during the process, your stool becomes harder and the process becomes more painful, which irritates hemorrhoids. The final result: It drops into the toilet like pellets rather than the S-shape we mentioned. The best ways to ensure smooth sailing are adequate water intake (so it's easy for the bowel to suck out fluid), physical activity (which helps speed up the process), and fiber (consuming prunes or psyllium, which will add bulk to your stool).

Your intestines are also responsible for the form of bad breath that comes from your body's basement—gas. Of course, as any newbie comic will share with you, gas comes in all forms, sounds, and smells. Whether it's spurred on by beans, beer, or your Gram's creamed spinach, all gas simply comes from the fermentation of certain foods by the trillions of bacteria in your digestive system. The bacteria love to process some food more than others,

> **FACTOID**
> We all produce one to three pints of gas daily. Less than 1 percent of it smells.

Myth or Fact?
Nuts cause diverticulosis.

Nuts can theoretically get stuck in those little pouches in your colon that are indicative of diverticulosis, but nuts don't actually cause it. In fact, there's never been a case where nuts have been implicated as the perpetrator. The real culprit is not having enough fiber and water in your diet.

which creates more gas. The average person passes gas about fourteen times a day (Howard Stern's guests were not included in the statistical analysis). So passing gas is really nothing to be ashamed of, unless it happens during your wedding vows.

Rectum

Though everyone has different digestive frequencies for different types of foods, the average time from start to finish for the whole process is about four hours. The last stop on the line occurs at the taboo center of your body—the place nobody likes to talk about. The rectum is the internal passage that leads to your anus—the sliding-glass doors of your body that allow your feces to make their entry into the afterworld. Anatomically speaking, your anus is a lot like your mouth (you can stop cringing now). It has cells inside the body that help transfer substances to cells outside your body. One of the most common problems you can experience at this locale is hemorrhoids, which are swollen veins in the lower rectum and anus. Causing a lot of bleeding, irritation, and pain, they typically come about when the veins swell under heavy pressure—which usually comes from having to strain when you're going to the bathroom. (Go ahead, get up and flush. Finish the rest of the chapter on the couch.)

Your Digestion: The Live Younger Action Plan

Nutrition is a lot like a class of high school kids. You have good foods—foods that do wonderful things for your body. You have so-so foods—foods that fall somewhere in the middle of the healthy and unhealthy bell curve. And you have bad foods—foods that essentially toilet-paper your organs, throw eggs at your insides, and pound your arteries with fat-cell spitballs. Yes, we all know how fun and exciting it can be to hang out with the bad crowd of burgers, fries, and shakes. But we also know the bad kids always cause trouble and their actions have long-term consequences, in the same way that bad foods do. Most of the things you can do to improve your digestive health revolve around the things that should go into your mouth and the things that shouldn't come near it.

Action 1: Eat Fiber— and Wash It Down

In any given day, lots of things enter our mouths—air, water, a piece of Bazooka. To prevent problems associated with your digestive system, these are the best things that can enter your intestinal pathway.

FIBER   Fiber is the community-service director of the major food groups—it's not a sexy job, but it sure does great things. Most important, fiber helps keep digested food bulky and soft—so it passes through the colon easily. Fiber makes it easier for the food to move through your intestines without much pressure being placed on your tubing. And that's important for avoiding such things as diverticulosis and hemorrhoids. Found solely in plant foods, fiber is largely indigestible as it passes through the digestive tract intact. It contains no calories but makes you feel full, which helps control overeating. Both kinds of fiber—insoluble and soluble—are good for you. Insoluble fiber doesn't easily dissolve in water and is not broken down by intestinal bacteria. (This type doesn't lower your cholesterol but still has an effect on your digestive system.) It's found in grapefruit, orange, grapes, raisins, dried fruit, sweet potatoes, peas, and zucchini, but especially in whole-wheat or whole-grain bread (it has to be whole-grain, not five- or six-grain bread, to have enough fiber). Soluble fiber does dissolve in water; it regulates metabolism and digestion and stabilizes blood glucose levels. And it's found mostly in grains such as oats, barley, and rye; in legumes such as beans, peas, and lentils; and in some cereals.

In RealAge terms, a man who eats 25 grams of fiber a day or a woman who eats 35 grams a day can be as much as three years younger than a person who eats only 12 grams a day (the average for American adults). Plus, one study showed that a 10 gram increase in the daily intake of fiber decreases the risk of heart attack by 29 percent—and makes you 1.9 years younger. These are the foods that can get you fiber quickly:

> lima beans (3 tablespoons): 13 grams
> buckwheat cereal (1 cup): 10 grams
> artichoke (1 large): 10 grams
> soybeans (½ cup): 10 grams
> almonds (24): 5 grams
> peanuts (30): 5.5 grams
> oatmeal (1 cup, instant): 3 to 4 grams
> Cheerios (1 cup): 3 grams

WATER (NOT SOFT DRINKS)   If you've ever been to a water park, you know the way water slides work. The water shooting down each sliding board "lubricates" it so that the rider moves faster. Without water, there'd be too much friction on the slide, and it would take someone twice as long to make a big splash. Water works the same way in your body—it's a natural lubricant that helps everything slide through your system. But it also has another great advantage: Water fights bad breath. As bacteria come up from your stomach to your mouth, they can become stagnant—which is what causes bad breath. Drinking water will help break up those stagnant bacteria and move them along, rather than having them greet people every time you say hello. Now, when we say water, we mean water—not any ole liquid. The empty calories and self-destructive ingredients found in soft drinks will leave you bloated, hungry, and fat. (Okay, if you like diet sodas, at least you won't consume the empty calories in the cola but we mean water here. And maybe the sweet taste of diet drinks encourages other sweet consumption—those who consume "diet drinks" are more likely to develop diabetes than those who consume black coffee, tea, or water.) Also, since the main cause of kidney stones is dehydration, it's essential to keep your body hydrated with sixty-four ounces (eight glasses of eight ounces) of water a day.

Action 2: Change How You Eat

Watch any hot-dog-eating contest and you know that there are as many eating styles in this world as there are actors waiting tables in Hollywood. You can have a positive effect on your health by making some subtle changes not just in what goes into your mouth but also in how you put it there.

AVOID LATE MEALS   If your idea of late-night entertainment is a party with a bowl of Lucky Charms, switch to lifting weights while watching Leno or Letterman (see Chapter 14). Lying down so soon after eating encourages the flow of acid back up your esophagus so you get that burning taste, which will intensify the symptoms of GERD. While you're at it, avoid GERD-promoting items like foods or beverages containing pepper or peppers, caffeine, and alcohol. Some pills can also cause GERD if you don't take them with water (these are individual to the person).

BUY NEW DISHES   Eat on nine-inch plates instead of traditional thirteen-inch dinner plates. Research has shown that the visual effect of eating is a powerful signal to your stomach to slow the digestion process. People who eat meals from smaller plates consume fewer calories—but still have the same feeling of satiety as people who eat off larger dishes. Finally a case where size matters, and smaller is better. Reducing portion sizes also has the effect of making you up to three years younger because it helps reduce arterial and immune aging.

TRICK YOUR DIGESTION SYSTEM   Many obese people have received attention for losing weight from gastric bypass surgery. After the surgery, people simply can't eat as much food because a major portion of their stomach has been excluded. But researchers recently found out that part of the reason why they're not hungry isn't necessarily because their stomachs are smaller but because the segment of the stomach producing the appetite-inducing ghrelin hormone was removed. But those hormones aren't just in the stomach; they're in the intestines, too. So one of the ways you can turn those hunger triggers off is by making sure you don't get to the point of feeling famished. The slower you digest food, the slower your stomach empties, the fuller you'll feel, and the lower the chance that you'll wind up with an aerial endorsement contract from Goodyear.

Fiber is one way to do that; here's another: If you have a little fat before your meal, you'll prevent your stomach from emptying quickly. Example: If you have tea and unbuttered toast in the morning, your stomach empties in about twenty to thirty minutes, leaving you craving a midmorning Doritos binge. But if you spread some peanut butter or apple butter on your toast, it takes about three and a half hours for the toast to leave your stomach. Feeling fuller slows everything down. We recommend eating a little fat before each meal, but especially before your most gorge-prone meal of the day—dinner. Eat about seventy calories in the form of healthy monounsaturated fats. That's about six walnuts, twelve cashews, or twenty peanuts. The extra fat also has another advantage: It helps absorb fat-soluble nutrients like the lycopene in tomatoes.

TRY DIFFERENT DESSERTS   We're a society programmed to end our meals with something sweet—a piece of chocolate, a cookie, or some mile-high fudge monstrosity. Besides the damage dessert can do to your waistline, ending your meal with sugary foods helps promote the buildup of bacteria on your teeth. Instead, think about other ways you can end your meal. Why not do what many Europeans do—and make salad the last thing you eat? Or even try an ounce of low-fat cheese or a handful of peanuts; they're foods that help clear harmful sugars and plaque away from your teeth. If you must have something relatively sweet, try having your glass of wine as your dessert.

Action 3: Really Feel What You Eat

Look, when it comes to health, nobody's perfect. But what's our goal here? To improve your health and to keep you young and active. So let's say your overall digestive health ranks 4 on a scale from 1 to 10; you don't have to get to a 10 to live better. An 8 would make your insides feel as if they're getting a Swedish massage. And you'll live longer and better because of it. If you're bothered, nagged, or even just mildly irritated by occasional rumblings in your gut, one of the best things you can do for your health is play mad scientist for a couple weeks. We don't know about you, but we always loved science lab. Mix and match ingredients, and you'll come up with the coolest concoctions that are customized to the needs of your body.

Since food has so much of an influence on our digestion, it stands to reason that you can change the way you live and feel by figuring out the foods that are causing you trouble. Since there are so many foods to choose from, the best way to experiment is through the food-elimination test (no, you won't be looking in the toilet again). In this test, you completely eliminate one group of foods for about three days in a row. During that time, you should take notes about how you feel with regard to energy levels, fatigue, and digestive regularity. Take notes when you go off foods and—just as important—how you feel when you reintroduce them into your diet. That way, you'll be in tune to those things that make you feel worse once you start eating them again. Here's the order of groups of food we'd suggest you eliminate from your diet at different times, just for two or three days:

wheat products
dairy products
protein
carbohydrates (including sugar)
fat
artificial colors

When you eliminate a group from your diet, you'll notice different things about the way you feel. For instance, you may have more energy when you eliminate the aging fats (saturated and trans) from your diet, and that'll help you stick to a diet low in saturated fat because you'll notice—and like—the changes. It's all about *awareness*—being in tune with which foods make you feel crummy and which make you want to sprint to the top of Mount Kilimanjaro. This three-day elimination plan is an especially good test because you may be able to identify subtle food allergies through this method. While some food allergies may be as obvious as a botched hair transplant, others may not be so clear. Low-grade food allergies can make you feel as if you have a touch of the flu—with a runny nose and headache. Through this experiment, you can help make a diagnosis and avoid some of the foods that make you feel less well. Best of all, this experiment trains you to do something that's good not only for your digestive system but for your overall health and youth: It teaches you to eat smaller meals by restricting some of the usual foods that you would toss in your mouth by habit. And that's good for everyone.

Action 4: Supplement Your Food

One big bowl of chili is enough proof that food can be very powerful, especially if you're sharing a tent. Still, you can make a few additions to help address this and other digestive issues.

MAKE YOURSELF PSYLLY   That is, the supplement psyllium (pronounced "silly-um"). It's a fiber supplement derived from a Mediterranean plantain, which has been shown to help bulk up stool and improve digestive flow by sucking water into the bowel. Take a rounded teaspoon per day, but make sure to add lots of water, or you'll feel as if you just ate concrete. Or add psyllium to your breakfast drink, as we do.

STOP PUSHING THE GAS   Though gas is natural, it simply doesn't go over well in the office elevator. You can help suppress it by taking an over-the-counter medication containing simethicone. Simethicone helps break down gas bubbles to reduce gas. You can also soak beans in water overnight before cooking: that breaks down some of the compounds that cause gas. Be sure to use fresh water when cooking them.

B SMART   As we grow older, we often have more difficulty absorbing B_{12} from food. In fact, B_{12} deficiency is one of the most common deficiencies—85 percent of us come up short of getting the necessary B_{12} from our diet. Absorption of B_{12} in food requires a substance from our stomachs called intrinsic factor, the production of which decreases with age. (The American College of Physicians assumes that no one has intrinsic factor over age seventy.) So you can either get B_{12} into your body through a shot or a crystalline pill form (unless you have more body piercings than a punk rocker, we assume you'd prefer the crystalline pill). We recommend 25 micrograms in supplements. Getting the daily dietary and supplemental intake of B_{12} can have a RealAge effect of making you up to one year younger.

Action 5: Spend 120 Seconds at the Sink

You already know to brush your teeth with fluoride, which helps kill bacteria, but you also can live a lot healthier by hanging out just a little longer in front of the mirror.

FLOSS Do it every day. It breaks up the more than five hundred kinds of bacteria that live in plaque between your teeth and helps reduce the inflammation associated with gum disease. (One note: It's normal to bleed when you floss after a long layoff, but if you still bleed following each floss after a week, it's probably a sign you have some level of gingivitis.) This is important. Brushing and flossing every day combined with seeing a dental professional every six months or so can have an effect of making you up to 6.4 years younger. Because of its ability to decrease inflammation in your gums and subsequently in your arteries, flossing will help you keep your heart pumping and your sex life thriving—not to mention your teeth intact. And it appears to help prevent cancer in other areas of your body. Pressed for time? Then follow this rule: Floss only the teeth you want to keep.

Another way to thwart inflamed gums: Eat fibrous foods like apples or chew sugarless gum, which helps build up saliva. That helps you avoid dry mouth, which is a common cause of gingivitis.

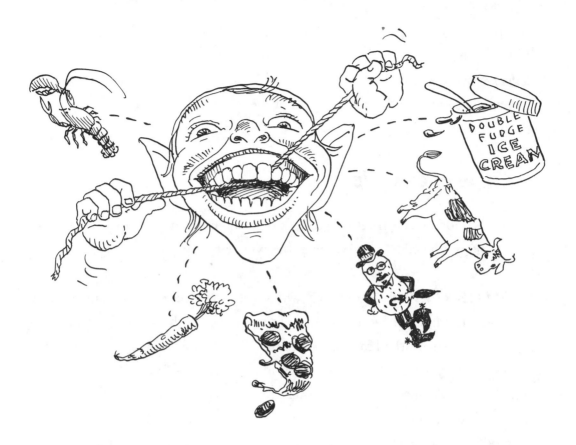

SCRAPE BY Many bacteria don't just hang out between your teeth; they lounge around on your tongue, too. Use a tongue scraper or brush your tongue while brushing your teeth to help remove some of the bacteria that cause bad breath.

SMILE Look at the front of your teeth. If they're flat (teeth should be like your nails—higher in the middle than the sides), it's an indication that you're clenching your teeth at night, which makes you more prone to TMJ disorders. Why? Think of your jaw as a three-legged stool with one of the legs being your front teeth and the TMJ on either sides being the other two. If you grind down your teeth, you shorten a leg and throw off the balance of the stool—and that causes jaw pain and headaches. To help ease the stress of the joints, take a cork from a wine bottle and hold it lengthwise between your front top and bottom teeth (without the bottle, Slugger). Now relax your jaw and mouth muscles around it for at least a few seconds (or forever is good). This helps ease some of the tension that's built up from clenching and misalignment.

Action 6: Clean Up

Dirt is good on construction sites and baseball uniforms, but it's generally not so great for your health. These two methods will help your bottom line.

STAY CLEAR OF TOXINS Anybody who's had a bad piece of meat or fish that led to a one-night stand with a toilet knows all too well the typhoon that swirls in your digestive system from a bad case of food poisoning. Responsible for twenty-five hundred deaths every year in the United States, food poisoning—caused by the invasion by foreign bacteria of your system—usually manifests itself with vomiting, diarrhea, and your promise to swear off the culprit forever. One way to avoid it is to make sure your food reaches the temperature of 165 degrees on the inside for at least fifteen seconds. (You'll need a food thermometer to confirm, since oven temperature doesn't correlate to the inside temperature of meat or fish.) Just because food isn't red or pink on the inside doesn't mean it reached the temperature, either.

Also, throw away your sponges. A sponge is like the back row in study hall—it attracts all the bad elements. In fact, bacteria grows on sponges, so every time you use one, you have the potential of passing bacteria from sponge to dish to food to mouth to one nasty day in the restroom. Instead, buy ten cheap dishcloths and get two buckets. Put clean cloths in a clean bucket. When you need one, take one from that bucket, then toss it into the second bucket, which should contain diluted bleach, after use. That bleach will kill anything that tries to grow. Then wash all of them once a week. (Though throwing sponges away is the best solution, you can also wash them in the dishwasher or nuke them in the microwave to kill bacteria.) And, of course, you already know not to leave Aunt Mae's macaroni out in the sun, because sun grows cultures of bacteria that secrete toxins. And that won't taste good, no matter how much relish she uses.

WIPE WET In Western culture, the theory goes, a man shakes with his right hand so he can't use it to grab his sword. You know what Eastern culture says? We shake with the right because we know darn well you just wiped yourself with your left. Besides Pilates, the best thing you can do for your bottom is to buy wet wipes. Why? If you accidentally got feces all over your hand, would you wash it off or wipe it off with dry toilet paper? Exactly. You'd run over to the sink faster than a sprinter in an Olympic qualifier. So why do we wipe ourselves with dry, sandpaper-like toilet paper after we go to the bathroom? It's also not the right cleaning system because it's irritating and increases the likelihood of getting hemorrhoids. While we're not recommending you install a bidet, you can get the same effect by simply wetting toilet paper in the sink before using it or using disposable wet wipes that are small versions of the ones you use on babies.

FACTOID

Vegetarians who haven't eaten meat in a long time don't like it if they try it again. That's because they don't secrete the right mix of enzymes from the salivary glands to the stomach's digestive enzymes and small intestine to optimally digest meat. That triggers a reaction when you do eat it: it feels heavy, you don't digest it as well, so you don't feel good and you don't enjoy it.

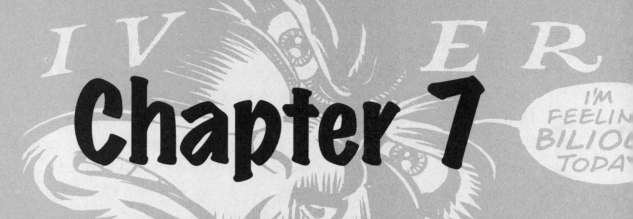

Chapter 7

In Your Trunk:
Your Liver and Pancreas

Major Myths About the Liver and Pancreas

Trunk Myth #1	Eating liver is good for your liver.
Trunk Myth #2	Fat is a bigger problem for the pancreas than for the liver.
Trunk Myth #3	Your liver is helpful only if you drink a lot.

If your organs were celebrities, you'd immediately know how they stacked up in terms of status and fame. The heart and brain reign as biological kings. They're the A-listers, the ones that get all the attention, the glory, the magazine covers, the best tables, and the medical paparazzi detailing every minute of their existence. Then there are the B-list organs, like the stomach, the lungs, the skin, and the sex organs. Of course they're on our radar, we know what they do, and we'd surely recognize them if we saw them out and about combing the malls. Lastly, there are the C-listers—those organs that we might know by name but couldn't tell you much about. Yup, they're the organs with serious respectability problems; no matter how much good they do, they can't get a lick of press. Specifically, we're talking about the Rodney Dangerfield of internal organs: the liver. Sure, you know a little something about it (filters your tequila, right?), but that's about it.

The reality is that few of us know much about the liver and its digestive neighbor, the pancreas. If you were to play medical word association (you do, don't you?), most of you would probably answer the same way.

We say liver? You say booze. We say pancreas? You say diabetes. We say liver and pancreas? You say get to the point already.

And you're right: Those two organs are associated primarily with alcohol and obesity. But to stereotype the liver and pancreas in that way would be like saying that your brain's only function is memory or the only thing your private parts are good for is eliminating the morning's coffee.

And that's a shame, considering the biological miracles that the liver performs every day. Consider this: The liver is the only internal organ that can regenerate itself. In fact, you can lose up to 75 percent of your liver, and the remaining parts can regenerate themselves into a whole liver again. Amazing stuff. ("If only hair worked the same way," says the bald man . . .)

As we continue our look at the digestive process, we need to examine these two organs. So let's peel back that fatty layer of digested mashed potatoes and take a look inside.

Your Liver: Break Down

If you allow us a quick diversion from medicine to mythology, we want to quickly tell the story of Prometheus. This poor fellow gave fire to the humans. His punishment from the Greek god Zeus for committing such a crime: He was chained to a rock, where a vulture would peck out his liver. Amazingly, the liver wouldregenerate overnight. How did the Greeks know of the liver's power? Maybe it was because they survived injuries to the organ in battle. While the Greeks were onto something, we're pretty certain that they didn't have as much insight into the liver as the scientific world does today.

Maroon and shaped like a boomerang, the liver is the second largest organ in the body (the skin always steals this glory). The reason why it's so vital is that it serves as your body's border inspection station. Virtually every nutrient we consume, whether it has a valid passport or not, must pass through the liver so it can be transformed into a different biochemical form. That transformation is what allows the nutrient to be used, transported to a different location in the body, or stored as an extra inch of blubbery goop on your thighs.

Structurally speaking, here's what you need to

FACTOID

There seems to be a relationship between having two or more eight-ounce cups of coffee (that's 300 milligrams or so of caffeine) a day and good liver health. This amount is less than the six cups needed to decrease the risk of Parkinson's and Alzheimer's diseases and the three cups to reduce the risk of type 2 diabetes. At the same time, you should also avoid having more than three drinks of alcohol a day — because of its toxic effects on both your pancreas and liver.

know about the liver (see Figure 7.1). It's located just below the right rib cage in the upper right side of the abdomen, above the pancreas and the small intestine. Your liver does three main things: helps digest stuff, make proteins, and gets rid of bad stuff.

All of the blood that has visited your small intestines flows through your portal vein into your liver, so almost all of the nutrients you eat have to pass through the gauntlet of the liver before passing to the heart for generalized distribution. Why "almost"? There's a little absorption in your mouth and under your tongue, but *almost* means 99 percent for the typical person. Your liver decides what gets kept out, what gets patted down and inspected, and what's allowed in to be distributed throughout your body.

Within the organ, there's a network of bile ducts; bile, if you remember from

FIGURE 7.1 **Love the Liver**   The liver, while known as the great detoxifier of the body, also plays a crucial role in breaking down the nutrients that you consume as they make their way through the rest of the digestive system. Bile from the liver is stored in the gall bladder until you eat, and then is released together with pancreatic juices into the small intestine.

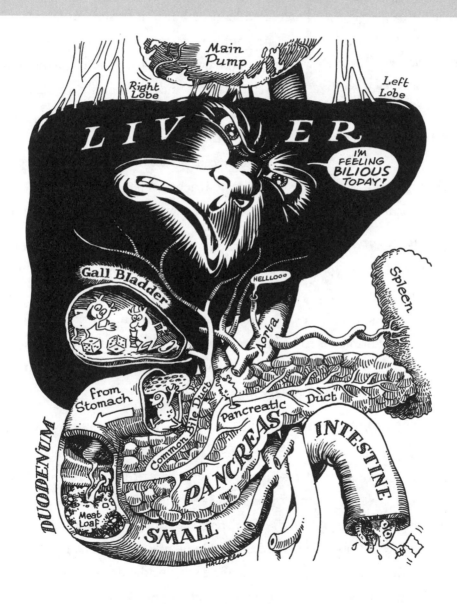

In Your Trunk: Your Liver and Pancreas ★ **209**

the last chapter, is the greenish liquid produced in the liver that helps break down fats. The liver also uses bile to clear bilirubin from the blood. Biliwhat, you say? Bilirubin—it's a substance that comes from the breakup of hemoglobin in dead redblood cells. An increased level of bilirubin results in jaundice (a yellowing of the skin and all mucous membranes—that includes the eyeballs, where the yellowing is usually detected earliest and most easily), a sign of many liver diseases.

The various functions of the liver are carried out by the liver cells, called hepatocytes (see Figure 7.2). They are responsible for the organ's ability to regenerate; hepatocytes act as stem cells that can re-form liver tissue. These cells work primarily to serve these functions:

NUTRIENT BREAKDOWN   We all may know that skim milk is good for your bones, fish is good for your muscles, and olive oil is good for your heart. But only a weird cartoonist thinks that your bones actually bathe in milk or there's a blood vessel that transports fresh olive oil through a side door in the aortic chamber. Everything we eat and drink has to be broken down into different chemicals before it can get to work on helping (or, in the case of some foods and drinks, harming) your body. And that's one of the primary jobs of the liver.

STORAGE AND CREATION   The liver, which makes protein and stores glucose, vitamin B_{12}, and iron, helps get nutrients to your body by processing all foods—carbohydrates, protein, and fat—into glucose that can be used throughout your body. Glucose is a fancy name for a specific and common sugar (yup, everything is turned to sugar). Iron stores in the liver are great enough for most people that iron supplements are not usually needed, except in people with iron deficiency anemia, which is the most common nutritional deficiency worldwide. The liver also serves as the initial source of glucose when you rush the hot dog stand at halftime (even be-

Figure 7.2 **Cell Plan** Liver cells—called hepatocytes—not only give the liver the ability to regenerate, but they also power the liver to metabolize or detoxify what we put in our mouth. The food passes from the intestines via the portal vein through the sieve-like hepatocytes and out into the central veins that feed the heart.

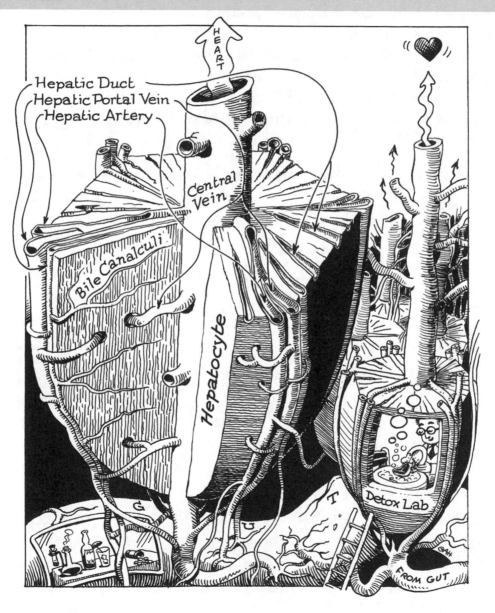

fore you get there), since the sugar in your blood provides only ten minutes of energy. It then does double duty to break down the nitrates from that hot dog in the detox function described below. This, by the way, is the reason why you don't burn fat immediately when you start exercising—it's because your body is using the fuel that's stored as glucose in the liver first.

DETOX   While we commonly think of detox as some thirty-day program for troubled celebs, the natural detox program happens inside your liver all the time. Here's how:

Most of what you put into your mouth isn't exactly pure. Plants are sprayed with chemicals, animals are injected with potent hormones, and lots of foods are genetically engineered with so much stuff that they make Frankenstein look as natural as a puppy. What's that mean to us? For one thing, it means that these toxins enter your body and can potentially destroy tissues or damage cells. So it's the liver's job to cope with these toxic chemicals as they travel from the environment via food into your body, almost like a drug smuggler trying to make it past customs.

How does the liver do this? Look at Figure 7.1 and you'll see rows of liver cells separated by space. Those spaces act like a sieve, which is where the blood flows. This sieve—like a customs agent finding out what illegal goods you're bringing across the border—removes toxic substances from the bloodstream. Those toxins can come in the form of everything from drugs and alcohol to chemicals and microorganisms. The way it does this isn't with drug-sniffing dogs but with special Kupffer cells, which eat up and break down the toxins. In short, these cells disarm the toxins by converting a dangerous chemical to a less harmful one or by packaging them for easier disposal through our bile or urine. The latter approach reveals how the sly liver doesn't always have to fight its enemies head-on. Instead it often uses a martial arts approach and paralyzes toxins by wrapping them in a water-soluble chemical so that they land in your toilet rather than in a vital organ.

The downsides? Two, mainly: First, some toxins cannot be packaged and hide in the fat part of the cells in your liver; others create damaging free radicals, which cause harmful oxidation in your body. These free radicals take a toll on the liver; that's why your body's natural antioxidants are essential to your frontline defenses and why vitamins like folate, B_{12}, B_6, and vitamins C and E are so important for liver health. Without these nutrients, the risk of failing to keep up our detox system shoots up and increases the possibility of allowing cancer-causing or atherosclerosis-enhancing inflammatory substances through the border patrol. As you'll see in our action steps below, a variety of foods and nutrients can ensure that you increase your natural antioxidants and that the detox process is as smooth as a freshly laid marble floor.

Your Liver: What Can Go Wrong

Most of us think we know the top three things that can destroy a liver: booze, booze, and more booze. While it's true that too much alcohol, either all at once or over a long period of time, can be as destructive to a liver as a baseball

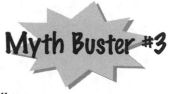
Myth Buster #3

Myth or Fact?
Detox diets work.

It takes a lot longer than a week for the liver to remold itself and recover from chronic injury, and studies repeatedly fail to show a benefit from short-term "detox" diets. The way that they can be beneficial? They reboot your taste buds and cleanse your intestines, so you can return to food free of allergies and with a heightened appreciation of simple and beautiful real foods. Processed foods wreak havoc on the liver, which has no way to understand how to metabolize them—except to treat them like toxins themselves.

to a window, alcohol isn't the only thing that puts your liver at risk. Here's a look at a few of the other potential problems.

OUTSIDE DESTRUCTORS One of the main liver diseases we see is hepatitis—an inflammation of the liver caused by viruses (but it can also be caused by autoimmune conditions, genetics, and some poisons). Hepatitis A is often in the news from bad food—for instance, a preparer who didn't wash his or her hands properly can poison food with the hepatitis A virus. Hepatitis B and C can be spread through sexual contact, IV drug use, and tattooing, with C being the virus more likely to transition to a chronic infection and cause cirrhosis, which is when scar tissue forms in the liver and replaces dead liver cells. Too much alcohol is a common cause of cirrhosis, but contact with other liver toxins can also kill off liver cells to cause cirrhosis. Think of this the next time you take one extra bite of Aunt Emmy's pecan pie. And, of course, your liver is also susceptible to cancer, although cancer in the liver often occurs when it spreads there from a primary source in another organ, like the colon.

GENETIC DISORDERS   As is the case with moral values and preference for sports teams, you can also get liver problems from your parents. They come in a lot of different forms, and rather than going into detail about all of them, we'll just briefly mention a couple of them so you're aware of them.

★   Gilbert's disease (which doesn't rhyme with Dilbert but, rather, is pronounced Gill-beartz) is a benign disease found in 5 percent of the

Should You Take BCAA?

Branched-chain amino acids (BCAA), a primary component of muscle, account for more than one-third of all amino acids in muscle protein. They're studied for a variety of purposes, such as aiding muscle recovery and decreasing effects of diabetes. Since researchers found that people with certain liver diseases may have decreased levels of these branched-chain amino acids circulating in their body, BCAA supplementation in liver patients has been studied. So far there's no evidence to suggest that they're helpful as a preventive means, but they could be helpful if you're suffering from advanced liver disease like cirrhosis.

population, who can't metabolize bilirubin normally. The main symptom, mild jaundice, most often appears after exertion, stress, fasting, and infections.

★ Hemochromatosis—a common genetic disorder present in about 1 in 250 of us and in the partial form in 1 in 25—causes people to accumulate and overload on iron. Eventually that iron overload can damage organs such as the pancreas, liver, and heart, which can result in diabetes or liver or heart failure. If you suffer from joint disease, severe fatigue, heart disease, impotence, or diabetes, it's worth checking what are called your transferrin levels to determine the levels of iron in your blood. That can let you know if you have the disease or may be a carrier.

DETOX DYSFUNCTION If the detox pathways in the liver become overloaded, the risk is that toxins will build up faster than sidewalk snow in a blizzard. And without a biological shovel to clear them away, there's a lot of liver trouble lurking. Why? Many of these toxins are fat soluble, meaning they wiggle their way into fatty parts of your body, where they may stay for years (or for your entire life!). And by fatty parts of your body, we don't mean your gut or your butt but fatty organs like your liver itself, brain, and hormonal glands. The effect: such niceties as cirrhosis (extensive liver scarring), brain dysfunction, and hormonal imbalances that can bring about infertility, breast pain, menstrual disturbances, adrenal gland exhaustion, and early menopause—not to mention an increased risk of many cancers.

Your Pancreas: Sugar Smack

The pancreas, the liver's backyard neighbor, gets attention primarily for its role in producing insulin. But that's not all it does. Looking like a strip steak with a fish head, the pancreas is about six inches long. Attached to the muscles and tissues near your back (which is one of the reasons why it causes back pain when diseased), the pancreas has two very different roles, with specialized exocrine and endocrine parts to carry out these tasks. (*Exocrine* implies that it secretes and has actions locally; *endocrine* means that it most commonly secretes into the bloodstream.) The exocrine role is performed by acini—grapelike bundles of cells that secrete pancreatic juice that are shown in Figure 7.3. When food hits the first part of your small intestine, these cells squeeze out juices to digest food so that it can be absorbed in the small intestine. The pancreatic juice also neutralizes the strong acids from the stomach so they don't damage the intestine downstream. This also explains the dangers of pancreatitis (discussed below), which is often caused by a blockage of the pancreatic duct. This forces these powerful chemicals to spill over and literally digest the pancreas itself.

The pancreas is also important because pancreatic enzymes play very specific roles in how protein, fat, and carbohydrates are broken down chemically so they can be used elsewhere in the body. The good news is that although the levels of digestive juice decline as you age, you usually die with your pancreas having considerable kick to do its digestive job, so you really never have to take supplemental

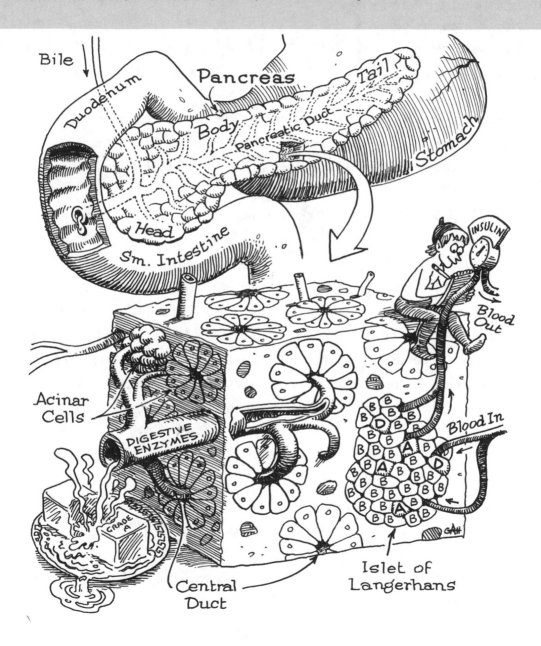

digestive enzymes unless you get a pancreatic disease or are born without them.

Now, you're probably more familiar with the endocrine part of the pancreas. This contains tissue that sounds like it belongs more on a map than in an organ: the islets of Langerhans. These islet cells constitute less than 2 percent of the mass of the pancreas, but they manufacture hormones like insulin. As you see in Figure 7.3, hormones produced in the islets of Langerhans are secreted directly into the blood by (at least) four types of cells. You can think of them as members of a Greek fraternity—minus the pledge paddles and hazing incidents.

BETA CELLS (65 percent to 80 percent of islet cells) These are the cells that produce insulin, the hormone that helps the body store and use glucose. Think of insulin as the U.S. Postal Service and glucose as the mail; insulin is responsible for delivering that glucose (sugar) from the bloodstream into muscle, fat, liver, and most other cells so that your body can use it for fuel. We wish insulin had a mantra similar to the USPS—neither blood, nor fat, nor DNA will keep insulin from delivering glucose throughout the body—but it doesn't quite work that way. Problems happen when either the pancreas doesn't make enough insulin or various parts of the body block insulin and prevent it from delivering glucose to those cells.

ALPHA CELLS (15 percent to 20 percent) Alpha cells release a substance called glucagon, which forces your body to make more glucose when you're exercising (and helps break down fat in this process). And you thought that huffing, sweating, and getting hit on were the only things that happened during exercise.

THE OTHER CELLS Three other types of cells round out the islet team. Delta cells are part of the feedback loop in the pancreas; remember that almost all biologic processes have a built-in "off switch" like this. These cells produce somatostatin, which among other actions turns off the alpha and beta cells.

PP cells may sound like code for preschool bathrooms, but these cells contain pancreatic polypeptide and prevent pancreatic enzymes from being secreted into the gut after a protein meal, fasting, and exercise.

Finally, a few epsilon cells contain the hormone ghrelin, which stimulates our hunger and very often causes us to eat like a bear in a stream of salmon.

Your Pancreas: What Can Go Wrong

As you've guessed by now, one little kink in any of the digestive organs can throw the entire system off track. It's no different for the pancreas. With some minor malfunctions in the digestive process involving the pancreas, you can experience problems digesting fat, which can lead to the ultrapopular side effect of fatty stools. (You know your stools have a lot of fat in them when they float; remember that fat always floats.) And you may also experience some pain when ducts get blocked by stones or thick mucus. But the main problems concerning the pancreas are these two:

PANCREATITIS Inflammation of the pancreas is usually caused by toxins, like alcohol, a virus, or a blocked duct draining from the pancreas. The good news is that the problem is averted by avoiding the toxin (caffeine, perhaps, or one too many double shots of whiskey) that may have irritated this sensitive organ, or the gallstones that block the duct. The toughest part about this condition is that it can be more painful than watching a twelve-hour awards show on TV. Why? Pancreatitis is caused by a malfunction of the digestive process in which the digestive juices spill back into the pancreas and then into the abdominal cavity and dissolve tissue. Because that tissue is located right above a big set of nerve cells called the celiac plexus, it's a wowie zowie kind of back throbbing that's some of the worst pain people can experience.

DIABETES   Essentially, people with diabetes have high blood sugar because they either don't make enough insulin (type 1) or because the inside of the cells that make up our muscle, fat, liver, and organs act as if they have shut the door on insulin and prevent glucose from being delivered inside (type 2). Obesity is the major risk factor in decreasing insulin's effectiveness, and the rise of obesity is the major reason why we've recently seen diabetes levels skyrocket. Of course, there are many problems associated with diabetes, including frequent urination, fatigue, impotence, nerve dysfunction, accelerated arterial aging, and even the development of vision problems that can cause blindness.

Your Liver and Pancreas: The Live Younger Action Plan

As you can see from this and the previous chapter, the digestive system is a lot like a car or a computer. A lot of things have to go right for it to work properly. And when one thing falters, the whole system can turn your gut into a tornado of trouble. Luckily, there are enough data about the liver and pancreas to show that you can help them function to their fullest potential to promote good digestive health and also to avoid the troubles that can come when things get out of whack.

FACTOID

In America, we eat licorice-flavored candy at the movies. In Japan, licorice extract is eaten for the liver. Specifically, licorice root extract is used as part of an herbal mixture for hepatitis. While there have been some studies investigating the use of licorice extracts for hepatitis, we don't recommend its use if you have liver disease, because of the lack of evidence and the potential of toxicity from high doses.

Action 1: Live Clean

While it's impossible to stay entirely toxin free throughout your everyday life, that doesn't mean you can't take steps to help reduce the pollution that pummels your body. Lessen the load for the liver, and you'll live longer. So what's that mean? Choose charcoal-filtered purified water over unfiltered tap water. Choose unrefined and unprocessed foods over the ones that spend more time in a factory than in the earth. Choose fruit over Froot Loops. Choose proteins like lentils, soy, beans, nuts, and seeds over red meats and the accompanying animal fats to avoid consuming the toxins that those animals were exposed to. And avoid eating any liver of any species that has been exposed to toxins (see "Live on Liver?" on page 208). Your liver—not to mention your heart, your brain, and your waistline—will thank you. Also, have protected sex and new needles and new pigment for tattoos, as hepatitis B and C are transmitted in these ways.

Action 2: Add the Crunchy Veggies

You already know that cruciferous vegetables (broccoli, cauliflower, Brussels spouts, and cabbage) are good cancer fighters. They've also been shown to help aid the detoxification processes of the liver. While you're at it, it's also important to have foods loaded with vitamins B (like whole grains) and C (like citrus fruits and leafy green vegetables) because they too have been shown to aid the detoxification process by helping your innate antioxidant system.

Action 3: Sprinkle On Some of This

Ginseng, cinnamon, coffee, and tea have been shown to help increase insulin receptivity, which can help lower the risk of aging from type 2 diabetes. Some studies have shown that one of the substances in ginseng berries (not the root) or a half teaspoon of cinnamon a day can increase insulin function by more than 50 percent.

Action 4: Get These Nutrients

These supplements have been linked to improved liver health; here's our take to help you manage the often-confusing store shelves:

Nutrients:

★ **Lecithin** (a supplement that contains 10 percent to 20 percent phosphatidylcholine, depending on the brand): Phosphatidylcholine is a necessary component of VLDL (very-low-density lipoprotein), which transports fats processed by the liver around the body. One component of the chemical, called choline, comes from the diet and can help replenish the needed levels of phosphatidylcholine in the liver to build VLDL molecules. However, when people are deficient in choline, these VLDL particles cannot form correctly, so fat builds up in the liver to cause damage. There are two ways to get choline or phosphatidylcholine: through a supplement or in food. A varied diet should provide enough choline. Men should aim for 550 milligrams and women for 425 milligrams a day. One large egg contains about 125 milligrams of choline, and one cup of toasted wheat germ contains about 175 milligrams.

★ **Zinc:** Zinc has been shown to help detoxify the body of alcohol. The optimum amount, especially for anyone who drinks alcohol, is 15 milligrams per day.

Supplements (take with the guidance of a doctor or herb expert because of their lack of standard dosing and potential interaction with other drugs):

★ **Milk thistle:** It's considered the safest and best supplement for liver health. Milk thistle's powerful ingredients, flavonoids, protect against inflammation and an unhealthy thickening of the liver. They also may help prime the body's immune system and antioxidant system. Though its use is not supported by the reams of data we like to see, the evidence does suggest some positive effects, as well as confirms its safety. The dose is 80 to 200 milligrams one to three times a day.

★ **Dandelion:** A member of the sunflower family, it's one of the most nutrient-rich plants there is. The whole plant is edible, but the herb is a source of

Hangover Helper

You don't have to be an MD to know the effects of an OD. Overdose on blueberry pie, and you're going to break the bathroom scale. Expose yourself to too much sun, and your skin is going to crinkle like a piece of bacon. And we all know what happens when you tip a few too many glasses of your favorite booze at the office party/happy hour/best friend's wedding. The outer effects from the morning after: Your head pounds, your stomach churns, and your whole world spins faster than a motorcycle tire. On the inside: Your liver has to work OT to handle the OD. While one to two drinks a day have been shown to confer many health benefits (including cardiovascular and longevity benefits), upping that amount can be risky for more than the obvious reasons of decreased mental and physical abilities that come with excessive drinking; it's also because the day-after hangovers are linked to memory impairment and decreased visual-spatial skills — making you more prone to accidents even the day after vodkafest. Some steps you can take on the off chance that you or your maid of honor needs a little help:

FOR PREVENTING THE HANGOVER (besides not drinking too much!) While you drink, eat foods with healthy fat such as avocados or walnuts. That will help to slow or delay the absorption of alcohol. Same goes for honey and tomato juice, which are both rich in fructose, allowing your body to metabolize alcohol more effectively. Also, choose light alcohol over dark alcohol. Darker drinks contain substances called congeners. They're what give flavor, color, and aroma to alcohol, but there's also a higher association with hangover headaches from drinks with congeners than from drinks without them. In short, vodka and gin trump whiskey, bourbon, and red wine.

FOR HEALING THE HANGOVER While no randomized studies prove it, hangover symptoms seem to be diminished by caffeine and water. So drink a lot of water or fluids that have minerals and electrolytes (like energy drinks) to help alleviate the dehydration associated with alcohol consumption. Caffeine can also help subdue headaches because of its effect on constricting your arteries — but remember to drink more water with it, as caffeine is a diuretic.

potassium, sodium, phosphorous, and iron, as well as vitamin A. The recommended supplement dose is 900 milligrams a day. Dandelion has a number of laboratory studies to suggest that it protects hepatocytes; however, good clinical data from humans are lacking.

Action 5: Don't Toxify the Detoxifier

Vitamin A can cause fat storage in the liver, chronic hepatitis, and cirrhosis. Patients with chronic liver disease should consume less than 2,500 IU of vitamin A per day in pill form (getting A through food seems okay). A list of other nutrients and supplements that have been shown to have toxic effects on the liver:

★   nicotinic acid (niacin; Nicolar)
★   pennyroyal oil
★   senna fruit extracts
★   valerian
★   iron
★   mistletoe

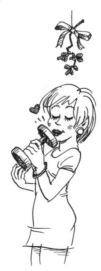

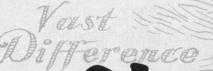

Chapter 8

Sex Marks the Spot: Your Sexual Organs

Major Myths About Sexual Organs

Sex Myth #1	Humans are consumed with sex because they're simply horny creatures.
Sex Myth #2	Only women have menopause.
Sex Myth #3	Older men will inevitably develop erectile dysfunction.

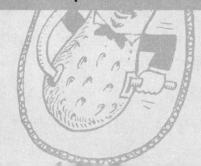

*D*ecorating isn't just something you do to birthday cakes and around the holidays; it's something that homeowners all over the world do to express beauty, whether it's pagodas in China, hand-painted tiles on Italian porches, or flags with football helmets on them in Philadelphia. The message from our house's exterior is our signal to the rest of the world that we want you to look at us—and we want to make the home warm, comfortable, and enticing.

That's one of the major roles of sexuality, too—to make us feel beautiful and to make us attractive and appealing to others. That's why we all employ unique ways of dressing up our anatomical exterior, so that others will be curious enough to take a tour of our psychological interior. We decorate our bodily homes with hair gel, nose rings, push-up bras, dragon tattoos, Speedos, tuxedos, manicures, five-figure wedding dresses, low-rider jeans, lipstick, leather pants, muscles, sunglasses, teeth-whitening strips. You name it—we have more ornaments than the mall on the day after Thanksgiving. And that's the beauty of being human; we can make our homes look different from anyone else's in the neighborhood.

While decorating a house serves an important aesthetic purpose, ornamentation serves a much more functional one in people. No matter what artificial tactics we use, we also have natural ornamentation that plays a major role in the mating dance. Ultimately, our goal is to seek a tango partner, and if all goes well, we do the tango to fulfill the greatest responsibility of our sex organs—to pass our genes to the next generation.

Considering the average woman thinks about sex every two or three days while the average man thinks about sex at least once a day, you'd think we'd be able to exchange thoughts about sex as easily as we exchange gifts. Truth is, despite what *Sex and the City* and Dr. Ruth have done for making sex a public issue, we're a private society when it comes to what transpires in the rich anatomical climate due south of the belly button.

Since sex is such an important part of our lives from a health and longevity standpoint, we shouldn't be embarrassed to talk about things like orgasm, ejaculation, and impotence. Recently, we have made some strides. For example, several spokesmen for Viagra said that they did it not for the money but because somebody had to come forward to talk about the problem of erectile dysfunction. And more high-profile people are being open about their battles with infertility. Why? Because they know that sex and sexual problems are nothing to be ashamed about. And they're right.

In reality, sex is one of life's driving biological forces and—at least anthropologically—why we are consumed with sex. We eat, we seek shelter, we procreate. From the most basic metabolic level, that's why we exist, and evolution commands us to do so. Think about this: After we pass prime procreation age—somewhere around thirty-five—we start experiencing the majority of age-related changes in our bodies that make us susceptible to disease. In essence, once the world gets what it needs from you (offspring), it's ready to inflict the mechanisms that discard you. You're finished procreating, your job's done, thank you, commence gradual artery clogging, game over. Okay, so biology isn't *that* harsh, but from an evolutionary standpoint, your genetic value is equated with your ability to procreate. After thirty-five or so, your genes no longer protect you. Of course, as humans, we know differently—that we value one another socially, spiritually, morally, and emotionally and we value the more mature members of society to guide the species to make smarter decisions. And as individuals, we have realized that sex doesn't have to stop as you get older (take the folks in Sun City, Arizona, where recently, there were at least a dozen reported incidents of seniors having sex in public places).

Myth Buster #1

To that end, it may help to break down some of our anatomy and look at it from a purely functional perspective. So let's extract the science from the sex to explain how humans are different from the rest of the animal kingdom.

Though one slang name for an erect penis may indicate otherwise, humans are among the few mammals that don't have a bone in their penis (many other animals have a bone structure called the "bacula" to help them achieve and maintain erections; humans don't have them because they're cumbersome and prone to injury, and because we've developed a better system). The human's penis works on a transportation system of veins and arteries that supply blood to make it erect (more on the details in a bit).

Because men don't have bony structures that could get in the way, they are able to have disproportionately large penises for their bodies. Really. Compared to many other primates, the human penis is larger proportionally than just about any other species. Evolution didn't just grant men the gift of girth so they could trash-talk gorillas at the zoo, but for this reason: Women are smart. In many other species, the male's job is to spread his sperm to as many females as he can. He's the king; he procreates. Mufasa fathers Simba, and a new king is born. Since humans are biologically—if not always socially—monogamous creatures, the male wants to find a partner who willingly accepts his sperm.

Women know that. While they may not say it or even think of it, women—on an evolutionary level—correlate penis size with potency. It makes sense, right? From a pure pitcher-catcher perspective, men could have much smaller penises. All they need to do in order to pass along their sperm is to penetrate the surface of a woman's vagina; even if penises were much smaller, sperm would still be able to swim up the path to get the job done. Faster, stronger sperm would be more crucial than a bigger penis.

Human males are larger not because of any kind of neighborhood competition among the men of the species (*My flamingo is bigger than yours, Fred!*) but solely because of its role in attracting child-bearing partners. But there's a trade-off: The human male's testes are tiny, especially when compared to other species like chimpanzees. When a female chimp goes into heat, she copulates with as many males as she can in order to ensure that she produces offspring. That child is then protected by all the adult males, since any of them could have fathered it. So the testes in these species need to be big to produce large quantities of sperm, because their sperm fights with other sperm for the right to the egg. Since humans theoretically don't have to compete with other men, their testes don't need to produce an oil rig's worth of sperm, which means their testes don't need to be as large (and thank goodness—considering how many times men's groins have been greeted by an errant baseball or an angry knee).

In the animal kingdom, if everything works out right, male chimp joins female chimp and baby chimp is born. Our sex lives are a little more complicated. We have sex for lots of reasons. Because we want to have kids. Because we want to express love. Because we want to have fun. Because nothing good is on TV. As with any of our body's organs, not everything works out exactly as planned. Our sexual culture is not only rich with love and lust but also filled with broken condoms, STDs, infertility, and erectile dysfunction. Problems associated with our sexual organs are complex and personal, which can make them difficult to talk about.

Above all, sex is one of life's greatest treasures—for your relationship, your spirit, and your health. But your sex organs are also fragile organs that are prone to many conditions that can make sex difficult, uncomfortable, or even impossible. So let's drop our drawers and take a closer look at what makes us function as sexual creatures—to see how you can live younger and better.

Your Sex Machine: The Anatomy

Let us ask you this: Where'd you learn about sex? Health class? The locker room? Pop's stashed magazine collection? Chances are, the extent of your initial sexual instruction came in about the same form as instructions for putting together a tricycle. Step 1: Insert rod A in slot B. Step 2: Enjoy the ride. No doubt, you've picked up a few pointers along the way and now know a lot more about sexual machinery than you did when you were eight. But since most people are as embarrassed talking about sex as they are about admitting to owning a Milli Vanilli CD, we thought you'd benefit from a spin through a more holistic instruction manual. To that end, we've combined male and female anatomy because, one, the male and female anatomy does have some not-so-apparent similarities, and two, because we believe it's important for each gender to learn more than a little bit about how the other gender works.

Anatomy of Attraction

Most of us know the relationship between the penis and vagina—the penis is the car that parks in the vaginal garage. But if the car breaks down in the driveway, you can't pull it into the garage. Ditto if the garage door is jammed shut. You need power to consummate the relationship. In the case of both men and women (especially men), nothing works without high-quality blood flow, and that starts with attraction.

Perhaps to the disappointment of fashion manufacturers and hairstylists everywhere, smell seems to be one of the dominant factors in attracting partners. Adult species release chemical compounds called pheromones that secrete smells that make us attractive to others. It's a chemical reaction more than a cerebral one, which is why we're attracted to some people and repelled by others without really knowing why.

Surely, love and lust are complex emotions that include a little bit of luck, a little bit of work, and a little bit of that intangible "chemistry." But from a purely biological standpoint, these chemical compounds send signals to your brain to put your love meter on high alert or to close the gate to all who try to enter. These signals bypass the thinking or logical part of your brain and go straight to your amygdala—the emotional part. And that's why strong attractions cause intangible sensations like butterflies in your stomach, tingling in your spine, and all-out, I've-got-to-be-with-you insanity.

The Vascular System

Now, when that chemical reaction is triggered in the brain, it hops on a downtown express bus to start a ticker-tape parade in the loins. How? In a man, the signals from the brain trigger a reaction that causes blood to rush into the penis like Class V whitewater rapids.

During stimulation, the muscles around the penis arteries relax so blood can be let in and absorbed by a spongy structure on the top side of the penis called the corpus cavernosum (see Figure 8.1). Because the blood rushes in, the veins in the penis are squeezed small, so the blood stays engorged in the corpus cavernosum (all the while, a soft structure on the underside of the penis, called the corpus spongiosum, remains relaxed to allow semen out during ejaculation). Without proper blood flow—meaning that arteries do not dilate appropriately because they are inflamed or clogged—men can't get an erection because they can't get blood in or keep it there. And that's one of the most common causes of erectile dysfunction—a condition that affects some 30 million American men.

From a broader perspective, the penis is the man's dipstick—it tells you how everything is functioning throughout the rest of your body. If the soldier stands at attention when called to do so, it's a good indication that you have good blood flow in other places. But if he decides to take a little R & R, it means that a man's arterial health is not as youthful as it needs to be. That's because the chemical mechanisms

Myth or Fact? About the time you retire, you're going to need Viagra.

Erectile dysfunction, like wrinkles and partaking in early-bird dinner specials, increases as you age. It affects 5 percent of men in their forties, up to 25 percent of men by the age of sixty-five, and over 50 percent of men who have reached eighty. And while half of men experience some kind of erectile problem between the ages of forty and seventy, it doesn't mean you have to be one of them, even after eighty—especially if you follow our guidelines for optimum arterial health in Chapter 2. In fact, more than 60 percent of men in their seventies report that they're swinging the clubs just fine, thank you very much. And there is no reason not to have the same pleasure till the very end.

FIGURE 8.1 The Male Dipstick

In order for the penis to develop hard erections, the large blood vessels from the heart (aorta to iliacs) bring blood to smaller arteries, which must relax to let blood into the dorsal artery. The veins then shut off the exit path so all the blood engorges the penis to form an erection.

Nerves around the prostate, which lies on the rectum, also help control blood flow but can be injured during prostate surgery. The two testes, which are typically different heights, lie outside the body so they can keep sperm cool to increase their survival. During copulation, special muscles retract the testes in preparation for ejaculation.

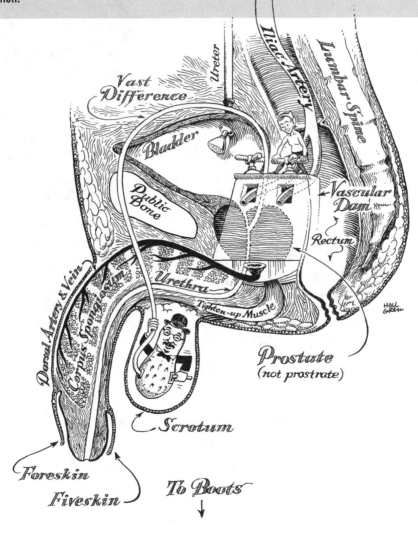

that work to get blood into and out of the penis are the same ones that help blood flow to and from the brain, heart, and kidneys. No matter the location of veins and arteries in your body, it's the same process of blood flow.

Of course, it used to be assumed that all erectile dysfunction stemmed from the psychology of sex—that men have total control over whether or not they can maintain and sustain an erection. But we now know that a man can't will his penis to an erection like a magician levitates an assistant. Many chemical factors play a role. Still, it's important to note that while good arterial health increases erectile health, the chemical reactions in your brain that come in the form of anxiety, stress, and depression can also be related to erectile dysfunction.

FACTOID

As we wrote in Chapter 2, all of our arteries—yes, even the ones that lead here—are dilated by a short-lived gas called nitric oxide. We continue to make this gas as quickly as it dissolves—unless damage to the inner layer of the arteries slows the process. Without enough nitric oxide, the arteries are unable to open up and feed more blood to make your sex organs hard (male) or engorged (female). So aging of your arteries is the leading cause of sexual dysfunction.

Hormones

We all know the role hormones have on gender differences. Testosterone is the substance that gives James Earl Jones his most famous attribute and estrogen is the substance that gives Dolly Parton hers. Because hormones do so many different jobs, it should be no surprise that another key reason for sexual dysfunction stems from testosterone deficiency in both men and women. Even though women produce only small amounts of the male hormone, a woman's testosterone levels help drive libido. Women lose testosterone as they age, and a large number of drugs, like beta-blockers and other medications to control hypertension, can negatively affect testosterone. One of the key physical outcomes for lack of testosterone in women is that it causes a lack of lubrication and a thinning of the skin surrounding the labia and nearby areas that makes sex painful. In terms of arousal, it's also important to note that while the glans penis is hypersensitive and what stimulates men, the clitoris is the equivalent and engorges with blood as well. The onrush of blood flow to it is what helps provide some of the stimulation that women experience during sex.

At the same time, women's estrogen levels also decrease as they age (just as men's testosterone levels do). In addition to having a lack of lubrication from testosterone, this estrogen drop causes the size of the labia to shrink. That makes the clitoris more exposed, which may lead to reduced sensitivity or unpleasant tingling. Add to the fact that the natural swelling and lubrication around the vagina slow after you age, and loss of libido is the female equivalent of erectile dysfunction.

There's really no way to quantify this kind of sexual dysfunction in terms of a so-called normal sex drive. Some couples are perfectly happy having sex five times a year, for instance, and some wouldn't mind doing it that many times at halftime. The real issue comes when one person in the relationship wants sex significantly more than the other. And that's a difficult issue considering that men reach their sexual peak in their late teens and early twenties, while women reach theirs in their late thirties or early forties. Another difference is that men are wired to have sex every third day—about the time it takes to produce the highest-quality sperm. When you consider the fact that one-third of women experience at least occasional bouts of loss of libido, then you have the makings of a sexual dysfunction that has at least one important remedy—communication (more on that in the Live Younger Action Plan on page 246).

Of course, hormones play a major role in many other areas of the reproductive process, such as menstruation. The hormones estrogen and progesterone change their levels to prepare for pregnancy, but they also change their levels when pregnancy does not occur. Those changes direct the process that prepares the uterus for the next cycle, when an egg will be available, by sloughing excess uterine tissue through contractions of the uterus. That's the process of menstruation, which causes vaginal bleeding, as well as hormonal changes that affect the way women deal with life and stress. Some women feel little effect, while others may use that time to register a saucepan as a deadly weapon. Oral contraceptives work by regulating the process to prevent a thick uterine wall from building up (and that seems to correlate with less bleeding, cramping, and saucepan throwing).

As the fertility process decreases (it is still debated whether this is signaled by the ovary or the endocrine control in the brain), women lose their ability to have sustained levels of estrogen and progesterone, until they even-

Myth or Fact? Bras or trauma to the breast cause cancer.

There's no evidence showing that things that could inhibit drainage from the lymphatic system—like bras and trauma—cause cancer. But at this stage, it's still difficult to deny conclusively.

Better Breast Health

While not technically sex organs, breasts certainly play a role after reproduction. Besides their function of feeding offspring, breasts—depending on your perspective—also play a role in sexual pleasure and sexual identity. The primary health concern—cancer—usually starts when a woman (or her partner) finds a lump in her breast. About 80 percent of these lumps are cysts—benign lumps that do not become cancerous. But they're hard to differentiate from cancers when they're first found (until a biopsy is performed). Cysts, which stop with menopause, are larger and more tender just before periods. A hormonal imbalance is the likely cause; to help prevent cysts, avoid methylxanthines, which are found in coffee, black tea, and colas. (See more on breast cancer in Chapter 12.)

One other note about breasts: Don't believe any hype about nonsurgical methods for improving breast shape. Like other extremities (nose and ears), breasts get larger and sag with time as we replace glandular tissue with fat (that's true for both men and women, by the way). Bras, better posture, and exercises that work the underlying pectoral muscle can improve appearance, but there aren't any nonsurgical methods for actually improving a breast's natural shape. Another reason to avoid cigarettes: They destroy collagen, which is important for maintaining breast shape.

Myth or Fact? Masturbation is good for men.

While some previous studies have made researchers believe that frequent ejaculation could increase your risk for prostate cancer, one major study of thirty thousand men showed otherwise. The study concluded that men who ejaculated between thirteen and twenty times a month decreased their risk of cancer by 14 percent—and men who ejaculated more than twenty-one times a month decreased it by 43 percent. In addition, many sex therapists believe that masturbation can improve your health—by relieving stress, for instance. What they do warn, though, is that masturbation should never be a substitute for sexual activity with your partner. On the other hand, there's no clear evidence showing a beneficial or harmful effect of masturbation on benign prostatic hyperplasia. And you probably won't go blind, either.

tually run into the time when they no longer menstruate. Menopause is signaled by many hormonal changes, which lead to a loss of some fullness around the vagina, hot flashes, mood and memory changes, and insomnia. (By the way, men can go through menopause also, but it's more gradual in its onset and not as clearly defined as it is with women.) To combat

Myth Buster #2

the problems associated with menopausal symptoms, hormone replacement therapy (HRT)—or, as it's now called, hormone therapy (HT)—became a popular treatment. Since we lose levels of hormones as we age, it was thought that ingesting hormones could be a way of keeping us young. The problem with HT is that it is linked to very serious side effects, including increased vein clotting, which can lead to a clot breaking off and traveling to the lungs (pulmonary embolism); cancer; and heart attacks. We can't recommend HT as a first-line therapy (see *YOU: Staying Young* for a more extensive discussion). For those within ten years of entering menopause who have significant symptoms, we recommend a 162-milligram dose of aspirin along with bioidentical pharmaceutical-grade estrogen and a micronized progestin such as Angeliq and Prometrium. For those without significant symptoms or who are more than twenty years postmenopausal, the risks at this time exceed the benefits—but talk to your doctor. (In any case, those women who are prescribed HT need to take aspirin to prevent potentially fatal clots.) Three substances—soy, red clover, and black cohosh—and paced respiration have all also been shown to work to reduce symptoms associated with menopause in about 35 percent of women. And eliminating all saturated and trans fats in your diet may end hot flashes, as that puts a halt to many of the extra constrictions and dilations of blood vessels.

What we want to concentrate on is that you don't have to view menopause as a sexual power outage. Sex doesn't stop after fifty. In fact, it never has to stop (just consider those seniors in Sun City, Arizona). Sixty-year-old couples have more sex than fifty-year-old couples (see Factoid on page 246). Sexuality is a major part of who you are. Embrace the fact that your body changes and see our recommendations later in the chapter for how to change with it. Because, really, just because you've lived in your house for a long time, that doesn't mean you let the weeds grow to the second-floor window or keep the same paints, fabrics, and furniture you had in the 1970s. You take care of and redecorate your home and your body, because there's a lot of satisfaction in feeling attractive to others—and to yourself.

Prostate and Cervix

FACTOID

Here's a breakthrough worth watching: Purified human milk, when placed on the HPV virus (wart), may be effective in killing the virus.

It doesn't take a *Sports Illustrated* subscription to know that the male and female anatomies are different in some pretty overt ways. Because of that, our internal anatomies have to have their differences as well. On the female side, one of the most important internal structures to think about is the cervix—the neck of the uterus that opens downward to the vagina. The cervix plays an important role in pregnancy; it lengthens to hold the fetus in the uterus and then shortens and dilates to allow labor and delivery. Cancer of the cervix, which develops from abnormal cells on the cervix, is perhaps the most detectable and preventable cancer. One proven cause is sexually transmitted disease—the most significant culprit being human papillomavirus (HPV), which causes genital warts. Because there are rarely any outward symptoms of HPV (though some women may experience mild irritation, burning, and itching), it's one of the stealth diseases that can attack a woman's sexual organs. HPV and cervical cancer can be detected early with a Pap smear. (Pap smears and pelvic exams should be regular after a woman becomes sexually active. That should include once a year for women with no signs of HPV and every six months for women who've had HPV treated.) While some forms of HPV seem to occur for no reason, more than 50 percent of all women have a chance of acquiring HPV with their first sexual encounter. This cancer can now be prevented (as can the infection) by immunization (like tetanus shots) to all girls between nine and eleven years of age or to women of any age, as long as they have not yet been infected with HPV.

In men, the prostate—the walnut-shaped organ that has the consistency of the water chestnut—governs the speed, strength, and frequency of urination and ejaculation. When men have prostate trouble (see Figure 8.2), they notice symptoms in such forms as frequent or painful urination or trouble ejaculating. Of course, the main concern men have with their prostates is cancer. The fact is, prostate cancer will hit just about every man if he lives long enough. It's a common disease in older men, but the concern really revolves around the aggressiveness of the cancer. Many men can live twenty years with slow-growing forms, which tend to occur in older men, while the aggressive form, which is more common in younger men, is more often deadly. But there's also another common prostate disease to be aware of— benign prostatic hyperplasia (BPH). Essentially, in men with BPH, their prostates enlarge around their urethras—the major road of fluid from the internal organs to the outside world. That enlargement causes the prostate to squeeze down on the urethra like a farmer's hand around a cow's udder to disrupt typical urine flow. People with BPH end up getting up frequently throughout the night to urinate, and they have difficulty initiating a stream of urine. As the disease progresses, the difficulty worsens—and you can never get all of the urine out of your bladder. (The fear is that

FIGURE 8.2 **Go with the Flow** The prostate regulates the flow of urine and semen into the penis. If the tissue within the prostate grows (hypertrophy), the narrow path is squeezed, making it difficult to initiate and maintain urine flow. When this happens, the bladder cannot empty itself completely, so the urine can back up (in the worst case) into the kidneys and cause infections and injury. Kidney stones, which are formed in the ureters next to the kidney or in the kidney itself, scrape surrounding tissues as they pass through the bladder and urethra.

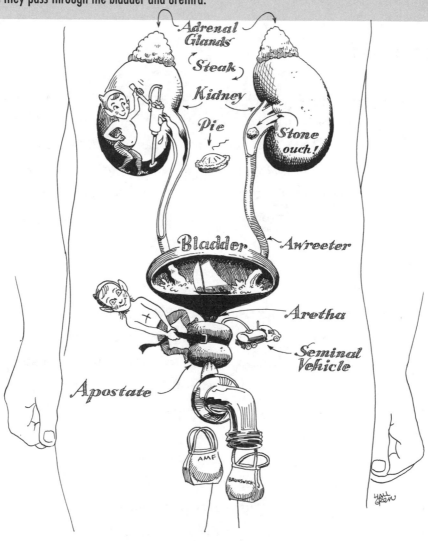

the urine can get backed up in the kidneys and slowly kill them over time—so keep getting up to urinate.) The way men decide to have prostate problems treated is very personal—some choose aggressive treatments that remove part of the prostate around the urethra, while some apt for more conservative approaches, like medication and alternative therapies that decrease swelling and help relax the muscle that's clamping the urethra down.

Sperm and Eggs

The reproductive process seems simple enough: See sperm swim. See sperm fertilize egg. See Missy ask for a pony for her fifth birthday. But conception is far from easy, and many couples who want to have children can't. Actually, the leading cause of infertility is the one that the fewest people think about: wrong place, wrong time; or not having sex at the time the egg is ready to be fertilized. In a system as delicate and intricate as the fertilization process, there are many things that can cause glitches along the way.

Every woman is born with the number of eggs she'll have in her lifetime. Some evidence exists that your stem cells can change this, but this has been accepted for many years. Those eggs live in her two ovaries. Every month—during ovulation— the ovaries usually release one egg cell (not one each, but one from one or the other of the two ovaries) from its follicle and send it on a very dangerous journey inside the body (see Figure 8.3). On the other side of the sheets, sperm begins the race when it hears the starter pistol (ejaculation). Before that point, sperm line up in a half mile worth of tubes through which they must travel before they get to the end of the penis (guys wish *that* was a half-mile long). With 300 million sperm contained in each man's ejaculation (that's the same number as the U.S. population), those sperm cells swim upstream with one gold-medal goal in mind—the egg. If unblocked by condoms or other barrier methods of birth control, they swim from the vagina and take the up escalator through the cervix to the uterus. With a lot of luck, a special

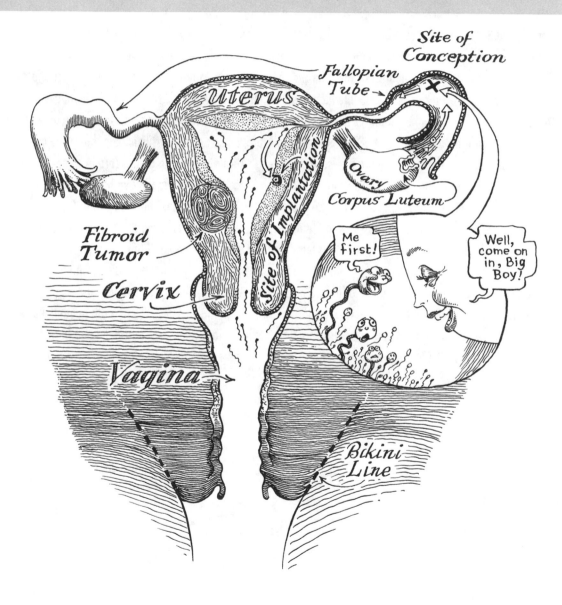

Figure 8.3 The Race Is On The ovary releases an egg that is grabbed by the Fallopian tube. If the egg misses this tube or stays in it, ectopic pregnancy can occur. As the egg passes toward the uterus, sperm try to fertilize the egg in a savage competition for survival, but low sperm count or motility (lazy sperm) can limit their success. After fertilization, the egg inserts into the wall of the uterus for development, but infections or fibroids of the uterus can inhibit implantation.

Myth or Fact?
Sperm that carries male chromosomes is faster than sperm that carries female chromosomes.

Yes, the male sperm is faster—because it's lighter, namely because it's carrying less genetic material. So while male and female sperm have equal muscular power in their flippers, the lighter one will go faster (just as a smaller cyclist will go faster than a larger one, if all other things are equal, because there's less mass to move). But if a couple has trouble having a boy, that doesn't necessarily mean it's the man's fault. Though you can blame a man for missing an important conversation because his eyes were glued to the TV, you can't pin this one on him. The sperm does dictate the sex of the fertilized egg, but there are a lot of mutual factors that contribute to it—such as the egg's receptivity to the male's chromosomes. Some couple may try copulating upside down or in other acrobatic positions because they've heard rumors that you can influence the gender of a child, but the process is a lot more complex than even that. For example, even if the male sperm outraces the female sperm, the male sperm will die off if the egg isn't in proper position for fertilization, leaving the female sperm clear for landing. While male sperm are faster, female sperm are like tortoises—they keep pushing ahead slowly, hanging out and waiting a few days. For boys, copulation around ovulation is critical, or the females will win. By the way, although the sperm is made by males, the receptiveness to sperm varies with females, which is why both genders have some role in determining the sex of the offspring. Another fact: More males are conceived and born than females, but they're the weaker sex when they're young, so there are more females alive in the world.

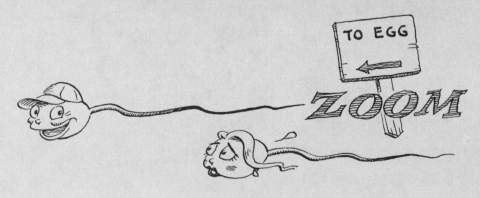

lining in the Fallopian tubes that contains small hairlike structures is sucking the egg downward at the same time, so the sperm, like Alaskan salmon, have to swim upstream. The thick-walled uterus, which is actually larger than a weight lifter's bicep, literally sucks on the penis and ultimately pulls the sperm into its chamber for fertilization. At that point, it's a dash to the finish to see which sperm cell can fertilize the egg first. But all sperm are not created equal. Like football players, some carry the ball and are supposed to score, while others block and tackle to allow the ball carrier to score. If one does, the fertilized egg reaches an area of the uterine wall (womb) where it gets implanted.

You'd think that with 300 million sperm entering the race, there'd always be one that makes it to shore, but infertility remains a major concern. While it affects only 7 percent of couples who are thirty years old, it affects 33 percent of forty-year-old couples and 87 percent of forty-five-year-old couples. That's because the journey isn't as simple as swimming a lap in a pool; it's more like crossing the English Channel without a wet suit—lots of things have to go right in order to get from one shoreline to the other. On the male side, two major things can cause infertility. Either a man's sperm count is low—meaning that without as many swimmers, there's a lower chance one will reach the finish. Or a man's sperm simply doesn't have the strength to make the entire journey (that's called a lack of sperm motility), and those cells die before they reach the Holy Grail. On the female side, women might have an infection that irritates the uterus so the eggs cannot attach to the lining, or maybe there's some type of chemical reaction that doesn't allow egg cells to mature well enough to be released by the ovaries. There could even be some kind of structural issue or blockage in the Fallopian tube that prevents the fertilized egg from traveling to its destination. Some women have fibroids—benign, spongy tissue that frequently distorts normal uterine or Fallopian tube anatomy;

> **FACTOID**
>
> In vitro fertilization takes place outside the parents. These are the cells that would be discarded to allow stem cell research (see more about stem cells in Chapter 10).

fibroids can grow to the size of grapefruit, and they can change the anatomy to make the uterus not as receptive to eggs. Stress—specifically, stress from not being able to get pregnant—makes conception even more difficult. While reducing stress, deep breathing, and other mechanisms we talk about can help, most infertility treatments are designed to make the sperm stronger or more plentiful, or to make the female swimming pool more hospitable, or to circumvent those blockages, like in vitro fertilization, in which the egg and sperm are harvested from humans so the fertilization can take place outside the body.

Your Sex Machine: The Live Younger Action Plan

Maintaining the health of your sex organs not only ensures your longevity but also helps support a rich and fulfilling life. Above all, the most important thing you can do is follow our guidelines throughout the book for decreasing arterial aging; a clear and well-flowing vascular system promotes blood flow to *every* part of your body. Maintaining good blood flow is one of the best ways to make sure erectile dysfunction isn't inevitable as you age. Of course, Viagra, a dozen roses, and picking up your socks every once in a while aren't the only things that may do wonders for your sex life. Just a few simple changes may be all that's needed to keep your sex organs in tip-top driving condition. So pull them in for a pit stop. We'll show you how to change your oil—and help keep your libidinal engines revved.

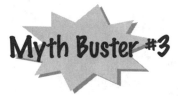

Myth Buster #3

Action 1: Have More (and More Thoughtful) Sex

The best prescription for your sexual organs isn't one you can find in a pharmacy. It's one you do in bed, in the shower, or on your weekend getaway. All the studies point to the fact that having sex makes you young. (By "having sex," we mean having stress-free sex, so that's safe sex, in which you're protected from STDs, and sex that doesn't induce stress, as an extramarital affair would.) What we know is that the more (for men) and higher-quality (for women) orgasms you have a year, the younger you are. If you are fifty-five years old, increasing the number of times you have sex from 58 times per year to 116 times has an effect of making you as much as 1.6 years younger, and having great-quality sex even more than that can have an effect up to 8 years (*Honey, let's get healthy!*). Though we don't know exactly how it works, it could be from relieving stress or by decreasing cardiovascular aging with frequent high-quality sex. Maybe just as important is the therapeutic value of sex, in that it promotes companionship and emotional satisfaction. It just *feels* good—on both physical and emotional levels. When you cuddle, you release the hormone oxytocin, which causes some of that feel-great feeling. Bonus: The data also imply that if a fifty-five-year-old has sex seven hundred times a year, it would make him or her sixteen years younger (unfortunately, the data sample on people who fit this criteria was approximately, uh, zero).

> **FACTOID**
>
> One episode of sex of twenty to thirty minutes can burn three hundred calories—the equivalent of running three miles. But the usual episode of two to six minutes uses only twenty-five calories (a quarter of a mile). If you cannot walk up and down two flights of stairs without stopping, it's a sign that you've got a problem that most likely will affect your sex life.

Of course, between seventy-hour workweeks and the fact that raising children is as draining as running a three-legged marathon, having time and energy for sex isn't always as easy as it sounds. Another complication: those rivaling libido levels.

When he wants it, she doesn't. Or vice versa. Luckily, there are ways to help improve your compatibility.

LINGER Men's orgasms are easy to understand—because they're external. But women's orgasms can be more mysterious than a Dean Koontz book. That's because many of us really don't understand what's happening physiologically. Essentially, when a woman is stimulated to the point of an orgasm, the uterine walls contract—and she can experience rhythmic, muscular contractions of the uterus, vagina, and clitoris. But every woman is different. For some, it may feel like a geyser. For others, it may feel like nothing more than a momentary flutter. But here's what many men have a hard time understanding: Because they can't imagine having sex without an orgasm, many men can't appreciate the fact that women can enjoy sex without having one.

So instead of trying to make the final destination a female orgasm, a man should concentrate on ensuring that his woman enjoys the interaction. Some women don't have to orgasm at all to enjoy sex, while some women can easily have multiple orgasms. Absence of an orgasm doesn't mean failure, but absence of arousal usually does. When you consider that the average man achieves orgasm in three to five minutes and the average women takes four times as long, you can also see why many women won't achieve orgasm in every sexual encounter. Add to that the pressure put on many women to have orgasms, and a sexual encounter can become more stressful than tax day. And that just about guarantees a woman won't have an orgasm.

It has been said that women fake orgasms because men fake foreplay. Therein lies one of the biggest problem between couples—lack of compatible levels of libido or arousal. To improve a woman's sexual desire, add more foreplay. Kiss, touch, hug, squeeze, nibble, stroke, brush, tickle, tease, add your own verb of choice. Whatever you do, just make sure you know this equation: Longer foreplay equals better lubrication, which equals more satisfaction.

To help add moisture, you can increase lubrication safely with water-soluble lubricants like K-Y jelly or lipid-soluble gels. And for some women, testosterone cream—applied directly to the clitoris twice a day—helps increase stimulation, libido, and intensity of orgasm. Testosterone is a driver of sexuality in both men and women. It naturally decreases as we age, and we'll discuss hormone therapies in depth in Chapter 11. But testosterone has been shown to be effective in men whose testosterone levels are judged as low. How do you know if you're in this category? Men should be concerned if they don't have to shave their beards once a day and women if they need to shave their legs less frequently (and not because of waxing).

FACTOID

About 85 percent of men and 60 percent of women aged fifty-seven to sixty-four report having had some sexual contact with another person in the last year, but the number dwindles to 38 percent and 17 percent, respectively, in people seventy-five or older. The reason for women is fewer partners. Among those sexually active in their seventies, about two-thirds had sex at least twice a month, and more than half continued that pace into their eighties. We have no data on unmarried centenarians.

EXPERIMENT Despite what the sex-toy industry might promise, there's no magic tool that can drive up desire instantaneously. Increasing a partner's desire takes experimentation, trust, communication, and a reasonable amount of risk taking. Some of the common problems that many women describe when they report a low sex drive include not feeling loved or the sense that sex has become routine or boring. Think of what your life would be like if you ate the same thing every day for breakfast, lunch, and dinner. Boring. You should approach your sex life with the same attitude. Add variety. Try new dishes. Sprinkle in some spice. Do whatever it takes to make your sexual palate satisfied (short of trying a new chef, if you're married). That includes trying new positions, initiating sex in different rooms of your house, or introducing some elements of fantasy into your bedroom.

Here's another way to amp things up: Schedule sex. Many people avoid scheduling sex because it seems as if it would be too forced and would remove the spontaneity that we assume all sex should include. Actually, planning sex can have the opposite effect. Knowing that you're scheduled for a rendezvous with your partner builds anticipation, promotes fantasy, drives up libido, and very often leads to a romp that's hotter than beach sand at noon.

GET SWEATY   Though sauna sex might sound enticing, we want you to sweat from exercise. Besides all of its other benefits, physical activity is also great on your sex life. Many species dictate desire through smells. For centuries, scientists have been looking for these chemicals and pheromones that increase sexual desire in women. Of all the things that have been tested, there's only been one that's been shown to increase female desire: male sweat (really). For men, there's perhaps an even more crucial reason to sweat. Men who burn at least 200 calories a day through exercise reduce the chance of impotence. Finally, since stress can be a contributor to erectile dysfunction and infertility, it's a great stress reducer. While you may not be able to alter the stresses in your life, you can at least alter your response to it through consistent physical activity.

STRIP   While body image can be a major obstacle in the sex lives of many couples, it's only when you become comfortable with your own body that you'll let others be comfortable with it. So get naked (go ahead, we'll wait). Now look in the mirror. Appreciate the body you have. You don't need to be a supermodel or an athlete to appreciate your body and be sexual.

Action 2: Use Your Mouth

Optimum sexual performance and health aren't just about the fruit in your looms; they're about the health of your whole body. Your brain and your arteries, for instance, play a major role in erectile and sexual dysfunction. So it stands to reason that you can improve the health of your sexual organs through many ingredients and nutrients, which, in terms of sexual conditioning, makes your pantry the second-most-important room in your house—because your stomach isn't the only organ that needs to feel satisfied. Our guide to the most important nutrients for your sexual health:

SELENIUM AND LYCOPENE Both have been shown to increase prostate health. Selenium is a mineral found largely in plant foods like garlic that absorb the element from the soil. In two studies in areas where there wasn't a lot of selenium in the soil (South Carolina and China), selenium supplementation of 200 micrograms a day decreased the risk of prostate (and other) cancers by 50 percent. The National Institutes of Health (NIH) is now looking into whether additional selenium helps people who already get some in their diet, because there's a risk of getting too much. Related research shows that the risk of developing prostate cancer is as much as 45 percent lower in

Myth or Fact? You're stuck with symptoms associated with PMS.

Every month women may experience hormonal changes that may make men want to declare permanent secession from the other gender, but that doesn't mean women have to be left with a Midol in one hand and a balled fist in the other. The cure is through fats—omega-9 and -3 types. Evening primrose and olive oil supplements provide the former (1,000 milligrams twice daily) and should be combined with a similar dose of flaxseed oil for the latter (one to two tablespoons of oil or ground mature seeds or twelve walnuts or two ounces of fish or three grams of fish oil or echium oil daily, or 600 mg of DHA supplements in two or three divided doses). Daily requirements of calcium (1,200 milligrams in two divided doses for people under sixty and 1,600 milligrams in three divided doses for those over sixty) have also been shown to decrease symptoms for women who experience PMS—and increase the happiness of the men who live with them.

men who frequently eat foods that contain cooked tomatoes, tomato sauce, tomato drinks, or tomato paste. For one, men who eat cooked tomato products ten or more times a week have a 35 to 45 percent reduction in severe forms of prostate cancer compared with men who eat tomato products fewer than two times a week. While the key ingredient may be something else, some believe the cancer fighter comes in the form of lycopene, a substance found in tomato products. But you can't just slice a few tomatoes into your salad to reap the effect; the tomato needs to be cooked in order to provide the most nutrients. Spaghetti sauce is actually the optimal food for lycopene; first of all, it's cooked, and second, for good absorption you need to consume a little fat with the lycopene, and tomato sauce contains that as well. To absorb the optimum amount (that is, 400 milligrams per week), you'd have to eat 164 raw tomatoes or 16 cooked ones—but you need only ten tablespoons of spaghetti sauce. Another bonus: Lycopene has been shown to reduce arterial aging. But pass on the meatballs. Saturated fat has been linked to the increase and growth of prostate-cancer cells.

VITAMINS, MINERALS, AND OMEGA-3S By now, you know the importance of working vitamins into your diet. It's no different for your sexual health. There are some data that show that vitamin E—especially mixed tocopherols—decreases the risk of prostate cancer. (But if you're taking a statin—and we know we're repeating, but it bears repeating—you shouldn't take more than 100 IU of mixed tocopherols or vitamin E because it inhibits the function of that statin by 40 percent.) For women, 800 IU of vitamin E has been shown to decrease the dryness of the vaginal wall to help with libido and arousal. Folate (800 micrograms a day) and the B vitamins in RDA amounts—as well as 3 daily grams of omega-3 fatty acids (in supplements, in DHA-fortified foods or pills, in twelve walnuts a day, or in thirteen ounces of nonfried fatty fish a week) and 15 milligrams of zinc—have been shown to help increase fertility as well by improving sperm mobility and by improving the hospitality of the uterus toward the implantation of the egg. Finally, good ole vitamin C also will increase sperm motility, which might prove useful, depending on whether you want more kids in your life.

SAW PALMETTO   The supplement saw palmetto has been shown to decrease the risk that benign prostatic hypertrophy will wake you up at night. But when you look for it, you need to check for ones with the ingredient beta sitosterol—the substance that's correlated with decreased swelling. Half of the saw palmetto products on the market don't contain any. Take 160 milligrams twice a day.

Men might also consider taking 2 grams of L-arginine, an amino acid found in pumpkin seed and other foods listed below, and 500 milligrams of L-citrulline twice a day. It's been rumored that taking these together (we wish the data were stronger than rumor) will increase nitric oxide production by the inner layer of your arteries, thus increasing blood flow, which can prevent erectile dysfunction as well as increase sperm count. These two twice a day just might (the data are not stronger than that) decrease all other forms of arterial aging, like heart disease, stroke, memory loss, peripheral vascular disease, and skin wrinkling. Foods high in these two substances: almonds, cocoa and real chocolate, garbanzo beans, peanuts, salmon, soy, and walnuts.

Action 3: Detect Intruders

As we explained in the introduction, this book gives you news you can use to live younger and better; we're going to avoid "see your doctor" advice the way skiers avoid trees. But when it comes to serious conditions that can affect your important sexual organs, you need regular checkups to detect the presence of viruses and other enemy invaders. So unless you have the schooling and the ability to bend like a paper clip, we don't think you can do these tests on your own. Men over fifty—or over forty, if there's a family history of prostate disease—need to have a prostate exam. It may be uncomfortable for just a moment, as the doctor inserts one well-lubed finger into the rectum (two, if he wants a second opinion) to feel the size of the prostate. But that check is the first sign of prostate trouble. And women need regular Pap smears and pelvic exams to detect the signs of HPV or the first signs of cervical cancer. We recommend one every year for most women, or every six months if you have a history of HPV or abnormal Pap smears.

Action 4: Don't Stop without a Second Opinion

Over 50 percent of all men and women have problems with erectile function, orgasm, or painful intercourse. Yet only 33 percent of men and 20 percent of women talk to any doctor about it, let alone consider a second opinion. It's too important not to seek professional help; don't be satisfied if the first doc doesn't help you solve the problem. More and higher quality are better in this game.

Chapter 9

Common Sense:
Your Sensory Organs

Hatrack

Cauliflower Ear

Inner Ear

Semicircular Canals
Center of Bala

Middle Ear

Eardru

Major Myths about the Sensory Organs

Sense Myth #1   Most eye conditions are dictated by genetics, not lifestyle.

Sense Myth #2   You should regularly clean your ears with Q-tips.

Sense Myth #3   The more you spend on making your skin look good, the more it will.

$9.95

ook out the window. You'll see kids playing, neighbors walking, Mr. Wonker pulling weeds in his boxers (again). Now look closer and notice the smiles, the flowers, and maybe more of Mr. Wonker than you ever wanted to see. Most of us take our windows—and the views we have from them—for granted, probably because we usually think about windows in terms of function. They let in light, they give us a fresh breeze, and they also let out not-so-fresh smells. But windows do something just as important as all of those things: They allow us a detailed view of the world's beauty. That's what your eyes—and all of your senses—do. They gather information from the outside world so that your brain can process it and decide what it wants to do with that information.

Some species survive on different senses (dogs on smell, bats on hearing, massage therapists on touch), but the sense that makes us most human is our eyesight. Roughly 80 percent of what our brains process comes from what we see. We may not always be feeling, smelling, or listening (many spouses can attest to that). But unless we're sleeping, meditating, or praying that the kicker makes the game-winning field goal, we're constantly processing information visually.

You may not know that the most active muscles in your body aren't the ones in your legs, back, or arms; they're the ones in your eyes. Your eyes have over 2 million working parts and the ability to process thirty-six thousand bits of information every hour (that's a lot of information; to put it into perspective, thirty-six thousand is about the number of people who fit in a sold-out Fenway Park in Boston). And they're always moving—even when they're not open (remember, REM sleep stands for rapid eye *movement*). That makes your eyes one of your body's most powerful tools. They're so powerful, in fact, that many cultures have used the eyes as symbols of power. There's the evil eye, which is described by many cultures as having such a mystical quality that you can inflict malice on someone through a gaze. There's the eye of a hurricane (while the *actual* eye of a hurricane is a relatively calm place, the most violent weather occurs right outside of it). And let's not forget the ultimate measurement of perfection for an archer or dart thrower—the bull's-eye. Still, your eyes aren't your body's only mechanism for processing information. Your whole sensory system is designed to work a little like windows—to pass along information to your brain. You hear a car horn to tell you not to merge left. You smell chocolate from the fudge store to trigger hunger. Your sense of touch advises you it's wise to step away from the cactus that's embedded in your arm.

The biggest difference between your sensory organs and other organs is that their malfunctioning doesn't have life-threatening implications—more like life-altering ones. If your heart or brain stops working, so do you. But we do understand that losing your senses would change many things about your life, and few people would volunteer to do so. In many ways, you do have a choice about maintaining their vitality, if you can take steps to protect your sensory organs from problems associated with aging. Your senses all act a little differently, so let's spin through your major sensory organs—your eyes, ears, skin, and pain receptors.

Your Senses: The Anatomy

Most of your other organs are related to function—they work so you can live. Your sensory organs do play functionary roles to protect you (you see a DON'T WALK sign, you smell smoke, you taste spoiled milk). And they're largely responsible for quality of life, so that you can enjoy such things as Tom Cruise movies, Shakespeare, grilled wasabi-crusted salmon, Gershwin, red-hot chili peppers (the food or the band), manicures, Saturday-morning sex. You love them because of how your sensory organs work—they allow you to marinate yourself in the experience by sending stimulatory signals to your brain.

Myth or Fact?
Your eyelashes are
mostly decorative.

They primarily protect your eyes against pollen and other items in the environment, but they also can sense when something is coming toward the eye, which gives you a microsecond to react—and close it. You grow new eyelashes every five weeks—and some medications actually make them grow.

Eyes

If you look at the evolutionary anatomy of eyes, you'll notice some major differences between humans and animals. For one, humans have their eyes set closer together than many other animals, which gives us wonderful depth perception. In exchange, we lose some of the great peripheral vision that protects cows. In a way, that makes us a species with blinders on—because we have binocular vision. The other interesting evolutionary element about our eyes is that little reddish-pink fleshy substance on the inside corner of your eye (it's called a caruncle, and this is an acceptable word in Scrabble). That's actually a remnant of the reptilian eye. Because reptiles have to see in fresh water (which can be irritating when it interacts with the salt in our bodies), a clear lid covers their eyes. Since humans don't need that flap to live in air, we lost it through evolution, and it became the remnant that we have today.

HOW THE EYE WORKS First, let's dissect your eyeball's anatomy. To give them their squishy shape, your eyeballs contain a lot of fluid. Without fluid, your eyeballs would collapse—almost like a beach ball without air. The fluid constantly circulates into and out of your eye and is filtered through a meshlike covering, like a window screen. Behind your eyeball, there's a lot of fat; that's what pushes your eyes forward.

To see, your eye essentially takes information from outside sources and passes it along to your brain. As you can see in Figure 9.1, information travels through the cornea, the clear covering of the eye, to the iris, which is the colored part of the eye charged with regulating the light that can hit the retina. Behind the iris sits the lens, which is shaped like a camera lens. This remarkable setup not only changes shape to

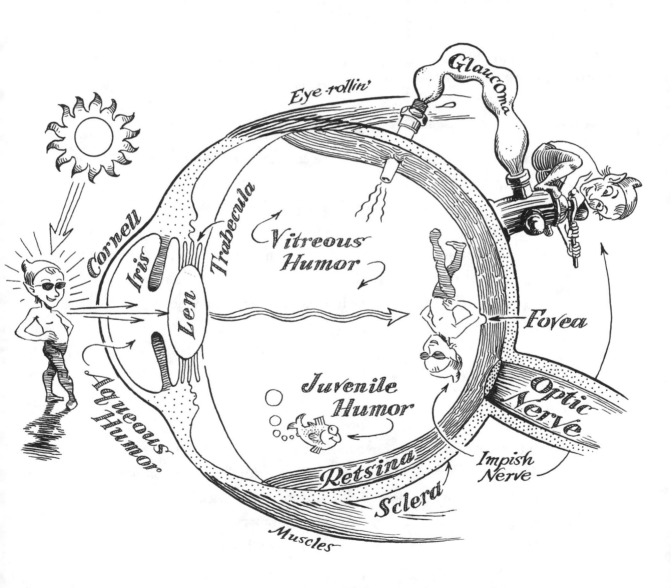

FIGURE 9.1 **You Have to See It to Believe It**   The resilient cornea protects the lens from getting scratched. The lens, which is prone to cataracts from sun exposure, projects a flipped version of what we really see onto our retina. In glaucoma, the trabecula that usually drains fluid from the eye can close, causing a buildup of fluid and pressure of that fluid that then damages the optic nerve. Fat bulging behind the eyes makes them seem more prominent and attractive.

focus light but filters out some parts of the light spectrum that may be harmful to the eye. The cornea and lens focus light to form an upside-down image on the back of the surface of the eye—your retina. Once it reaches the retina, it's then sent through the optic nerve and rotated another 180 degrees so your brain can determine what you're seeing right side up.

That's actually only one of the ways that animals refract light to see. Flies, for instance, have multiple solar plates on their corneas, and each one of them focuses light. That gives them a very fragmented view of the world; they don't see anything well, but they see everything panoramically. And that makes sense; flies don't need to focus on calculators and classified ads; they just need to see well enough to avoid a flyswatter or horse's tail. Spiders see like we do, but their systems work a little differently. They move their retinas to focus; if they want to see farther away, they push their retina closer, while the lens stays fixed. One of the key differences in animals is that hunters have binocular vision to focus on prey, while the hunted have peripheral vision to better locate potential predators.

What Can Go Wrong

Lots of things can make windows ineffective—they can break, they can fog up, they can be painted shut, they can come out on the losing end of a collision with a baseball. With your eyes, lots of things can tinker with the process of vision, too—some will fog them up and some will cause an all-out break. No matter what the cause of the problem, we usually think of the primary long-term effect of optical problems: blindness. Though Jose Feliciano shows his appreciation for his other senses, many of us still fear that losing sight would mean that you'd no longer be able to view the beauty in birds and beaches, in family and friends, in art and sports. So while you can certainly live without one of your senses, we also know that all of us would prefer to preserve our eyesight. As you age, these are the major things that can contribute to the decline in vision.

REFRACTIVE PROBLEMS It's said that Nero would look through an emerald to help focus on gladiator fights, and that's thought to have been one of the first inventions of eyeglasses. Simply, refractive problems like nearsightedness (when you can see only close things) or farsightedness (when you can see only faraway things)—stem from that process where light comes in. The normal eye is a perfect sphere, where the cornea and lens focus light to form the image on the retina. In nearsighted people, the eye is too long from front to back, so when the light travels through, it doesn't focus on the retina but on the middle of the eye. Now, your vision can change for several reasons. For instance, you may notice worse vision in the morning—but that could stem from dehydration of the cornea, not from true re-

fractive problems. Your eyes need to be well lubricated to focus; they stay lubricated through your three-layer tear supply and by blinking. With blinking (it's a process in which the upper lid moves but the lower one doesn't), your tear film is evenly distributed over the surface of the eye, particularly the cornea. (Winking does the same

> ### FACTOID
> You've heard of having a sixth sense, but you also may have a third eye. Eastern religions sometimes portray people with an eye in the middle of their forehead. Turns out, that's located in about the same spot as the pineal gland in your brain. That pineal gland actually senses light the way your eyes would. Some animals can change their skin color when they sense different light—even if their eyes are closed—because the pineal gland actually "sees" the light. In humans, the pineal gland may work the same way but through other mechanisms that sense light. (One interesting note: If you remove the pineal gland in rats, they then have an adversity to alcohol—and that may become a breakthrough that will help humans deal with addiction and control cravings.)

thing but has a side effect of increasing your risk of sexual harassment suits.) In either case, the movement of your eyelids has the effect of spraying Windex on your windows. Dry eyes are a little like dry mouths; you produce fewer tears as you get older. Keeping well hydrated by drinking water can help, but you may need to use artificial tears as well.

Eyeglasses were certainly the first wave of treatment methods for refractive problems. Though they don't *cure* vision problems, they address eye conditions in such a way to help you see a clearer picture. Nine out of ten people can improve their eyesight with a corrective form of treatment, like glasses (Ben Franklin invented the first bifocal). Later, contact lenses were developed. Essentially eyeglasses that you place on your eyeballs, contacts have evolved from large glass pieces that had to be removed with a small plunger to soft lenses that perfectly fit on the eyeball. New waves of contacts will become even more sophisticated—some lenses may detect levels of blood sugar, so diabetics will know when their blood sugar changes based on the color change of the lenses (yes, you would need a mirror).

Now, of course, we have many varieties of refractive surgery, like photorefractive keratectomy, Lasik, and others, which can permanently correct the refractory problem by reshaping the cornea back to perfect—so that the light focuses on the retina. Lasik has become a very fast and relatively precise process—one in which the eye is numbed, a corneal flap is lifted off the eye, then a computer calculates the amount of tissue that needs to be changed. Within seconds, light beams are sent to cut and reshape the cornea, which allows light to hit your cornea at a different angle so that your vision is improved. Of course, some people need corrective lenses at a young age, but eyes change with aging—even though the speed of that change varies, so some people never need glasses.

MACULAR DEGENERATION   As you know, the retina captures the light entering your eye. It changes the light energy into an electrical signal that travels along neurons to the brain area, where the signals are interpreted. You have two types of structures that capture the incoming light: rods control black-and-white images, and cones control color images. The center of the retina, called the macula, is the most active part of the eye and processes the light signals that allow us to do fine work like reading and recognizing facial detail and beauty.

The macula, which contains many cones but also some rods, can deteriorate as we age—making it the most common cause of age-related vision problems. This degeneration comes in two forms. One is the more common dry form. Although the exact cause is unknown, we know that those who smoke, haven't consumed many omega-3 fats (specifically DHA), and have high blood pressure are most affected. "Wet" macular degeneration occurs when abnormal blood vessels form under the retina. The vessels eventually leak blood elements and damage the retina. In some instances, laser treatment can improve or slow the progress of wet macular degeneration. We also know that multivitamins can delay or in some cases prevent early wet macular degeneration from becoming "eye blinding" in some people. We know that macular degeneration isn't as much of a genetic condition as it is one of lifestyle. So making lifestyle choices that keep your arteries young will reduce your chances of developing both forms of macular degeneration. Yes, genetics do play a role, but lifestyle can control those genes in most cases. Genes are a lot like the land on a three-acre piece of property; you can't do much to change the way the land looks and works. But you certainly have control over what kind of home you build on the property—and that's

Myth Buster #1

Myth or Fact?
Those spots you see floating around in your eyes are dangerous.

If you have enough of them, it seems as if you can see a planetarium in your line of vision. Though those little black dots can be disturbing the first time you notice them, they're actually harmless unless they're increasing in frequency. They're little specks that float around the vitreous fluid in your eye and are usually caused by some form of trauma (like a car accident), or through a lifetime of optical wear and tear—lifting, straining, and rubbing your eyes.

the way it is with lifestyle choices. It's also the case with cataracts and glaucoma; you can control how fast they develop and whether they'll cause you to lose your eyesight. With genetics, you've been given your piece of property, but that doesn't mean you can't make your own changes to it.

CATARACTS If you boil a pot of pasta by the kitchen window, the window's going to steam up so you can't see out of it. That's what cataracts do: cloud the lens of your eye to cause blurry vision. Many things, including UV light, cigarette smoke, and extra glucose in people with diabetes (things that accelerate arterial aging), can increase the risk of cataracts. And the clouding can get worse over time. Though cataracts don't really cause a total loss of vision, they can worsen to the point of making you legally blind (you're legally blind if you can't read the big letters on a vision chart from a distance of twenty feet). They can be removed and a synthetic lens implanted to correct the problem.

GLAUCOMA With glaucoma, the draining system of your eye clogs up (think of a bathtub drain being covered by hair). The fluid can't drain out, which creates a lot of pressure on the optic nerve, which leads to blindness. You can have either acute-angle glaucoma (which is a sudden problem with drainage) or wide-angle glaucoma (which is a more gradual, chronic problem). Think of the optic nerve as a fiber-optic cable bundle, containing more than a million fibers, like those used by phone and cable companies. As we age, a few of these fibers die. In people with glaucoma, these fibers drop out at a higher rate than normal, often because of high pressure in your eye. Since it is the pressure difference between arterial blood and fluid in your eye that matters, low blood pressure in the vessels serving your optic nerve, perhaps brought on by too much blood pressure medication, can starve these delicate fibers. That's one reason why so many people who have high blood pressure are also on glaucoma medication. When enough (about one-third) of these fibers die, we begin to lose parts of our visual field. As further fibers die, you become aware of loss of your side vision (probably by this point, over half of the nerve is gone). Eventually, with untreated glaucoma, all fibers die and you lose sight completely.

Finally, there's a theory that toxic substances you take in from the environment can lead to damage to the eye so that the blood can't reach the optic nerve. Smoking, for instance, can lead to a slow clogging of the drain that allows fluid to leave your eye—again, like hairs in a bathtub drain. This is a problem not deep in the plumbing but at the surface of the drain, which can accumulate over time. But with glaucoma, you probably won't notice early signs, because it affects more of the peripheral vi-

Looking In: Insight to the Eye

Most of us assume that our eyes are just for looking out. But just like windows, they can just as easily be used for looking in. Your eyes are actually a link to your brain—doctors can see representative brain cells in the optic nerve when they look into your eyes—making them a window into your brain. Thus, by doing so, doctors can usually detect diabetes, high blood pressure, and plaque in your arteries and can occasionally detect multiple sclerosis, brain tumors, stroke, leukemia, and many other conditions. That makes your eyes one of the best ways to have your brain personally audited for many bigger problems that can affect you down the road.

sion at first, rather than the center. Ophthalmologists can detect glaucoma early and treat it with a combination of eyedrops, laser, and occasionally surgery. Only regular eye examinations can diagnose glaucoma early enough for proper treatment. The better you take care of your general medical health, the better your chances of preserving vision if you develop glaucoma.

Ears

You're most familiar with the outer structures of your ears, and you know the many purposes they serve. They hold up glasses and provide a nice backdrop for gold earrings. They also let you hear the sweet sounds of Beethoven, the comforting words of a partner, and the activities of the newlyweds in the next hotel room. The outer fleshy part of the ear, in essence, serves as a funnel for sound. It directs and localizes sound (that's actually why we have two ears—so you can determine the direction from which the sound is coming). Once sound enters your ear canal, your brain can make decisions based on the sounds you've heard.

In order for you to hear, sound travels down an assembly line of structures—each with its own role in producing sound (see Figure 9.2). The outer ear contains your eardrum; its role is to convert sound waves into mechanical vibrations that vibrate the three bones attached to the inner

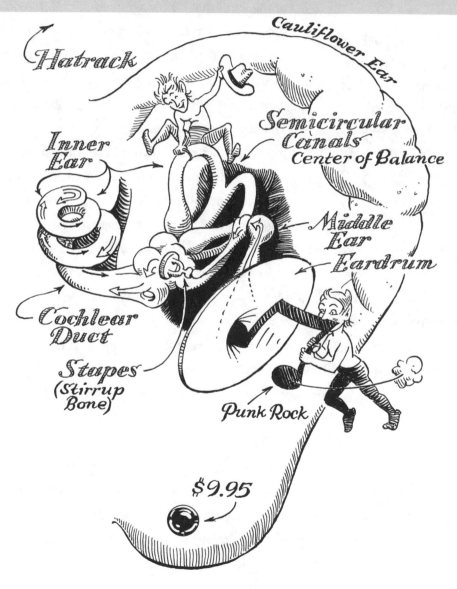

ear, which is filled with fluid and nerves. At that point, a sloshing motion is produced in the inner ear when the fluid is vibrated, moving tiny hair cells in the ear. The nerves recognize that final step as an electrical connection to send signals to the brain—and that's how we hear sound. If you have too much wax, it can block the sound waves from ever reaching the drums, which prevents the bones from moving, ultimately restricting your ability to hear. Essentially, your ear is taking sound waves—a form of mechanical energy—and converting them to electrical energy so your brain can understand it. That's right; our ears convert an analog world into a digital one. Your ability to hear also depends on the hairs on the cochlea. If your hair cells die, you suffer hearing loss—most likely because of loud noises or less blood supply. And you have two frequency ranges with which you usually hear sound. High-frequency ranges, which people lose first, help you hear things like leaves rustling and whispered consonants, while low-frequency ranges help you recognize speech.

About 60 percent of people over sixty-five will experience some loss, and 40 percent need some amplification (about 10 percent of male patients with hearing loss are referred to a doctor because their wives get annoyed their husbands don't hear what they're saying). The condition is so common that one of our colleagues says hearing loss doesn't run in families—it runs in humans.

The biggest threat to your hearing is LOUD NOISE. MUCH RESEARCH HAS SHOWN—sorry, didn't mean to shout . . . Much research has shown that being exposed to loud noises over a period of time can lead to significant and permanent hearing loss. Later in the chapter, we'll explain what some of those things are (remember, even the noise of snoring is about 85 decibels). Of course, hearing loss can

What Is a Decibel?

Your ear is one of your body's most sensitive organs, as it can hear even the softest of sounds—a fingertip brushing against skin, milk swishing in your mouth. More likely, though, it's exposed to the ever-present loud sounds in our world. To determine their strength—and the damage they can do—we use the decibel scale. On the scale, the smallest audible sound (near-total silence) is the baseline—0 decibels. A sound ten times more powerful is 10 decibels; a sound a hundred times more powerful is 20 decibels; a thousand times more powerful is 30 decibels; and so on (a jet engine is 1 trillion times more powerful). Any sound above 85 decibels can cause hearing loss (the trick: if you have to raise your voice to be heard by somebody else, the sound you're trying to talk over is more than 85 decibels). Eight hours of exposure to 90 decibels or more can cause damage, and any exposure to sounds over 140 causes immediate damage. Here's how some of the noises in your life stack up (all are ratings taken while standing near the sound; levels decrease with distance):

Near silence:	0 decibels
Whisper:	15 decibels
Normal conversation:	60 decibels
Snoring:	85 decibels
Lawn mower:	90 decibels
Car horn:	110 decibels
Rock concert or jet engine:	120 decibels
Gunshot or firecracker:	140 decibels

occur for other reasons as well. A relatively simple and treatable infection can develop if water gets trapped inside your ear (a common occurrence in children). Without quick treatment, it can lead to hearing loss.

As opposed to not hearing enough, some people experience chronic ringing in their ears—a condition called tinnitus. That's a disorder related to the function

Myth or Fact?
Music is bad for your ears.

Well, certainly loud music is. But in some cultures, music has a healing impact. Some cultures believe that music has vibratory energy that can have a therapeutic effect and change the way your body interacts with disease.

of the cochlea—a circular structure in your ear containing tiny hairs called cilia. When they are working correctly, sound outside your body hits the eardrum and vibrates the fluid inside the ear, which shakes the cilia. The cilia transform the sound wave into electrical energy so the cranial nerves can conduct the information to the brain. If the cilia are inefficient, your ears ring. Typically, people with tinnitus are more prone to hearing the ringing when they're by themselves because it's usually drowned out by all the buzzing and hissing around them when they're with others.

Next to the cochlea resides a vestibular labyrinth—three serial canals all on different axes from one another. They are responsible for rotational movement—specifically in terms of giving you the information about where you are in space. It's one of the four things that make up your balancing system (the other three are your vision, which helps correct balance problems; proprioception, which is responsible for telling you where your body parts are relative to space; and your cerebellum, which integrates all the other parts to give you balance). This is great redundancy, but if two of the four systems don't work, you'll live life as if you'd just finished your third bottle of wine—staggering, dizzy, and feeling all out of sorts. Balance problems increase as you age, and 70 percent of us experience some type of dizziness problems. In fact, more than 2 million Americans see a doctor because of dizziness every year.

Within your ear canal, glands secrete wax. We've figured out all kinds of beautification purposes for wax, like cleaning cars and stripping off back hair, but ear wax has a more important function. Acting like a Venus flytrap, ear wax traps dust and repels water that can enter and damage your ear—making it the perfect system for when man lived outdoors. After it traps foreign substances, the wax is

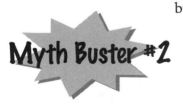

pushed to the outer area of the canal, where it dries up and is supposed to tumble out of your ear. One of the worst things you can do to your ears is use a Q-tip, fingernail, or fishhook to pull wax out of your ear. Anything you put in your ear acts as a ramrod and shoves the wax in deeper (not to mention risks puncturing your eardrum), which can hinder sound waves from making it to your main auditory processing center.

Skin

Just like the paint on your house, skin comes in many colors and is exposed to all of the elements of the world. While it seems as if the main purpose of skin these days is to sell girlie magazines, its primary purpose is to protect your insides. Though skin is literally only skin deep, it does offer many insights into the way our inner system works. Covering seventeen thousand square centimeters in the average person, your skin is your body's largest organ and, in fact, is more than just a physical body or armor. Skin also:

★ Protects against infections. Infections from the outside world travel to our inside world via three places—through our lungs, our intestines, and our skin. Since our skin has the most interface with the outside world, it has a protective quality to it; the top layer of skin is a dead layer, which acts as a shield against outside invaders.

★ Sends important signals to our brain. For example, if you burn yourself and it hurts, you're receiving the message to step away from the campfire (that's good). If it's painless, it means you may have killed the part of the skin with pain fibers. The effect? Not only wouldn't you get the message, but you also wouldn't be able to heal properly.

★ Helps us develop. Of all the senses that we can be deprived of during development, the one that causes the most damage if it's missing is touch (we know this from baboon studies, but it also appears to be true in humans). Take this a step further, and we know the importance that touch can have therapeutically—such as from massage used as a healing mechanism and even sexual touch for emotional well-being.

★ Helps us heal. That's what scabs do—they provide a layer of protection and moisture to allow skin to fuse together over the wound. (Picking a scab interrupts and slows down that healing process because the healing cells are pulled off when you peel off the scab.)

FACTOID

Contact dermatitis is associated with blisters, redness, and itching—but only at the site of exposure from a direct toxin or allergic reaction. You can figure out the trigger by doing your own detective work. Think about a recent change in soap, laundry detergent, new jewelry (could be caused by nickel in jewelry), new perfume. To diagnose the problem, remove the potential trigger and see if you're still affected (it's what the doctor will tell you to do, too). It's just another condition in which paying attention to your body—and how it reacts to the world around you—can let you be the world expert on your body.

To understand the skin, which is made by stem cells, you have to look at it like layers of coating on the outside of your house. You don't have just one coating of robin's-egg-blue paint; you probably have several layers, including the primer and a couple coats of paint. In your body, your skin is also divided into layers. The outer layer of your skin (as seen in Figure 9.3), called the epidermis, covers the layer called the dermis. The epidermis actually doesn't have any sensory fibers, so that's not the layer that feels pain; it's the dermis that has those fibers that make you react when

FIGURE 9.3 Let's Show Some Skin Skin senses pain with nerve endings in the dermis. Elastin fibers within the dermis work like rubber bands to keep our skin tight and young looking. Sun damage and arterial aging from things such as smoking destroy the elastin and eventually cause wrinkles. The sebaceous glands secrete lubricants to protect our skin and provide chemical messages to the world around us (some folks are attracted to your smell and others aren't). Sweat glands release fluid that evaporates to cool us during exertion.

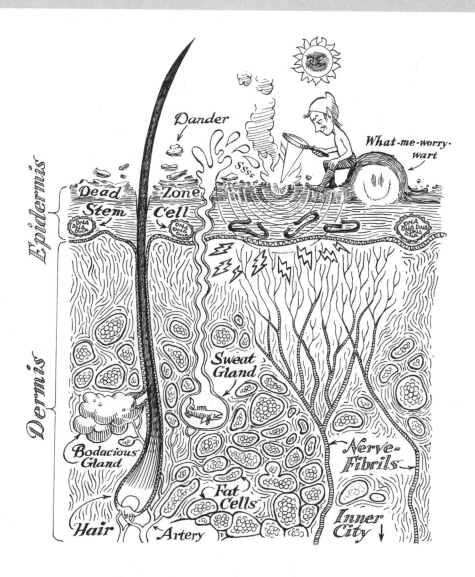

Myth or Fact?
Sweat stinks.

Whether it was in the high school locker room or on a subway in August, you've surely had to hang around people who sweat a lot. But the fact is, sweat doesn't smell. It's actually sterile, just as is urine (which gets contaminated only when it comes in contact with bacteria after being expelled). You actually have two types of sweat glands that produce stuff that looks and feels like sweat. Most of this secreted fluid serves a beneficial purpose by helping to flush toxins out of your body. It's only the apocrine sweat gland that secretes the odor—the smell that produces part of our identity, attracts mates, and makes you pick the treadmill at the other end of the gym. These glands are located in predictable locations—including armpits and around genitals.

your partner scratches your back. Underneath the dermis, there's subcutaneous tissue—such as hair follicles and glands that make solutions like sweat—making the skin the largest sensory organ in your body.

Though anything from cat claws to razor blades can disturb the structure of your skin, the greatest enemy, when exposed to it in large amounts, is the sun. We'll deal with skin cancer in a later chapter, but in terms of aging and appearance, most people associate aging skin with wrinkles—and wrinkles are caused by prolonged exposure to the sun. Ever seen a wrinkled butt? Probably not—that's because most buttocks never see the sun (thank goodness), so the unexposed skin stays baby smooth and baby young for a lot longer than more exposed parts of your body. What happens with wrinkling relates to the collagen fibers that lie below the dermis. Those fibers are like little rubber bands; when they're injured by the sun, they get stretched out. That causes scarring of the tissue, leaving the babylike skin to retract and form wrinkles (aging of your arteries denies nourishment to these rubber band–like fibers, producing the same effect as too much sun). Typically, it takes thirty years for sun damage to appear, so the damage you did in your twenties will start showing up in the form of wrinkles during your fifties. In fact, most of your skin damage will occur before the age of twenty, so get the kids to pay attention. If you're one of those people who spent adolescent summers in the sun without wearing sunblock, it's possible you'll end up with more wrinkles than a teenager's bed.

SENSING PAIN   Within your skin, you also have a very important mechanism dealing with the sense of touch—pain fibers. If you have ever crashed a bike or burned your hand on the stove, you know that your skin is directly connected to your pain receptors. But you also know that pain has more levels than the Mall of America. You can feel muscular pain, you can feel emotional pain, you can feel throbbing or stabbing pain, you can feel it in your back or your head, and you can ignore it or treat it. In our society, we typically think of pain as a negative thing, right? We don't like pain, and we want to live without it. While we do want you to live pain free, we also want you to realize that pain is a healthy thing. Pain is like your body's smoke detector—it's the mechanism in your body that alerts you that you could be experiencing something dangerous. While everyone knows that a house without a smoke detector is hazardous (in fact, not having one ages you by half a year), the same holds true for you. A body without pain has no warning signal that a potentially danger-

ous fire is brewing somewhere in your body. You have two kinds of neurofibers that deal with pain. One set carries messages that trigger a sense of dull pain or an annoying sensation (such as a cold room or a snake slithering up your leg); they move over slow-traveling pain fibers (C fibers for trivia fans). The other set works to convey pain quickly—such as the pain of being stabbed or punched.

Fifty percent of all visits to physicians are for pain. Nobody likes to live with pain of any type, and one of the most worrisome things about pain is its association with depression. Depression increases pain and sensitivity to pain, and it can become

> **FACTOID**
> Excessive sweating—a condition called hyperhidrosis, which affects 25 percent of Asians—comes from a malfunction of the sympathetic nerves that causes an inappropriate amount of sweat from your extremities. Though it can now be treated permanently with a minimally invasive thorocoscopic procedure that divides the culprit nerves, it's actually one of the reasons why many cultures don't shake hands but bow instead. If you have excessively sweaty armpits, Botox injections have been shown to help in 90 percent of people (for context: 36 percent also saw benefits from the placebo—saltwater injections).

Here's the Skinny

One of the first places we notice aging is in our skin. We see aging in wrinkles, in skin cancer, in liver spots. Generally, what's good for your inside is also good for your outside: protecting your skin with a 4 or more star UVA blocker and an SPF 45 on all exposed spots all the time and avoiding cigarettes (ten cigarettes a day can double facial lines). Many people also consider water an effective way to hydrate skin and keep it healthy. Though it's unproven in this realm, drinking water is worth doing for its many other benefits. Here are some of the common cosmetic skin problems associated with aging and some insight about treating or preventing them:

★ Liver spots: Fading creams that bleach can soften their color.
★ Eye bags: They're hereditary and caused by a collection of fat around your eyes. Lack of sleep and too much alcohol exaggerate the problem.
★ Fine lines. Fine wrinkles caused by frowning can be reduced with glycolic peels used over a period of several months.
★ Wrinkles, crow's-feet, facial lines: A number of cosmetic procedures including fat, collagen, and Botox injections have been show to reduce wrinkles and lines.

The bottom line in all this? There's no sense in worrying about every line or wrinkle; you'll only make those forehead furrows permanent if you frown about them.

a vicious cycle. The more pain, the more depressed you feel because you're unable to do the things you used to do; the more depressed you become, the more pain you feel. Thus, treating pain is important to keeping you living younger—and enjoying life. And while pain commonly comes from skin receptors, simply breaking the pain cycle with an analgesic does not correct the cause of the pain any more than applying paint to a ceiling fixes a leaky roof. So getting younger involves not just treating the pain sensation, which is very important so you can live in a house that looks and feels good, but finding and treating the real *cause* of your pain.

Your Senses: The Live Younger Action Plan

Part of living younger isn't just about making sure your arteries stay open and your lungs stay filled with air; it's also about *feeling* younger. Few things make you feel older than the decline of your senses—especially your hearing and sight. This action plan is about maintaining—and improving—your quality of life so you can continue to enjoy all of the wonderful sensations of the world.

Action 1: Practice Preservation

We live in a world that endorses preservation. Museums house artifacts from generations before us, mothballs (we don't approve) save sweaters, and you can keep canned beans in your pantry until the year 3072. You can preserve your body, too, with the proper care.

SKIN As you get older, your epidermis makes new cells more slowly, and sun damage thins living epidermis from twenty to two cells deep over time. One of the ways you can help make your skin younger is to trick your skin—to make it think it needs to produce new cells. Use glycolic alpha hydroxy acid (AHA), a substance found in many skin creams. It works by increasing skin turnover—that is, it irritates your epidermis, removing dead cells, causing your skin to think it needs to rejuvenate and produce new cells, which has the effect of making your skin look younger. But you don't need to spend a lot of money on

Myth Buster #3

expensive face creams to do it; any product that contains AHA will work; the expense of some products comes from other ingredients—not the ones that do the work. Remember the adage—feed your skin at night, and protect it during the daylight.

EYES   Long or intense exposure to sunlight is potentially harmful because certain wavelengths of light can damage the lens and retina. Skiing and water sports aren't dangerous just to your knees but also to your eyes because of both direct and reflected light. Glasses that filter out the "bad" light spectrum (ultraviolet A and B) are essential for those who frequently work or play outside. UVB rays are usually filtered through your cornea and windshield, but UVA rays are not—and exposure to those rays correlate with development of cataracts and macular degeneration. Check labeling to make sure your sunglasses block UVA rays (inexpensive glasses can block them), or invest in a visit to your optometrist or optician to have the UV protection in your glasses measured to make sure the coating is adequate to block out harmful rays.

EARS   We're going to whisper this one to you: Keep quiet. Nothing damages your ears more than loud noises (and maybe a pro boxer). Luckily, your ears are able to reset themselves, so the loudness has to be sustained all at one time in order for you to feel the effects of any damage. The scary thought is that anything over 85 decibels can lead to permanent hearing loss (to get a frame of reference, rustling leaves are 0 decibels and whispering is 15). At 90 decibels, a hair dryer or a lawn mower can cause damage after just two hours—which is nonthreatening for most of us (unless you have a big lawn or Rapunzel-esque hair). But it's very threatening for hairdressers and landscapers, who are exposed to those noises all the time. And the louder a noise gets, the less time it takes to inflict damage. A rock concert, at 120 decibels, can cause permanent hearing loss in forty-five minutes (but three minutes is considered the safe maximum for continuous 100-decibel noise). Avoiding loud noises or protecting your ears with plugs when exposed to them is the single best thing you can do to preserve your hearing.

TOUCH It used to be that people had this mind-set when it comes to pain: Deal with the pain, live with it, and maybe it'll eventually subside. But just because you have pain doesn't mean you have to suffer through it. In fact, it's imperative that you don't—that you find ways to remedy the pain. See, when you have pain, your pain receptors have heightened awareness—they expect pain, so the pain you feel spirals up. The more you live with it, the more you feel. It's almost like rewarding a toddler who whines by giving him what he wants. If you do, you're reinforcing that whining is okay, so he'll just whine more. If you tell your body it's okay to be in pain—by not doing anything about it—you're reinforcing the message that pain is okay. That's why it's imperative to reset your pain fibers and live pain free for at least six hours at a time. That way, the next pain you feel won't feel as severe as previous bouts. If you don't reset pain fibers, you risk the pain becoming permanent—especially in cases of chronic pain that lasts more than three weeks. Resetting your body is like putting new batteries in your smoke detector.

There are many therapies that help interrupt pain so your body can reset—such as ibuprofen and even creams made with capsaicin (the ingredient found in chili peppers; it binds with pain receptors to help manage chronic pain). Another option is acupuncture—the Eastern style of medicine that focuses on the concept of energy meridians that pass throughout your body. By focusing on specific areas of pain, acupuncture resets your pain thresholds and redirects pain through your body's pathways. If you do consider acupuncture, we urge you to see someone who is accredited and licensed. You can check with the American Academy of Medical Acupuncture at www.medicalacupuncture.org for a list of therapists in your area. Massage therapy can also be very effective for treating muscular and skeletal pain. To find a certified massage therapist in your area, check the American Massage Therapy Association at www.amtamassage.org.

Artificial Audio: How to Decide Whether You Need to Give Your Ears a Hand

As you get older, it's typical to expect some changes in your body. While your lifestyle choices can dictate how much or how little you sag, slump, or slow down, one of the most common changes understood over time is for your biological volume control to be turned down a few notches. And here's the thing: Most people think that hearing loss—which affects 16 million baby boomers—is as normal as a perfectly groomed TV anchor. So what's that mean for people suffering from it? They live in a cycle of complacency.

First, they accept life—with all of its beautiful melodies—as a garbled world that sounds more like a garbage disposal than anything else. Then they insist nothing's wrong, do nothing about it, and end up treating hearing loss with the same medical attention as they would treat a blister. Now they can't hear well, and the cumulative effect of missing conversations and shying away from people in general ends up having a huge impact on the strength of their social networks—all of which play a role in how well and how healthy they live. What started as missing a one-liner on *The Simpsons* spirals into a major disruption in life—and a deduction in the quality of it.

The truth is that you don't have to live with hearing loss. Even if your hearing has been damaged through years of exposure to high noise or through genetic means, the technology of artificial hearing devices has changed so much that they're truly life-changers for people who use them.

Now, what you choose to use depends on a couple factors—one of them being which part of your hearing system is damaged. If you remember back to the way we convert the analog world to the digital world (see page 268) you know that the hearing process requires sounds to vibrate against tiny hairs in the ear that are finer than phonograph needles. They're what transmit analog energy so that it can be converted to electrical energy through nerves to the brain. Hearing devices can help restore that broken system in a couple of ways. The options:

Hearing Aids: It used to be that hearing aids were simply amplifiers that you'd stick in your ear. Simply, they made all sounds louder. Fine in theory, but that doesn't help much if, say, you've lost the ability to hear high-frequency noises. In that case, the static you'd hear would become only louder static. Newfangled aids, which feature a device that goes behind the ear, with a small tube that travels inside the ear, get at the problem a different way. Inspired by spy technology that lets listeners pinpoint the person they want to eavesdrop on, new hearing aids are adjustable, so that you too can focus in on one person or one sound. That lets you weed out the muddle (say, background noise from a party or train station). For these aids to work, those hairs we just talked about still need to be intact. So if your hairs are excessively damaged, you'll need another auditory option, like cochlear implants (see below). Tip: Always buy a hearing aid from a company that allows you to return or exchange it within three months; that will give you enough time to fiddle and futz with it to make sure you can tune it to your own needs.

Cochlear Implants: Implants on a burlesque dancer may mean higher wages, but implants in your ear could change your life. Cochlear implants work differently than hearing aids; they actually allow sound to bypass those hairs and do the conversion to electrical energy themselves. Intended for people who have lost virtually all ability to hear, cochlear implants work by sending tiny electric impulses directly to the inner ear. The advantage is that they help users better determine where the sound is coming from, but they're still not so hot in allowing you to distinguish noise from desired sound (though technology will improve that over time). There is some thought that for people who suffer from excessive hearing loss, an audio cocktail of sorts—a combo of hearing aid and cochlear implant—can really improve sound quality and the ability to hear and decipher speech.

Action 2: Use Protection

It's the mantra used by high school health classes when talking to students about safe sex. For your purposes, it's all about having safe sun. In some ways, getting sun is very important. Getting ten to twenty minutes of sun exposure every day helps you convert some forms of inactive vitamin D into a precursor that becomes active vitamin D—which has a huge beneficial effect on your cardiovascular and immune systems. And that has a RealAge effect of making you more than two years younger. But you have to limit the time you're exposed to protect yourself from skin cancer as well as wrinkling. Doing both—getting the right amount of sunshine and not too much—can make you up to three years younger. If you're in a position where you're going to be exposed to a lot of sun, like working in an outdoor job or going on vacation, it's imperative to use sunblock to keep damaging UV rays from reaching your skin—especially between ten A.M. and four P.M., when the UV rays are most powerful and dangerous. Always use both a 4-star UVA blocker and SPF 45 or more (the 45 means that you get forty-five times the amount of protection against UVB rays that you would get if you wore no sunscreen at all). And you should use SPF 45 routinely (that means *every day*) on every exposed surface of your body—hands, face, neck—no matter what.

> ### FACTOID
>
> For computer fatigue, set the computer lower on the table or use a portable computer so your eyes look down when you work. That way, the opening between the lids stays small, which reduces the risk of developing dry eyes.

Action 3: Pamper Your Eyes

Your eyes do a lot for you. They help you enjoy scenic routes, admire Monet, and read gossip columns. It's payback time—time to thank your eyes for all the good things they've done. So we recommend you reward your eyes with this optical spa package.

DRINK WATER The tear ducts in your eyes aren't just active when you're cutting onion, watching Meg Ryan movies, and seeing the Cubs lose; as you know, they're also responsible for keeping your eyes lubricated. Dry eyes—a very common problem—result from an inadequate amount of fluid coming out of those ducts. The best treatment isn't to keep your eyes wet with another viewing of *Titanic*, but by drinking enough water throughout the day.

> ## FACTOID
> When it comes to your eyes, Popeye trumps Bugs Bunny. While good for your eyes, carrots aren't as powerful as spinach. Research shows that more protective benefits come from the lutein found in spinach than the beta-carotene found in carrots. That's what's up, doc.

SNOOZE As you know, sleep recharges your whole system—including your eyes. And it's the best answer for tired eyes. Sleep helps retinal membranes by allowing them to recharge from a hard day of seeing. You need at least five hours of sleep to help your eyes.

WALK AWAY If you sit in front of a computer screen all day, it's important to take a ten-minute break from it about every two hours. The light energy that comes from your screen can make your eyes ache. You can also help relieve some irritation by changing the flicker rate on your computer screen to seventy or above.

Action 4: Use Taste to Help Your Other Senses

Food isn't just to be enjoyed by your taste buds. Eating the right nutrients will benefit all of your sensory organs. These are the top nutrients for your sensory system.

LUTEIN It's a substance that's found in corn, spinach, and other leafy green vegetables, and it's been found to be one of the substances most beneficial for maintaining sight and improving the health of your eyes. We're not sure how many choices work to slow or reverse aging, just that they do—and lutein is one of the things that falls into that category. Some think it works by preventing oxidative damage to your retina, but we really don't know how it does its good deeds. You can also take it in supplement form—1,000 micrograms twice a day.

VITAMIN C AND BIOFLAVONOIDS   They've been shown to be helpful for your immune system, but they're also helpful for protecting against cataracts. See Chapter 10 for a list of the foods that contain powerful flavonoids. Many fruits and vegetables contain C and bioflavonoids, and there's evidence that eating a diverse diet that includes just four servings of fruit a day can make your RealAge as much as four years younger. Specifically, a recent study showed that people over age fifty who ate at least three servings of fruit a day were less likely to develop macular degeneration than those who ate one and a half servings.

DHA-OMEGA-3s   As we age, our fat cells in that third layer of skin thin out and get a little bumpier. That's part of what causes the raisin-like appearance of older skin. Somehow, the fatty acids (DHA specifically) in fish oil and salmon help make that layer a little thicker and smoother, so that wrinkles go away and the skin becomes fuller. (As always, you'll want to avoid saturated and trans fats because the heavy oils associated with them can promote acne.) Another reason DHA is so good: It helps your eyes. See, your retina is a very membranous structure, and

> ## FACTOID
> Stopping smoking will help not only your lungs but also your skin. Giving up cigarettes actually makes your skin younger, and it can prevent the wrinkles that even middle-aged smokers get around their mouths. When you smoke, it prevents the inner layer of your arteries from making the very short-lived chemical nitric oxide, which helps your skin retain its flexibility. So when you stop, the blood vessel lining is able to make and deliver the nitric oxide, which dilates and opens your arteries and allows your skin to regain flexibility, rather than retain wrinkles.

your whole eye is covered in a soft double layer of membranes (think two layers of cellophane with jelly in between). Because of that, your eye is very dependent on the liver because the liver helps metabolize fat-soluble vitamins that feed and maintain those membranes. If you're deficient in a substance called DHA (docosahexaenoic acid, the ultimate form of omega-3 fatty acid in humans), it can delay the conductor system that converts light energy to neural energy in the retina—a process that's faster than a computer chip. Take 600 milligrams of DHA a day in algae, pills, or fortified foods to help prevent macular degeneration. There's also some evidence to suggest that omega-3s can help improve dry eyes.

THE EYE COCKTAIL A large study sponsored by the National Eye Institute of the NIH found that certain vitamins—when taken together—can help prevent vision loss for those who actively have age-related macular degeneration (it wasn't studied to show preventive powers for those who don't have the disease, and it did not prevent dry macular degeneration from becoming wet macular degeneration). The study found that those people who already had wet macular degeneration had a more than 25 percent reduction in the risk of vision loss if they took (every day in divided doses) 500 milligrams of vitamin C, 400 IU of vitamin E, 15 milligrams of beta-carotene, 80 milligrams of zinc, and 2 milligrams of copper. The study is being repeated with lower doses of zinc and beta-carotene.

> **FACTOID**
>
> As hormones surge at puberty, acne becomes more of a problem because the extra oil generated by the skin leads to infections. Besides washing the face and using antiacne medications, your diet can have a major role in reducing acne. Eliminating oily (saturated and trans fat–laden, but not healthy fat) foods is important. Because of the lack of oily foods and saturated fats, the Owner's Manual Diet is a wonderful anti-acne diet as well.

Action 5: Test Yourself

We know you don't have expensive diagnostic tests at your disposal, but that doesn't mean you can't get some idea of how your senses are doing. Try these periodic self-tests to measure where you stand.

BALANCE TEST   Stand on one leg with your eyes closed (and hands to your side); have someone time you to see how long you can stand without having to put the second foot on the floor. If you're over forty-five, doing this for more than fifteen seconds is very good. If you can't, it can signal a loss of balance—something that will make you more vulnerable to accidents as you age. One way to improve your balance: Lift dumbbells instead of using weight machines. Having to balance the weight yourself forces you to work on motor skills that involve balance.

SIGHT TEST   Want a tip-off about whether you need to see an ophthalmologist or an optometrist? There are a couple of things you should look out for to determine if your eyes have been deteriorating:

★   If you experience eye fatigue quicker than usual when you're doing some activity that you normally do, whether it's working on the computer or reading the rest of this chapter

★   If your eyes get tired earlier in the day—say you can't read in bed anymore, though you used to read before you fell asleep

★   If it takes your eyes a little longer than normal to recover from bright lights you see at night (say, seven to ten seconds as opposed to three); this is especially evident when you're driving

HEARING TEST   You can do preliminary tests on your hearing by asking yourself a couple of questions:

★   Do others complain that you watch television with the volume too high?

★   Do you frequently ask others to repeat themselves?

★   Do you have difficulty understanding young children?

★   Are you unable to understand when someone talks to you from another room?

If you answer yes to these questions, you should have your hearing checked. You can also have someone whisper or rub his fingers together—first in one ear, then in the other. If you notice a difference between the levels, it's a sign that you could be experiencing some high-frequency hearing loss—the part that people lose first. If you do determine a difference, a doctor will want to see if it's being caused by excessive wax or fluid before determining it's some kind of age or noise-related loss. Considering that age-related hearing loss occurs in 25 percent of people between sixty-five and seventy-five and up to 80 percent of people over seventy-five, having your hearing checked can improve your quality of life. You can do a self-prescreening test on your hearing by calling 800-222-3277. You'll listen to and count a series of computerized tones; after the test, you'll be told whether your hearing meets normal standards or whether you should seek further testing.

Musician Quincy Jones says he feels decades younger now that he can hear again with the newest hearing-aid technology. Years of playing in bands hurt his ears, and he couldn't hear friends in clubs anymore, which made him feel old, especially as a musician. Restoring his hearing changed everything, so you shouldn't be bashful about seeing someone to have it checked.

EAR TEST   Look at your lobes. If you have a diagonal crease in your lobe, it's a sign that you might be experiencing arterial aging. In fact, it's one of the first signs of arterial aging, so follow our suggestions in Chapter 2 for things you can do to keep your arteries young. By the way, as long as you are examining your face, yellowish plaques of cholesterol deposits around the eyelids (xanthelasmas) are another warning sign.

PAIN TEST   Take a needle and close your eyes. Rotate the needle so you don't know which is the blunt side and which is the sharp. Now lightly prick yourself on the foot and see if you can tell which side is which. If you can't, it means you may have lost some of the fast sensory fibers, the slow fibers, or both. This deficiency means that you need to get yourself to the doctor to determine the underlying cause of such, reverse what can be reversed, and prevent further loss of pain sensation from occurring.

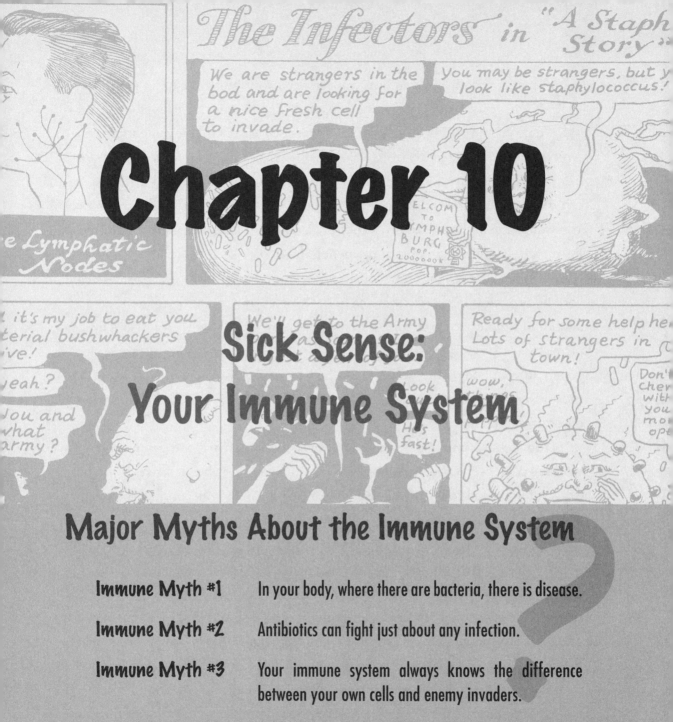

Chapter 10

Sick Sense: Your Immune System

Major Myths About the Immune System

Immune Myth #1   In your body, where there are bacteria, there is disease.

Immune Myth #2   Antibiotics can fight just about any infection.

Immune Myth #3   Your immune system always knows the difference between your own cells and enemy invaders.

Immune Myth #4   Once the symptoms of an infection fade, stopping antibiotics avoids complications.

Depending on where you live, you can keep your home secure in many ways. Some apartment buildings use doormen. Some houses have fences. Got a castle? One moat and an arrow-flinging army, please. Or you can choose other typical home-defense mechanisms, like deadbolts, electronic security systems, or a frothing pit bull named Rocco. No matter what your barrier method, there's a reason why you punch in a pass code, chain the door, or opt against neutering Rocco. You want a top-notch security system to protect all the valuables inside your home—from photo albums and stereo equipment to heirlooms and children.

All throughout your body, you also have your own security systems to defend your body against intruders. Skin and bones protect your internal organs in car accidents and from errant golf balls, hair protects your scalp from UV rays, and eyelids protect your eyeballs from finger-poking friends. But the most important security system in your body is the stealth one—the one that you can't see or feel but the one most responsible for protecting you from invading illnesses and for helping you recover from them.

You use your immune system every day, though you may not even know that it's working or how it works. Your immune response kicks in when it senses something evil lurking around your body, like bacteria or viruses. When you consider the fact that your hand alone may contain germs numbering 200 million (the U.S. population in the late 1960s), it's likely that your body is infected with bacteria right now, and the cells in your immune system are currently working their little fannies off to fight them.

Perhaps the reason why immune diseases are so complicated is that there are such a wide range of things that can cause infections in our bodies, so many ways our bodies respond to them, and such difficulty figuring out how to beat them. While it's easy to know when to stitch a cut or place a cast to stabilize a broken bone, immune problems have a wide range of solutions (medications work for some and not for others, for example). And that makes your immune system one of the more complex ones in your body.

As an example, let's look at a common form of bacteria—staphylococcus, a quick-growing bacteria that causes pimples. You can also follow along in Figures 10.1 and 10.2.

Your body's cells are a little like your taste buds in that they know exactly what they like and what they don't. When it encounters staphylococcus, your body recognizes it as a foreign substance, just as a guard would notice an unwanted intruder on a surveillance camera. When your body spots the intruder, a type of white blood cell—called a macrophage—finds the bacteria, engulfs it, and digests it, sort of like the way the security guard would stop and question that intruder. At that point, the macrophage gets on its walkie-talkie and calls for backup. The message—the chemical equivalent of *"Help! Help! Intruder! Pimple forming on tip of nose! Prom's tomorrow night!"*—is an SOS to other cells so they'll immediately respond to the area by traveling through the bloodstream (that's why skin beneath a scab is red—it's made up of the additional blood supply).

At the same time, the macrophage takes down information about the foreign cells so that the immune system can recognize it. Essentially, that information is what puts the bacteria on your body's Most Wanted List, as the macrophages let other cells know what to attack. As all of this information is being relayed, the backup immune cells are starting to arrive on the scene of the infection. They'll look for the code—the mug shot—to identify and obliterate harmful bacteria. As you can see in Figure 10.2, the immune cells attack in different ways. The T cells directly at-

FIGURES 10.1 AND 10.2 (FOLLOWING SPREAD) **In Sickness and in Health**
An invader into the body is ingested and processed by macrophages that send chemical messages (cytokines) that attract other white blood cells. (The cytokines can sometimes also cause fever, headache, and muscle pain.) Responding white cells attach to the macrophage so they can learn more about the invaders and develop specialized defense mechanisms—in the form of calling T cells and B cells to the area. The T cells directly kill the invader or help coordinate the immune response. The B cells create antibodies that act like bullets to destroy the invaders. When done, the excess white blood cells kill themselves (apoptosis) so that they won't kill our own healthy cells by mistake and cause an autoimmune disease.

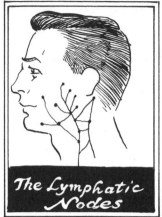

The Lymphatic Nodes

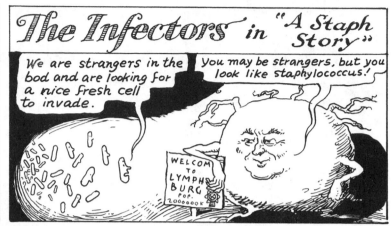

The Infectors in "A Staph Story"

We are strangers in the bod and are looking for a nice fresh cell to invade.

You may be strangers, but you look like staphylococcus!

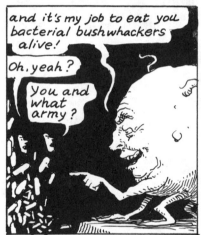

and it's my job to eat you bacterial bushwhackers alive!

Oh, yeah?

You and what army?

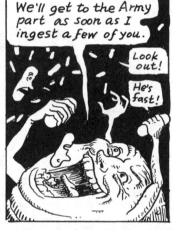

We'll get to the Army part as soon as I ingest a few of you.

Look out!

He's fast!

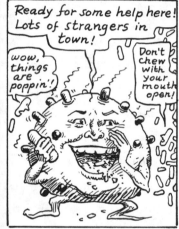

Ready for some help here! Lots of strangers in town!

wow, things are poppin'!

Don't chew with your mouth open!

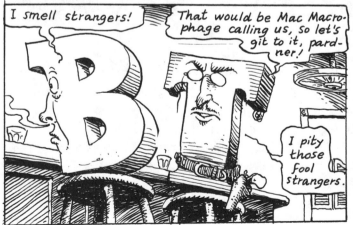

I smell strangers!

That would be Mac Macrophage calling us, so let's git to it, pardner!

I pity those fool strangers.

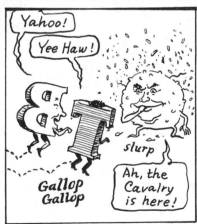

Yahoo!

Yee Haw!

Gallop Gallop

slurp

Ah, the Cavalry is here!

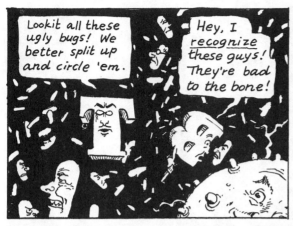
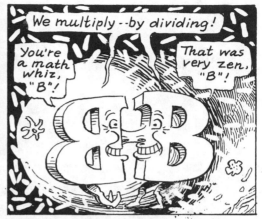
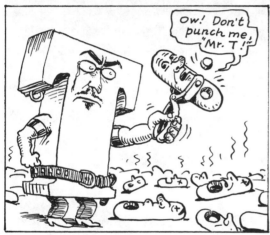
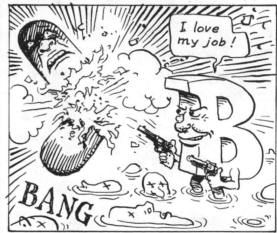
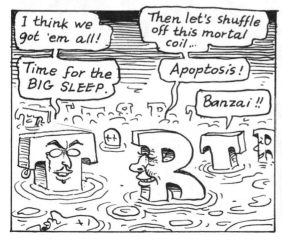
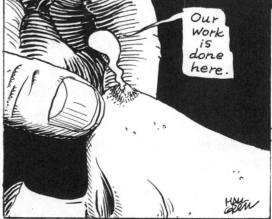

Sick Sense: Your Immune System ★ 293

Myth or Fact?
Popping your pimple speeds healing.

Popping pimples can be dangerous, but if done correctly, it can save you pain (and maybe some embarrassment). Self-grooming is common among all primates, including humans. But squeezing your pimples with your fingers damages the skin around the pimple and can worsen its appearance. Instead, sterilize a needle with alcohol or boiling water and literally pop the white head at the top of the pimple until the pus drains out. Here's how: Lance the pimple at the top by putting the needle parallel to your skin. Insert it on one end of the top of the pimple, and slide it through to the other end. Then pull away the top. It'll drain freely and won't hurt because it's dead skin. Warning: Do not attempt if you've had tremors (or more than one martini). Don't dig at it, either; besides hurting, it'll make it look worse. Also, avoid popping pimples above your nose since the surrounding veins drain directly into the brain and you can push bacteria inside if you squeeze down. If pimples in that area persist, get professional help. By the way, popping one appropriately does speed healing.

tack and digest the offending bacteria, while the B cells create immunoglobulins that act like bullets and blast through the covering of the bacteria.

Finally, that battle leaves the bacteria dead, but it also kills the T and B cells, leaving a pool of waste behind (it's called apoptosis—the T and B cells self-destruct so they don't destroy healthy cells). This pool of waste builds up pressure under the skin, creating redness from new blood supply lines coming to battle and pus from the white blood cells responding to the scene. Like a volcano, the waste material rises to the surface to form the pimple.

That's how the immune system is supposed to work, but it doesn't always run as smoothly as that. Just as there are different threats to your home—from neighborhood egg throwers to silver-seeking burglars—there are different levels of immunity threats to your body, as well as different ways your security system reacts to those threats. And your immune system seems to be less effective as you get older if you do not take care of it. As you age, your ID system becomes full, and some of the older information gets deleted so that you have space for information on recent intruders. Your B cells also slow down or malfunction, leaving you less powerful to fight bacteria as you age. Another obstacle: There are also crooked cops in your immune system—cells that go out and destroy good cells, rather than the bad ones.

Before we explain the ways that you can upgrade your own security system, let's take a closer look at how this intricate department of defense really works.

Your Immunity: The Anatomy

Besides cheese Danish and Marlboros, millions of other wannabe invaders threaten the health of your internal organs. Since you can't fight an enemy you don't know anything about, here's the backfile on the way your immune system is supposed to work, as well as the ways it can malfunction.

The Response Centers

There are usually only a few ways into and out of your house (doors, windows), and the same holds true for your body. Invaders like viruses and bacteria can break through the typical entranceways, like the mouth, nose, genitals, and, of course, skin. And just as burglars can snoop anywhere in the house, viruses and bacteria can go anywhere they want. Your security system, however, has only a couple locations in your house—the control panel on the wall, for instance, which provides the main communication with the entire system. In your body, your immune response system is housed in a few key areas.

THYMUS   It may sound like the name of a mythological Greek god, but the thymus plays a crucial role in your immune system because this is where your T cells mature. T cells are those helper cells that come in and add reinforcements to the initial emergency call. Some convince other cells to enter the fray and spread the news of battle. Some directly destroy the intruders and are aptly named natural killer cells. When you were a child, your thymus, which is located in front of your heart, was actually the size of your heart. (In fact, it was so big that when doctors do heart surgery on children, they have to fight through the thymus just to find the heart.) In adults, the thymus is much smaller—it actually shrinks dramatically as you age, until it is barely noticeable in eighty-year-olds. Presumably, this shrinkage is because you need a stronger immune response as a child, because you haven't yet been exposed to many of the viruses and bacteria that can make you sick. As you get older, you have more exposure and thus more resistance. There is some speculation that smaller thymus size can also mean that you're more prone to immune-related disorders that feature bacteria and viruses that your body doesn't recognize.

BONE MARROW   It would be unwise to house all of our protector cells in one area, so the bone marrow—the inner portion of the bone throughout the body—produces the young generations of immune cells that go to battle. In particular, the B cells respond to infections by creating antibodies—the small molecules that ram themselves into the side of bacteria and virus-infected cells. Once their protective shields are broken, these cells burst like swollen balloons. Small protein bullets called immunoglobulins work under the direction of white blood cells to hook up to infected cells and kill them.

SPLEEN   Chances are that the only time you've ever heard a spleen mentioned is when George Clooney said someone needed one removed on *ER*. But the spleen, a fundamentally important immune organ, is the coffee shop of your body—it's where all the T cells get together to talk to one another. In a sense, it's a hub of immunity, where blood flows and information can be exchanged about infections that need to be fought. You most often hear of a spleen needing to be removed because it may have been injured in a car accident, but taking one out reduces the ability of T cells to communicate, which makes you more prone to some types of infection.

LYMPHATIC SYSTEM   From your first sore throat, you were well aware of your lymph system—when your mom or doctor would feel under your jaw. That's because they were looking for swollen lymph nodes. Your lymph system is where all the immune activity takes place. It's like an old paddy wagon—it hauls off all the waste material (the bad guys) from the infection and drains it from your system. Now, the lymph system has hubs, or precincts, throughout your body—under your jaw, in your armpits, in your groin, and in many other places. So if you infect a fingernail, for instance (stop biting them, would ya?), the closest hub—say, in the elbow—swells with white blood cells. One by one, they figure out where the infection is and go out to fight it. Then the leftover remnants of the infection flow into the lymph drainage system and are broken down, and the useful parts are recycled.

The Threats

You already know a lot of things that your body welcomes—water, vitamins, daily foot massages. And you're surely familiar with some of the things most destructive to your body—cocaine, tanning beds, and bacon-and-sausage sandwiches. But there's a whole family of invisible threats to your body that are out to make your life miserable, or worse.

BACTERIA   Though their reputations are worse than those of crooked politicians, bacteria are a necessary part of our lives. In fact, we can't live without bacteria—they help us digest food; they add nutrients to our food choices

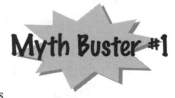

before we even eat them; and good bacteria help keep the bad bacteria out. And bacteria grown at pharmaceutical companies have been trained to help make many substances, like beer, and useful drugs, like human growth hormone. But just as with breakfast cereals, as many bad kinds as good kinds are out there. Bacteria, which are single-cell organisms, are neither plants nor animals. They're actually prehistoric organisms that lack the subtle architecture of human cells—namely, they don't even have a nucleus (the brain of our cells). In terms of size, about a thousand bacteria fit into 1 millimeter—about the thickness of a dime. Bacteria have the ability to replicate themselves—and that replication is what causes an infection. The result, like pimples or strep throat, can be treated with antibiotics designed to kill the bacteria (a throat culture or rapid diagnostic test can often determine whether a sore throat is caused by a bacteria or a virus). Bacterial infections can also be sexually transmitted, as in the case of chlamydia—one of the most common bacterial infections, which actually has no symptoms in 75 percent of people who have it. Any bacterial infection left untreated or undertreated, even if you have no symptoms, can cause chronic inflammation as our body aggressively responds—and that promotes aging of your arteries and your immune system. The other worry with many of these kinds of infections is that, if left untreated, they can wear down your immune system and cause more permanent damage to your organs. Uncontrolled strep infections, for example, can lead to abscesses in the tonsils and associated breathing problems, as well as cause long-term damage to the heart and kidneys.

VIRUS Many people distinguish between bacteria and viruses by treatment: bacteria respond to treatment with antibiotics; viruses don't. But that's not entirely true—there are many antiviral medications for AIDS. The main differences between the two types of organism have to do with their structure, size, and function. Bacteria are complex cells that have the ability to replicate themselves; viruses are about a hundred times times smaller, much simpler on a cellular level, and without the tools to replicate themselves. Viruses, which can be transmitted by hand-to-hand or mouth-to-mouth contact (the common cold) as well as sexually (HIV), need you to replicate. A virus works by invading one of your cells and hijacking it—essentially taking over its genetic code. When the virus uses the good cell's replication machinery, it's like the virus has gone to Kinko's and made millions of copies to send all throughout your bloodstream (the so-called e-mail viruses have been thus named because of this property—some are able to send a message to all your friends in your address book).

The most common virus is the one that causes the common cold, which is actually caused by several different families of viruses. Even though you may experience upper-respiratory symptoms associated with a bacterial infection, most cases of the common cold are not caused by bacteria—making antibiotics useless against the fight. If the illness

Myth Buster #2

persists, you might have attracted bacteria secondarily as a result of the virus weakening you; the typical sign of a secondary bacterial infection is producing unusually thick, colored mucus or sputum from your nose or throat when you cough or blow your nose. The vast majority of viral cold infections do run their course and exit your body via the portholes most associated with blowing, sneezing, and coughing. Antibiotics—when taken for viral infection—can actually have a negative effect by killing only the susceptible bacteria and allowing the more dangerous resistant strains to gain a stronger foothold. This reinforces the point that you should stop pestering your doctor for antibiotics if you're told that your condition is a virus. While it may have some sort of placebo effect, it's actually not helping you—and may even harm you, unless you actually have a bacterial infection on top of your viral one.

The flu virus, like a high school friend who wants to crash on your couch, makes your life miserable for a few days and then hightails it out of there. Others, like mononucleosis, which makes you extremely tired, take a little longer to run their course. Still others, like the herpesvirus, figure out a way to survive and be quiet within the body but then flare up occasionally (cold sores come and go). Even stranger: shingles. Even though you may have had chicken pox as a child, this virus (it's the same one) can affect a nerve root in your spine many years later to cause the intense pain associated with this weird ailment. Get the vaccine if you're over fifty.

Other infections change the way you live. The Epstein-Barr virus, for example, attacks your liver and causes infectious mononucleosis with a spleen swollen with immune cells ready for battle. One of the weaknesses of viruses is that in order for a virus to invade a cell, it needs some mode of transportation—it needs a chemical transporter to take it there. The latest therapies for viruses focus on blocking the transporter so the virus can't get into the cells. It's one of the reasons why Magic Johnson has lived so long with HIV but has not developed AIDS—congenitally, he's missing one of the receptors that would normally help the virus to invade his cells.

OTHERS Two other organisms that challenge your immune system are parasites and fungi. Parasites need another organism to live off of, so they require something from you to survive and to replicate themselves. In the case of tapeworm, it lives in your intestine—and can grow up to twenty-two feet long (about the height of a two-story building). Parasites are most common in unsanitary food and poor water supplies and are responsible for 4 billion cases of diarrhea around the world every year—bad news for everyone (except maybe Charmin). Fungi, which are about a hundred times bigger than bacteria, are actually primitive vegetables; they're small plants without chlorophyll that can't make their own food but can get it from other organisms, like your toenails. Some fungi we eat, like mushrooms and the yeast in bread. And since their natural enemies are the bacteria, they naturally produce antibiotics such as penicillin that we can take to protect ourselves. But some

Is It Strep?

If a sore throat is caused by a virus, you don't treat with antibiotics. If it's strep throat, then the bacterial infection can be treated with medicine. We used to tell the difference by looking down your throat. If there was white pus on the tonsils, it indicated a bacterial infection. But we now know that some viruses can produce pus and some bacterial infections do not. While a strep test will tell you for sure, you don't want to run to the doctor every time your throat feels like a matchbook. The measure some docs use: If your sore throat doesn't feel better within forty-eight hours, it's worth getting a diagnostic test to rule out a bacterial infection. To relieve symptoms, gargle with salt water. The salt can kill bacteria and numb the throat so you won't feel as much pain.

can also cause ailments like athlete's foot and vaginal infections, both of which can be treated with medication that kills or renders weak the infection-causing fungus.

The Malfunctions

Let's go back to the security guard questioning a possible intruder. In many cases, the guard can recognize someone suspicious (nylons over the head is a dead giveaway). But let's say an intruder is disguised as a delivery person or claims he's just visiting an aunt; then it takes a lot more skill and investigation to determine whether that person is a threat or not. That's one of the ways your immune system can go haywire—by not recognizing a potential threat. When you're immunized against mumps early in your life, your body actually gets the information about what the mumps virus look like. Your immune system then stores that info in its memory data bank; later, if you are ever exposed to mumps, your body will pull out the file on mumps, immediately recognize those cells as intruders, and send out the right defense in order to thwart an attack—without your ever having to be affected at all.

Now, when your immune system doesn't know what a potential intruder looks

Where Does It All Stem From?

One of the hottest political issues of the last few years has revolved around stem cell research. Stem cells are the initial cells from which all other cells can be made—they have multiple potentials: A stem cell can turn into a heart cell or a brain cell or a blood cell. But stem cells are more than a political issue; they're an aging issue as well. If you lose your normal tissue, adult stem cells (cells that can regenerate new heart or skin that persist in your heart or skin when you are an adult) living in your tissue come to the rescue and rebuild the damaged areas. Now, as you use up those precious cells, you lose the ability to repair tissue. The fact is that you lose adult stem cells as you age (which is why, in fact, there's so much attention put on getting them from embryonic sources)—meaning you're at more risk for age-related diseases. Though we don't know all the reasons why we lose them, we do know that some toxins like chemotherapy and radiation can damage your stem cells. So what do you do? Well, it's still early to know definitively all you can do to preserve your own stem cells. We know that meditation, physical activity, and DHA seem to preserve stem cells. And we hope (and believe) that if you take the steps that we've outlined in this book, you're taking steps to preserve those stem cells as well.

When damage has already occurred, receiving appropriate stem cell therapies could prime the pump of recovery of function. The moral dilemma is where to get the stem cells from, since the best sources today are from unused in vitro fertilized eggs that the biologic parents can no longer use. Deciding when life begins is a very personal issue, but many scientists appreciate the potential benefits of continued exploration in this field.

like, you have problems. If your body has no data on file—no record of criminal activity of sorts—your immune system has no ability to respond to that particular intruder. And as your immune system ages, it loses files. In the case of a typical flu virus, your body knows parts of it (it mutates every year, it seems, so you know only a part of the newer strain unless you've received a current flu vaccination) and is able to fight it off.

But when a virus is new—as in the case of the SARS virus—it doesn't display the same markers indicating that it is foreign to your body. Without that prior file, your immune system doesn't respond as quickly; the virus is then free to rummage through your things and destroy whatever it chooses: part of your nervous system, respiratory system, or something else. We feel the effects of the invaders when they produce toxins or when we produce substances that try to kill the offending agent. Those toxins or substances cause fever, chills, and aches. Fevers sometimes are good, because they're very dangerous to invading cells but not to your resilient cells.

Even worse is when a portion of the bacteria or virus looks just a *little* different from something else in your body—say, heart cells. Your body may kill the invader but may also initiate an attack on the normal tissues of your body that simply look like the invader cells—that is, your own immune system may actually start attacking your own body and destroy your own heart cells. This dangerous friendly fire is called an autoimmune response. So not only will it kill the foreign substance, but it will also kill the cells you need to function properly. In worst cases, that can lead to organ failure, but it can also lead to other autoimmune diseases such as lupus, inflammatory bowel syndrome, and rheumatoid arthritis. (By the way, an allergy is just an immune response to something like dust or detergent that you don't want an immune response to—it's like when your security system signals the fire department because the toast is burning.)

Myth Buster #3

The last important thing that can go wrong is actually fighting *too much*—or overreacting to an infection. In order to build the best immune response, it's as important to be able to shut it off as it is to turn it on. Why? Think about our security guard again. Let's say he sees an intruder at the front entrance and calls for backup. What happens if the whole department comes out to handcuff the intruder? Right—there's nobody left at the precinct to handle a problem at another house.

Your Immunity: The Live Younger Action Plan

No doubt, your apartment building has rules—no pets, no loud music, and no jumping into the pool from the third-floor balcony. Maybe your neighborhood does, too—no solicitation, no high fences, no plastic flamingos. Certainly, we live in a world where government is crucial to establishing order within a society—whether it's as big as a country or as small as a household. But when it comes to the things that threaten your body, bacteria and virus don't believe in rules. They believe in anarchy. They believe in rioting through your organs and creating chaos, only to leave your body in a pile of rubble.

The scoundrels need to be stopped. It's true that your body has an elite way of fighting attackers. In some ways, you need to trust your body to take care of you. But that doesn't mean you have to sit back and do nothing. In fact, it's up to you to call your anatomical city council meeting to order and establish some system of immunological government. When it comes down to it, you've got the power to establish some repercussions for the viruses and bacteria that think they can come over and play in your neighborhood. These are the ways to bolster your defense system:

Action 1: Trust Mom

Though you may not be able to tell by the fat-laden meat loaf she makes, your mom wants to keep you healthy. Let's face it: though she may have been wrong about rock music, she got things right a lot of times. These are her best prescriptions for staying germ-free.

"TIMMY, WASH YOUR HANDS!" Bribes, high fives, and love notes aren't the only things that pass from hand to hand. Germs do, too. In fact, they travel through your hands like a Ping-Pong ball. They're constantly being passed from one person to another through shaking hands and touching objects that other people have touched. It's the most common way infections can be passed—you touch someone or something, then your hand touches your mouth, nose, or eye. Now, we're not suggesting you lock your hands inside your pockets and never touch a thing (a definite downer on your anniversary).

Stop a second and think about how many things you touch that other people have touched immediately before you—sink faucets, door handles, gas pumps, money machines, other people's hands. The best thing you can do to prevent spreading (and receiving) germs is to wash your hands regularly. Discovered in the 1840s by an Austrian doctor who found that bacterial infections decreased with hand washing, the habit we take for granted is actually one of the most powerful things you can do to protect yourself from viruses, fungi, and bacteria. Soap and water will separate bacteria from your hand and keep it from entering your system the next time you touch your mouth or nose. For those times when sinks are hard to come by, it's a good idea to keep some antibacterial gel in your car, purse, or briefcase. Rub in a dime-size squirt to kill bacteria. While we want you to stay healthy, we also don't want you to be paranoid or antisocial when it comes to fighting off germs. Just don't limit yourself to washing hands before meals and after using the bathroom. The more you keep your hands clean, the more you'll be rewarding your immune cells with well-earned vacation time.

"TAMMY, DON'T DRINK THAT!"   Mom never liked it much when you'd stick your mouth in streams, under spigots, or on the park water fountain. She wanted you to drink the pure stuff. While it's easy to tell you not to drink lake water, we also want you to rethink your use of tap water. A lot of people can get low-grade infections from bacteria in local water supplies—and that can lead to such symptoms as bloatedness, itchy eyes, stomach cramping, and fatigue. And you'd have no idea what even caused the problems. You don't need to blow your 401(k) on bottled water, but it's a smart idea to use a water filter for any drinking water you use out of the faucet. Designed to remove bacteria and/or impurities from water, filters come in many types. The simplest is a pitcher fitted with a charcoal filter. You pour tap water into the pitcher; by the time the water seeps through the filter, it's been cleared of many impurities. High-end filters use reverse osmosis—a system that's under your sink or basement and pulls water across a membrane that cleans water for the whole house. And ultraviolet water filters irradiate water between your tap and the cup to destroy many bacteria.

"TOMMY, TAKE ALL OF YOUR MEDICINE!"   Typical scenario: You get sick. You call the doctor. You get medicine. You take medicine. You feel better in two days. You stop medicine. That's a mistake. Antibiotics aren't really designed to make you feel better, though that's a darn nice side effect. They're designed to kill or incapacitate the enemy. So while you may feel better in two or three days, it's important to take the whole course of antibiotics—even if it's ten days or two weeks—to make sure you've killed all of the enemy. If you take medication for only half its course, you may only weaken the remaining bacteria without finishing them off completely. And weakened bacteria actually come back stronger than before, worsen the infection, and spread it deeper into your body—which results in a greater threat to your cardiovascular and other systems.

Myth Buster #4

Unless you're longing to meet that new physician who specializes in infectious diseases, take the full course of medication. When you're fighting persistent little suckers like bacteria and viruses, you need to land the knockout punch, not just the meager hooks and jabs. By the way, antibiotics can kill not only the bad bacteria but the good as well.

Action 2:
Call in Nutritional Allies

T cells, B cells, and white blood cells pretty much have things under control and keep your home secure. But it never hurts to call in reinforcements—specially trained nutrients that have been promoted to the rank of immune booster. The best nutrients for keeping your system secure:

VITAMIN C   Take 500 milligrams twice a day every day to boost your immune system (so it can produce more bullets to kill the invaders). You can take it in supplement form, as well as through foods such as oranges and other citrus fruits, 100 percent natural orange juice, tomatoes, and bell peppers. Vitamin C, for all its power to keep your immune system and arteries young, can make you up to one year younger.

YOGURT   Yogurt that hasn't been pasteurized contains *Lactobacillus acidophilus*—a healthy bacteria that turns milk into yogurt and fights off fungus-related infections. Or you can take acidophilus in supplement form of 20 milligrams twice daily. It works by helping to prevent the overgrowth of fungi that shouldn't be able to grow in your body. Other alternatives: any probiotic (such as Digestive Aide or Sustenex) that has *Bacillus* coagulans. Another great fungicide: garlic.

FLAVONOIDS These vitamin-like substances (they work like vitamins but aren't essential for life) have been shown to decrease the rate of arterial and immune aging. They seem to allow your memory bank to maintain the memory of old foes longer and more intensely. If you eat a diet rich in flavonoids—about 31 milligrams of them a day—you'll have a significant effect on your RealAge, making you up to 3.2 years younger. Here's how to get there:

Oats (3 milligrams per cup)

Onions (4 milligrams for one small)

Broccoli (4.2 milligrams per cup)

Tomatoes (2.6 milligrams for one small)

Apples (4.2 milligrams for one medium)

Cranberries (8 milligrams for one eight-ounce cup)

Strawberries (4.2 milligrams per cup)

Cranberry juice (11.2 milligrams per eight-ounce glass)

Tomato juice or tea (7.2 milligrams per eight-ounce cup of tomato juice or brewed nonherbal tea)

Grape juice (3 milligrams per one five-ounce glass)

Red wine (3 milligrams per one five-ounce glass)

PUMPKIN SEEDS   They contain zinc—one of the ingredients that's been shown to help reduce the average length of the common cold.

Action 3: Know the Big Three

Look, if you live in this world, you're going to catch a cold. That's part of the trade-off of inter-acting with people: talking to them, shaking their hands, sharing subway poles with them. Germs will spread. So if your mission is to prevent colds, then your only real answer is to pack your boxes, say good-bye to the family, and move to the woods. If you come into contact with other people, you're going to spend some time sneezing, cough-ing, blowing, and sniffling. In fact, most American adults catch two to four colds every year. Just because it's a fact that you will catch a cold doesn't mean you have to live with all the consequences. Everybody seems to have his own remedy for what helps cure a cold, but the truth is you can't really cure a cold; you can only speed up its course. And there have been only three things that have been shown to have a real effect on speeding one up—chicken soup, zinc lozenges, and vitamin C (though we don't know why they work, research has shown that they do). Take regular doses of any of the three at the moment you start feeling symptoms—that's 500 milligrams of vitamin C four times each day with plenty of water immediately at the start of cold symptoms and for the next two or three days, or one zinc lozenge every six hours, or a cup of chicken soup four times a day at the onset of symp-toms. That can reduce the average time that a cold lasts from roughly five days to three.

Myth or Fact? You can catch a cold by being cold or wet.

It's an old wives' tale that you can catch a cold by running around in the cold without a hat on. Research shows that being chilled or wet has no effect on whether or not people catch the common cold.

Myth or Fact? Starve a cold and feed a fever. Or is it the other way around?

Doesn't matter, actually. Whether you have a cold or a fever, you should eat normally (unless normally means the grease-soaked buffet). The important thing for both is to stay hydrated—especially if you have a fever. Lots of fluid will help flush your whole body of infection. And rest, rest, rest—it helps T and B cells prepare for the fight.

Action 4: Call in Human Allies

It doesn't matter what kind of fight you're in—a bar fight, a fight with the mechanic, a family food fight—you always want someone else to take your side. Simple math shows that the more people who are on your side, the better your chances. The same goes for your health: creating a strong social network is paramount and raises the level of your immune system. How? Depression has been linked to infection, presumably because depression inhibits the fighting ability of your T cells. It's not just forgetting to activate your burglar alarm; it's not caring whether it's activated or not. Group participation works, too—religious groups, social groups, and work groups are all beneficial.

Action 5: Manage Stress

Though we don't have a lot of data about the mechanisms that link stress and aging, we are brought up to believe that stress is correlated with infections. In fact, stress is perhaps the greatest ager of them all. The more you're stressed, the greater the risk of accidents, infections, and arterial aging. It's not really the stress we're worried about, since everyone has it; it's more your *response* to stress. It seems that when you're in high-stress mode—working your tail off at work, for example—you're cruising along fine. But when you come off that stressor, you get sort of a rebound effect where you're a lot more prone to infections (your T and B cells go into hiding to avoid a fight and are slow to come back to help you). In terms of stress-reduction techniques, one person may like playing basketball to blow off steam; another may like sitting in steam. Some may like listening to Mozart; others may like listening to Metallica. But there's at least one thing that everyone can do in the face of stress: Remove yourself from a stressful situation immediately, whether it's by taking a walk around the block or simply moving to the next room. That momentary time-out gives you a chance to breathe and react rationally. Whatever it is, you need some sort of backup plan—some technique that removes you from the emotions of a stressful situation. It may be taking ten deep breaths or even scrunching your face up for fifteen seconds. Whatever it is, you can make your RealAge up to six years younger by developing a backup plan for reducing stress when your first lines of defense fail.

You should also change the way you think about some of the nagging stresses in your life—a demanding boss, the broken screen door, the cable company that never seems to get the bill right. Look, few people are trying to be jerks on purpose. What's stressful is the reaction to the situation or the action. That may not help you get your screen door repaired any faster or correct the cable bill, but when you remember that stress comes with the situation and action, not so much from malice, then you're better able to have a manageable response to otherwise stressful situations—and that's a healthier way to deal with them.

FACTOID

If you've ever crashed a skateboard or peeled a hangnail, you're sure to know about nature's Band-Aids. One is the scab, which covers the wound almost immediately. A scab is formed when proteins that help coagulate blood come out of the bloodstream to protect the wound—and actually accelerate the healing process. Pus, on the other hand, is a collection of white blood cells that congregate at the site of an infection where bacteria replicate and multiply. The presence of pus means that the white blood cells are trying to ingest and kill the infection. When they don't do it quickly enough, that draws more and more white blood cells to the area, which increases the amount of pus. Pus is also a sign that the battle is continuing and you are not healed yet.

Chapter 11

This Gland Is Your Gland: Your Hormones

Major Myths about Hormones

Hormone Myth #1   Hormones control our emotions.

Hormone Myth #2   The mind-body connection has not been proven with "hard" science.

Hormone Myth #3   Blood pressure below 140/90 is acceptable for you.

DANGER

HIGH-TEST ADRENALIN

CORTISOL

FULL-STRENG

Most of us think of our houses as inanimate objects. After the two-by-fours, a bucket of nails, and some slabs of drywall, you throw in a wind chime and a plastic deer, and you're all set. In the crudest forms of housing, that's the case—homes act as shelter from rain, wind, sun, and BB-gun-toting neighbors. But when you consider the modern American home, you realize how much your house really *lives.*

The water, air, and electricity that snake through your house act as the lifeblood for everyone inside. Those necessities, however, don't work unless you regulate them. The thermostat controls whether you feel cold or hot. The handles next to the faucets determine whether your shower feels soothing and warm or hotter than pelting lava rocks. Now think about all the dials, switches, and controls that give you the power to regulate virtually every system in your house. And think about this: The same emotion that flavors the furniture, artwork, and moose on the wall also makes your regulators work (you regulate because you *care* about your home). Most times, everything functions fine, and you barely even notice how your house works. But what would happen if your regulators failed—or if you ignored them? You'd experience all different levels of problems. At best, you'd sweat through a July heat wave (without AC), run up your water bill (without faucets), or scorch the salmon (without temperature control on the oven). In your house, all of these systems release essential elements to keep your house running smoothly—whether it's heat, water, or power—and you living comfortably.

That's really the job of your endocrine system: a system of glands throughout your body that releases essential hormones to keep your body fine-tuned to function well—and comfortably. Most of these hormones do Grandma's work; they perform good deeds without anyone ever noticing, and you live a good life because of all they do. These glands regulate themselves, so you rarely have to worry about switching anything on or off or turning any knobs (except in the privacy of your own bedroom). That doesn't mean that you should ignore your hormones; in fact, there are many ways to help regulate the hormones in your body.

Myth or Fact?
Hormones control whether we cry.

Just as sweat removes excess salt, urine removes waste, and mucus traps bacteria, tears serve a purpose. Basal tears are produced continuously to keep our eyes lubricated, which is important in preventing damage by air currents and bits of floating debris. Irritant tears are produced when the eyes are hit by wind or sand (or insects or rocks). They both have the same goal: protecting the eyes. Emotional tears are secreted in moments of intense feeling—sometimes joy but more often sorrow. They contain much more than basal or irritant tears; they carry stress hormones as a way of getting rid of them. But are the tears caused by the stress hormones? One major hormone that increases with stress is also associated with crying: prolactin. Levels of prolactin in the body correlate positively with frequency of emotional crying; as a whole, women cry more often than men (perhaps four times as often, according to one study) and also have a whole lot more prolactin (60 percent more). One more thing about crying: emotional tears are rare or nonexistent in other species. Discounting a few unverified tales of weepy gorillas and elephants (which may well prove, someday, to be accurate), it seems humans are the only ones to cry. Maybe we have more developed emotional processes, and emotional tears appear a way of conveying profound emotions. Although crying may embarrass you, it signals that you have reached a level of stress that is detrimental to your health and that you should let it out. It's okay to cry.

While most of us tend to associate hormones with teenage boys and posters of bathing beauties, hormones play a role in everything we do—how we handle stress, how we absorb fat, and how we reproduce. In truth, our hormones and the glands that secrete them are all part of a pretty complicated process. (If this were a medical textbook, the chapter would be filled with more four-letter acronyms than a government phone directory.) When these hormones go haywire, that's when things can get scary.

Though all hormone problems are different, many hormones have several

Actually, it's the other way around—emotions control our hormones through biochemical changes in the brain. Fear, for instance, is accompanied by the production of one set of brain chemicals that can make us alert and ready to flee, while pleasure triggers the release of other chemicals that soothe and calm. Here we can learn from the animal kingdom. Stressed-out mother baboons have more problems producing healthy offspring, presumably because the stress causes a sustained production of stress hormones, which in turn damages the hippocampus. That hippocampal damage causes defects in learning and memory. So even though baboons may not commute, do their boss's dry cleaning, or root for the Red Sox, they suffer very similarly from the scourge of stress.

Myth Buster #1

common characteristics. For one, they regulate some of the under-the-radar feelings that don't have an obvious physiological explanation—things like fatigue, sex drive, and whether you prefer hot or cold weather. But the second and often overlooked reality is the role that blood pressure plays throughout your endocrine system. In the case of most endocrine glands, high blood pressure plays a role in the dysfunction of that gland, or the dysfunction of that gland leads to an increased risk of high blood pressure. The correlation between the two shouldn't come as a surprise. That's because, as we've stressed throughout the book, arterial aging—and the effect it has throughout your body—is one of the greatest influences on your health and overall aging process. To understand how blood pressure plays a role, it's a good idea to take a closer look into your land of glands.

Your Hormones: The Anatomy

Normally, the word secretion makes you think of things like pus, mucus, and blood. They're certainly not Monet-worthy images, but there's no reason why secretion has to be associated only with things that belong in horror movies or in a tissue. That's because you are full of organs and glands that secrete substances, nutrients, and hormones all through your body. As anybody who's stepped on a just-used treadmill knows, the most visible glands you have are sweat glands. You can see the secretion, wipe it, and wash it. But just about everywhere else, your hormone-secreting glands do their jobs internally. We know this is a tough concept to wrap your brain around, which is exactly why we want to start this discussion here: in the brain.

In Chapter 3, we dissected the anatomy of the brain, but we intentionally ignored the pituitary gland. That's because the pituitary has less to do with what we traditionally think of as brain function (like memory), and more to do with its regulation of other endocrine organs.

As you can see in Figure 11.1, the pituitary gland is a small oval organ, about the size of a pea, and has two sides—the posterior and the anterior. The anterior (front portion) comes up from the back of the mouth and grows up into the brain, while the posterior (back portion) protrudes down from the hypothalamus in the brain to sit on a bone called the "Turkish saddle." It's a bone that sits at the base of the skull and holds the pituitary—almost like a ball resting in a socket. Although the posterior secretes a couple of hormones, the anterior gets all the glory for secreting hormones you probably recognize, if not by name, by their function. These include:

> ## FACTOID
>
> Growth hormone is—you guessed it—what lets children grow. A child who makes too little of it won't grow to a normal height, while a child who has too much could find himself in *Guinness World Records*.

- ★ luteinizing hormone, which plays a part in menstrual cycles and pregnancy and tells men when to release testosterone
- ★ prolactin, which helps women produce milk and plays a role in maintaining immune system cells in both genders (women have a lot more prolactin at all times than men)
- ★ thyroid-stimulating hormone, which stimulates the thyroid gland to produce more thyroid hormone that helps regulate metabolism and blood pressure
- ★ adrenocorticotropic hormone, which stimulates the adrenal cortex to produce cortisone, which helps regulate metabolism, blood pressure, and response to stress; aldosterone, which helps regulate water metabolism and blood pressure; and the sex hormone it produces (such as testosterone for women—see Chapter 8)
- ★ growth hormone, which, uh, helps you grow

Pituitary Gland

The pituitary has an important relationship with the rest of the body, not just with the entire endocrine system. Some people scoff at the notion of a mind-body connection in medicine, chalking it up to some wacky Eastern philosophy that has no more effectiveness than a placebo. But the pituitary is the physiological link between the blood and the brain. Situated in the brain, the pituitary serves as the central commander role of endocrine function—by sending out signals to glands throughout the body to release different hormones that dictate how you *feel*. It's how your mind is connected to your body, in that all the different ways you can feel are psychological, physiological, and chemical reactions. Now let's explore what parts of the endocrine system fall under its command.

Myth Buster #2

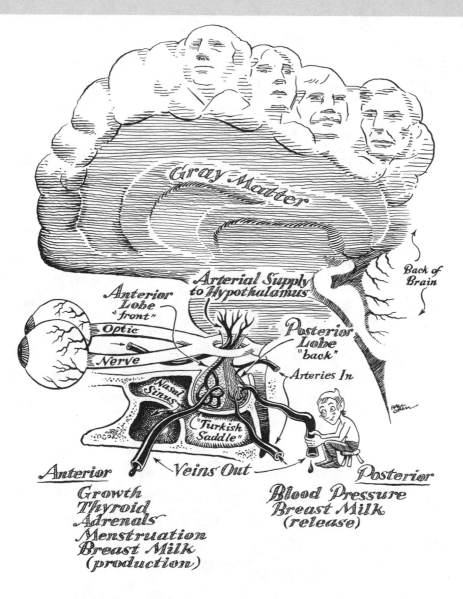

Gray Matter

Back of Brain

Arterial Supply to Hypothalamus

Anterior Lobe "front"

Optic

Nerve

Posterior Lobe "back"

Arteries In

Nasal Sinus

"Turkish Saddle"

Veins Out

Anterior
Growth
Thyroid
Adrenals
Menstruation
Breast Milk
(production)

Posterior
Blood Pressure
Breast Milk
(release)

Thyroid Gland

Located at the base of the neck on both sides (Figure 11.2), the butterfly-shaped thyroid gland produces, ta-da, thyroid hormone after receiving chemical signals from General Pituitary. The main function of the thyroid hormone is to regulate the metabolism of your cells—that is, the chemical changes in your cells that cause them to live, grow, and die. You can think of your metabolism as a little bit like your utility bill. From neighbor to neighbor, no two utility bills are alike. Some people keep their AC at seventy-six; some keep it at sixty-eight. Some take twenty-minute showers; some hop in and out in twenty seconds. We all use and consume energy a little bit differently in our homes, and we all use and consume it a little differently in our bodies. And that plays a key role in weight management; some of metabolism is genetic, in that you're predisposed to have a quick-working metabolism or a slow-churning one. That regulation comes, in part, from your thyroid hormone.

Still, guillotines and tightly knotted bow ties aren't the only things associated with your neck that can be harmful to your health. A thyroid gone wild can, too, and that's called hyperthyroidism, which occurs when the thyroid gland releases too many hormones. There are many things that can cause hyperthyroidism, including inflammation, pregnancy, and noncancerous growths on the thyroid. Think of hyperthyroidism as an influx of spring breakers on a quiet coastal community. The town's used to operating with a certain infrastructure fifty-one weeks of the year to support the small group of yearlong residents, but when tens of thousands of partiers descend on its destination wearing thongs and carrying bottles of Jack, the infrastructure isn't prepared to handle the mass of hysteria and hyperactivity. To put it mildly, the traditional townies go into a tizzy. Sure, the town will live through the season, but not without its share of arrests for noise violations, underage alcohol consumption, and indecent exposure.

When your thyroid sends out a surplus of hormones, your body goes into a bit

FIGURE 11.2 **Pain in the Neck** The thyroid, which is plastered against the trachea (windpipe), partly regulates your metabolism. A hyperthyroid gland secretes too much hormone and makes our body overactive with fast heartbeats, tremors, brittle hair, sleeping troubles, and irritability. A hypothyroid gland leaves the body with too-low metabolism, resulting in symptoms like weight gain, dry skin, depression, fatigue, and coldness. The thyroid can also have nodules or large goiters, which need further evaluation. Four tiny parathyroid glands lie on the thyroid and regulate calcium in your blood and bones.

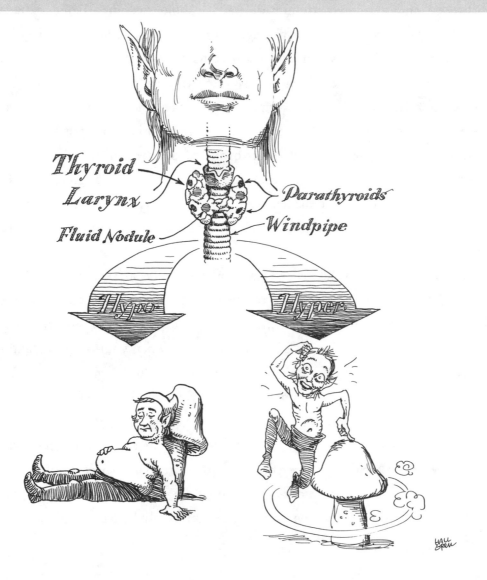

of a tizzy, too. It tolerates the surge to some extent, but not without some problems. Hyperthyroidism won't destroy your body immediately; it will send signals throughout that you're not operating optimally and, in turn, will rev up your metabolism as if it were a dragster. So you may experience rapid weight loss, an increased appetite, brittle hair that breaks, intolerance to heat, and fatigue—not life-threatening problems, but ones that make you feel all out of sorts. A lot of folks complain of being short-fused and develop a tremor or have trouble sleeping—being exhausted throughout the day is a major warning sign of hyperthyroidism. But the abnormal and occasionally very, very fast heartbeats of hyperthyroidism can be life-threatening. With all these common symptoms, the real question is: How do you know if your thyroid is the real culprit? Fifty percent of the time, if you were really observant, you would probably also notice an extra bump or goiter on your neck—a nodule of thyroid that goes off on its own, independent of other controls, and causes the overproduction of thyroid hormone. Ultimately, a thyroid function blood test reveals hyperthyroidism, and treatment can be handled with medication or, in some cases, closing the town to all spring breakers by removing the thyroid gland altogether.

On the other end of the thyroid equation is a small coastal community that decides life has passed it by. The core of residents has long since moved away, so only a few people are left. Eventually, they pick up and leave, too; businesses close and the infrastructure goes unused. That's hypothyroidism—when your thyroid gland fails to produce enough hormones to keep your metabolism moving. Everything slows down. Hypothyroidism causes symptoms like unaccounted-for weight gain, depression, dry skin, intolerance to cold, joint or muscle aches, fatigue, and small bumps on the throat (which usually can't be seen or felt). It's the most common of all thyroid problems—affecting one in ten people, with more than 60 percent of people affected over age sixty. It can be caused by the failure of the pituitary to secrete the hormone that stimulates the thyroid or, more commonly, by a disease in which the immune system attacks the gland to slow production of the hormone. For these people, medication to replace the hormone can help regulate metabolism and other affected functions back to normal.

Adrenal Glands

These are triangular-shaped glands located on the top of your kidneys; they look almost like a beret or even a two-colored plastic hat you'd put on the top of Mr. Potato Head (see Figure 11.3). But don't mistake their odd appearance (and eraser-like texture) for lack of importance; a slight tip of the hat would lead to a hormonal riot in your body. These glands are hormonal workhorses. They produce the stress hormone cortisol, as well as hormones that turn into both female hormones like estrogen and progesterone and male hormones like testosterone (especially in women, testosterone is thought to have a substantial role in libido). The inner part of the gland (the medulla) produces important chemicals, too, like adrenaline, the chemical that fires you up to win the tennis match or enables you to lift cars during times of extreme crisis.

Just like in other endocrine glands, problems happen when the adrenals produce more or less of a hormone than they should. Let's use cortisol as an example. The pituitary secretes adrenocorticotropic

FACTOID

Your adrenal glands also produce norepinephrine and epinephrine, levels of which rise when you get excited. In normal daily life, your levels of epinephrine hover between 200 to 800 nanograms per milliliter. You know that feeling when you narrowly avoid a car accident—when your face feels flushed, your heart races, and you swear at the incompetence of no-look mergers? In that case, epinephrine levels rise to between 1,500 and 2,500. In times of crisis for people with adrenal tumors, the level can reach 300,000—and force their blood pressure readings literally off the scale. Imagine feeling that way—like having a close-call accident—all the time. That's how people with adrenal tumors feel. Typically it's eight years before organized medicine diagnoses the tumor. Another interesting finding: 50 percent of people with these tumors are alcoholics, presumably because they use alcohol to calm themselves from that intense stress.

FIGURE 11.3 **Dunce Hats on the Kidneys**   Sure, the kidneys remove toxins and excess water from the blood for excretion in the urine, but they also regulate blood pressure. In fact, blockage of the kidney artery causes hypertension. Sitting like a dunce cap on top of the kidneys are the adrenal glands, which are signaled by the pituitary in the brain to secrete steroids and the sex hormones. Inside the adrenals are stores of adrenaline that are released in time of crisis.

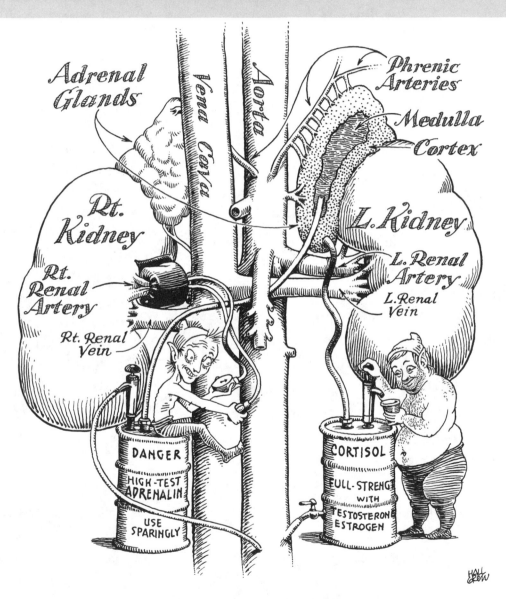

hormone (say that ten times fast) in response to stressful situations to trigger the well-known fight-or-flight response through cortisol secretion. When *excess* pituitary secretion happens, the adrenal glands respond by secreting *excess* cortisol. (The process is like a game of hormonal dominoes; one secretion triggers a chain of others.) Cortisol also controls the way the body processes carbohydrates, fats, and proteins, and helps the body reduce inflammation. When there's too much cortisol, it can lead to the classic signs of Cushing's disease, including weight gain, acne, a buffalo hump (collection of fat between the shoulders), increased urination, and the growth of facial hair (see the character at bottom right of Figure 11.3). Medication can be prescribed to treat it, but Cushing's is often caused by a benign tumor on the pituitary that needs to be surgically removed.

Now, if you produce too little cortisol, you may feel extremely tired and develop low blood pressure. Although infections can cause this problem, a leading culprit is autoimmune disease, where your own guard cells attack and kill the adrenal. Replacing the missing cortisol addresses the problem, but the pill must be taken daily.

Kidneys

Sure, the kidneys' day job is removing water waste from your body, but they double as key hormone-producing organs as well. Your kidneys are responsible for producing a hormone that stimulates the production of red blood cells by preventing their premature death. This hormone also helps preserve other cells, like heart and brain cells that have been injured by lack of blood flow. So the kidneys' hormone secretion plays a key (even if indirect) role in delivering oxygen to every one of your cells. They're like a Mafia boss in the movies—you never see the boss, but you know he has an oversized effect on the way other people function. Your kidneys also play a very traceable and key role in regulating blood pressure because they are ideally positioned to measure the pressure of blood pushing into them. If the pressure head is low, like after our ancestors were bitten by a saber-toothed tiger, they hold on to fluid to maintain our blood pressure. But when they overreact or are misled into thinking we need a higher blood pressure, the kidneys can readjust quickly. These organs are the ultimate fine tuners of your vascular system.

Gonads

You probably haven't heard the word since it was the punch line in a fifth-grade joke, but the gonad glands are your sex glands, with each gender carrying its own set. Let's start with the male system, since it's a little simpler. The testes are the two reproductive organs housed in the scrotum. They're responsible for reproduction because they make sperm, but they're also responsible for men's ability to grow beards, talk in deep voices, and boast that they can find their way around a new city without a map. That's because (once they get the signal from the pituitary gland) the testes make most of men's testosterone. When they're young, men need testosterone for strength (making tackles) and survival (making babies). As men get older, however, the games change, and they need testosterone for other things—namely to maintain things that influence quality of life. Despite the fact that some people think men's brains suffer from testosterone poisoning, men need testosterone to maintain libido, erections, and muscle strength. Now, a mild decrease in testosterone might not have much of an effect, but worry centers around an all-out testosterone deficiency (as defined by less than 300 nanograms per deciliter; for you lab rats, testosterone usually peaks in your twenties between 900 and 1,200). While many of the effects of low testosterone affect quality-of-life issues, having a testosterone deficiency has also been shown to accelerate coronary artery disease—which can be reversed with replenishment of the hormone. Appropriate testosterone replacement is one option in helping restore libido, erections, and muscle strength, but there's still research that needs to be done to determine whether replacement testosterone correlates with prostate cancer (speculation is that it does).

In women, the gonad glands are the ovaries—the glands that produce eggs. As women age, they enter a period when the ovaries stop releasing eggs ready to be fertilized. Not only does menstruation stop during this menopausal period, but the body produces less estrogen and progesterone—the hormones responsible for giving women secondary sex characteristics and helping during the pregnancy process. Typically, there's a gradual loss of hormones, and in those cases, the accompanying symptoms can be mild, but menopausal symptoms vary from woman to woman. That hormonal fluctuation causes many women to experience hot flashes, night sweats, insomnia, decreased sex drive, decreased lubrication, and severe mood swings. Menopause can also lead to bone loss—because of the lack of the bone-strengthening estrogen—which can cause osteoporosis.

We want to stress that menopause isn't a disease; it's a natural process that the body goes through as it ages. And it's not something you necessarily need to treat—depending on the level of your symptoms. That is, are they bearable or do they destroy your quality of life? The latter definitely need treatment, while the former do not, depending on the effect on your quality of life. One of the most controversial forms of treatment is hormone therapy (HT)—that is, the addition by pill or patch of estrogen and progesterone to help alleviate some of the symptoms associated with menopause. Initially, it was lauded as a wonderful tool to deal with hormonal loss, but the Women's Health Initiative and other studies scared many people away because of a correlation with such things as breast cancer and stroke.

> ## FACTOID
>
> You can't see a hormone deficiency the way you can see a bruise, goiter, or kitchen knife sticking out of your thigh. But this self-test may give men an indication about whether they have a health problem. While shaving rituals are as much cultural as they are physical, a man should look at his shaving habits as one indicator of low testosterone. If a man notices that he used to shave once a day but now has to shave less often, it's a sign that testosterone is not stimulating a great deal of beard growth, which is a sign of low testosterone levels. As long as a man hasn't changed cultures, not having to shave daily is probably a sign of a testosterone deficiency. And the same goes for a woman and her leg-shaving frequency.

Myth or Fact?
Sex cures depression by elevating hormone levels.

Semen contains powerful — and potentially addictive — mood-altering chemicals, including testosterone, estrogen, prolactin, luteinizing hormone, and prostaglandins. Some of these are absorbed through the walls of the vagina and are known to elevate mood. Though research shows that women who do not use condoms during sex are less depressed, that doesn't mean you should practice unsafe sex. Studies have found no correlation between high-risk sexual behavior and lower rates of depression. So while we can think of no better mood elevator than great mutually monogamous sex, high-risk sex does not have the same benefits.

Where do we stand? We think that there's an answer somewhere in HT. If you have disabling or even significant symptoms, we recommend that you consider a bioidentical estrogen and micronized progestin like Angeliq if you are in the first ten years after menopause. If your symptoms aren't disabling, try deep breathing and avoiding all saturated fats to reduce symptoms. Of course, many women do, and will, still use HT; in that case, we advise that if they want to use hormone therapy they should also take aspirin (162 milligrams with a half glass of warm water before and after the aspirin) every day to help reduce the risk of clotting.

Your Hormones: The Live Younger Action Plan

In many ways, hormones are your body's regulators. They regulate your energy supply, water supply, and heating levels. They regulate your ability to handle stress. They even regulate the ability to conceive and the desire to have sex in both men and women. But even small deviations from normal levels can make you feel weak, tired, and uninterested in doing the horizontal tango with your spouse. It's one of the body's most mysterious equations. Hormones control some of the under-the-radar aspects of our body—the qualities that we often take for granted.

Of course, medicine is busy perfecting ways to tinker with hormone levels artificially to make sure that you live as comfortably and happy as you can. And we think there's a great future in the use of these methods. That's not to say you can't do a little tinkering yourself (and we're not just talking about your gonads here). Certainly, if there's one thing we want to stress, it's that hormonal deficiencies aren't just things you need to accept. Not only are being tired, having less sex, or gaining weight quality-of-life issues, but they're also health issues. All of these symptoms make you more prone to aging. Certainly, some hormonal problems (like diabetes) have stronger long-term health implications than others, but remember, the one overriding thing that ties your endocrine system together is that your hormones are connected to your brain. So here's something to think about: Without optimal hormonal levels, you won't have optimal brain function. While you have less control over your hormone regulators than you do over other parts of your body, you can still take many steps to keep your hormonal levels as balanced as a tightrope artist.

Action 1: Control Your Blood Pressure

You'd think that a discussion of blood pressure belongs in the chapter on your heart and your arteries, and it does, since blood pressure is all about the volume and pressure of blood traveling through your arteries. But it also belongs here, because it has such a huge effect on how your endocrine system works. High blood pressure magnifies the aging and symptoms associated with diabetes, causes kidney failure and many other hormone-related conditions, and may be triggered by thyroid, adrenal, or kidney problems.

Optimally, you want to keep your blood pressure at 115/75. That's the level at which you'll see the least aging. Of course, there are many ways to lower your blood pressure, including medications, physical activity, and diet. A great approach that also helps your whole endocrine system is to lose extra weight. Being

Myth Buster #3

overweight not only increases blood pressure, it also puts you at risk for diabetes. Historically, obesity protected man against long periods of famine, so the body could call on excess fat to live; in most societies today, that's no longer a problem, so the body doesn't need to protect against starvation (see Factoid below).

If you've gotten this far in the book, then you already know how essential physical activity is to your heart, bones, and whole body. It's also paramount for your endocrine system—especially for people at risk of developing diabetes. Not only will exercise help control blood pressure, something very important also happens during that hormonal process: the sensitivity of your muscles to receiving glucose increases. When you exercise, your endocrine system releases insulin to transport that glucose-based fuel to your muscles and makes the insulin work better in getting glucose into your cells so that the glucose can be used—rather than leaving it at high levels in your bloodstream. In fact, it's rare to find people who exercise who don't decrease their blood sugar levels at the same time.

The best news is that you don't need a dramatic loss from the start to see the ef-

FACTOID

If you think America has a weight problem, pity the poor Chinese. Because they went through long periods of famine, they developed the genetics to prevent starvation so well that just a small fraction of the weight gain that causes diabetes in Americans causes diabetes in the Chinese. (At the same BMI of 27, the Chinese are sixty times more likely to have type 2 diabetes.) That's attributed to starvation genes. As you eat less and less food over days, your metabolism slows to the point that your body adjusts to not getting enough food—so it doesn't burn calories at the same rate. That change protects you from withering away after long periods of famine. (Typically, your body will lose a pound if it burns 3,500 calories more than it consumes. But in periods of famine, it will slow down in order to protect itself, so it takes more to burn that pound.) If it weren't for our ability to store fat, our ancestors would never have survived to make us. It's your karma.

fects. If you lose just 10 percent of the weight you've gained since you were eighteen—that's only four pounds if you've gained forty pounds—you can make yourself up to five years younger. By extension, that same 10 percent weight loss will usually decrease your blood pressure by levels of 7 mmHg from the systolic (the top number) and 4 mmHg from the diastolic (the bottom number), which can have the RealAge effect of making you more than two years younger.

Action 2: Know Your Meds

In this book, we've spent about as much time on medication as most men spend during foreplay—roughly twenty-three seconds. That's not a critique of med-

Myth or Fact?
When it comes to hormones, higher levels are better.

Judging by the size of fast-food meals and the number of X-rated Internet sites, more seems better. A number of quick-fix companies are trying to capitalize on that mentality by hawking extra hormone as the solution to all kinds of health problems—from weight gain to weak muscles. But because our hormone system is more complicated than a calculus workbook, the more-is-better philosophy doesn't fly. You can't just turn on all the faucets in your house, ratchet up the heat, or flip on all your switches—or you'll overload your systems and cause everything to go haywire. Anytime you try fiddling with your hormones on your own with anabolic steroids or fixes for weight loss or other ailments, you're causing your body to go haywire. For example, we often read about athletes who take androgenic steroids or supplements that get metabolized through to testosterone. This excess testosterone can lead to very aggressive behavior—as in, don't give that man a gun or even an argument—not to mention all the side effects like cardiovascular and kidney problems. If you do try to supplement your body with hormone replacement products, the best thing that can happen to you is that you only lose money.

Myth or Fact?
A blood test will easily determine hormone levels.

Yes, that's how hormone levels are determined, but getting perfectly accurate readings is a little like trying to find a paper clip in beach sand. In reality, hormones are bound in the blood with small proteins. Once bound, they often do not have the same physiologic benefit. Ideally, we need free (unbound to proteins) hormone values in a specific setting, but these are often more difficult for a laboratory to analyze.

ication (though it is one of our foreplay customs); in fact, the development of pharmaceuticals is one of the most important medical developments in history. For the most part, though, we're here to show you methods for prevention—ways to beat the problem before you need to worry about medication. Hormone problems are a little bit different: most of them are easily treated with medication, and hormones are a very subtle, fickle part of your body. How you take hormone medication can have a major effect on how your body reacts to it (for example, for those requiring thyroid hormone, consuming iron, calcium, or soy less than four hours before taking the thyroid medication can mean the thyroid medication won't be absorbed). That's why it's important to review a few things about hormone-related medications.

ESTROGEN Though there's much debate about HT, it does appear that dermal estrogen—that is, estrogen applied to skin—is safer than oral (pill form) estrogen. It also appears that the pill form goes into the liver and has some effect in clotting proteins that can make you more susceptible to closing off arteries; the dermal form, on the other hand, does not get metabolized as quickly in the liver. If you choose HT therapy to deal with menopausal symptoms, it seems that human estrogen—not plant-derived estrogen—is the most effective. Why? Plant estrogens have 150 isoflavones that interact with estrogen receptors in your body; some stimulate estrogen, while others block it—so you don't really know which are having an effect and which aren't. Last, remember to take aspirin if you're on HT.

CORTISONE Cortisone—a steroid used to treat all kinds of inflammatory conditions like skin rashes, arthritis, asthma, and lower-back pain—works by decreasing the inflammatory response and inflammation. But taking too much cortisone can also have a negative effect, by increasing your risk of elevated blood pressure, increasing your risk of infections, and thinning your bones. If you're worried about the potential side effects of taking cortisone, you should talk to your doctor about taking it every other day (or taking a small dose one day and the regular dose the next). When you alternate days, your potential for side effects can decrease by more than 80 percent. By decreasing the inflammation with steroids, you can often decrease the pain associated with the inflammation.

Myth or Fact? Plant hormones are natural.

Natural hormones are not ones that grow in the ground or in animals but rather those that we produce in ourselves. Everyone thinks plant hormones are better, but there's no proof that they're physiologically superior to others. Because of complex feedback loops, we need to be precise in how we signal our body's hormonal systems.

BLOOD PRESSURE TREATMENTS INCLUDING MEDS Since blood pressure affects so much of the endocrine system, it's worth noting some tricks to finding a treatment program that works best for you. To lower blood pressure, you need either less fluid in your arterial pipes, a less forceful pumping of fluid into your pipes, or larger pipes that can open even wider when the blood is pushed in. A common first step before trying medications is to reduce salt intake in your food since the salt traps water in the body. But only a few people with hypertension are extremely salt-sensitive, so this approach often fails to correct the problem. Instead, the salt can be chased out of the artery wall—and thus the body—with long-term (years of) salt restriction in the diet or regular use of a water pill or diuretic (parsley is a natural diuretic). Beta-blockers are commonly added to the diuretic because they decrease the rate and the force of heart contractions. Both actions push less fluid per minute into the pipes. But they stimulate hunger. ACE (angiotensin converting enzyme) inhibitors prevent one of the hormones that are produced in the kidneys from being processed into a substance that contracts and spasms the arteries carrying blood; with these drugs, your arteries can relax and dilate into larger pipes. Statins, while not a blood-pressure-lowering medication, lower the lousy LDL cholesterol and raise the healthy HDL cholesterol—to help keep your arteries flexible so they can open up to accept extra blood from the heart during stress. But many of these drugs have side effects, like lowering libido (and that's related to hormones, remember?), so it's important to find the medication that works best for you. It's likely that ten years from now most people who turn sixty will routinely be prescribed a blood pressure medication—like an ACE inhibitor or beta-blocker, to help prevent the damage that can be done to the body by having high blood pressure—as well as an aspirin, a statin, and a twice-a-day multivitamin.

Action 3: Eat to Feel Better

There are about as many reasons to eat as there are flavors of Ben & Jerry's. We eat because we're hungry, because we're bored or stressed, because it's the bottom of the ninth, because there's no need to leave an empty plate of nachos. Ultimately, we should eat for nourishment—to provide our body with the necessary nutrients to make it run like a fine-tuned engine (see Chapter 13 for the Owner's Manual Diet). To that end, we should also eat not only to reap long-term health but to regulate the hormones that can make us feel better every day.

SPA FOODS   Okay, so that's not technically a category of food, but it might help you in terms of thinking about what to eat. At spas that focus on healthy eating, you'll find foods with powerful ingredients. One of the ways food can play a role is to help your body process estrogen. A couple different categories of foods can help. Cruciferous foods like broccoli, cabbage, cauliflower, and Brussels sprouts contain compounds that help produce estrogen-like activity and protect against breast cancer. And isoflavones—a compound found in plants—have been shown to work similarly. Foods that contain the effective isoflavones include soy products like tofu and soybeans, as well as garlic and onions. Also falling into this category is the Mediterranean-type diet—a diet rich in olive oils, fish oils, calcium, and fruit, which we outlined in Chapter 2—for its beneficial effects on your arteries. Massages not included.

POTASSIUM AND MAGNESIUM   Studies have shown that increased potassium intake can decrease the incidence of some forms of arterial aging. Potassium is an electrolyte—an electrically charged particle needed for proper cellular functioning. Potassium specifically helps in carrying an electrical charge to help a nerve or muscle contract, and it helps regulate blood pressure and allow the heart and kidneys to function properly. (Adding the potassium equivalent of three bananas a day can make your Real Age as much as 0.6 years younger.) The recommended amount is 3,000 milligrams a day (in a balanced diet, you probably get about half that). One banana contains about 450 milligrams, and an avocado contains about 1,000 milligrams. Magnesium, essential for helping regulate metabolism, helps lower blood pressure by dilating arteries. Eating a magnesium-rich diet—400 milligrams for women, 333 milligrams for men—can make you nearly one year younger. It's usually found in whole-grain breads and cereals, while soybeans and lima beans contain 100 milligrams per serving and most nuts contain 100 to 300 milligrams per serving. Avocados, beets, raisins, and dates also contain magnesium.

Action 4: Speak Up

Many doctors are like detectives. The solution to whatever is bothering you—your anatomical crime—isn't always evident. So a doctor needs to piece all the symptoms together to try to make an assessment of what's wrong. In some cases (a broken leg), the problem is pretty clear. In other cases (back pain), it's not quite so clear. Once you bring in the endocrine system, diagnosis is murkier than a muddied creek. That's because the endocrine system is sneaky. You may feel certain symptoms, but you don't necessarily account for them when assessing your health; you may even chalk them up to being your own fault or to being a result of fatigue or stress (that is, not something that's *medically* wrong). That may mean you withhold important clues from your medical detective. So it's important to mention all symptoms you're having—no matter how inconsequential they may seem. And you should even take the liberty of saying, "Hey, Doc, you think it could be my thyroid?" These subtle problems very easily fall under the typical diagnosis patterns of many good physicians. Besides speaking up, you also should take responsibility for having certain important levels checked regularly. If you experience loss of libido, impotence, or other sexually related symptoms, it's a good idea to have your testosterone or estrogen and progesterone checked. Otherwise, follow these guidelines:

★ Blood pressure: every year after age sixteen.
★ Thyroid: once at age thirty-five, and every other year after that (unless you notice thyroid-related symptoms).
★ Blood sugar: once at age twenty, once at age thirty-five, and then every five years after that.

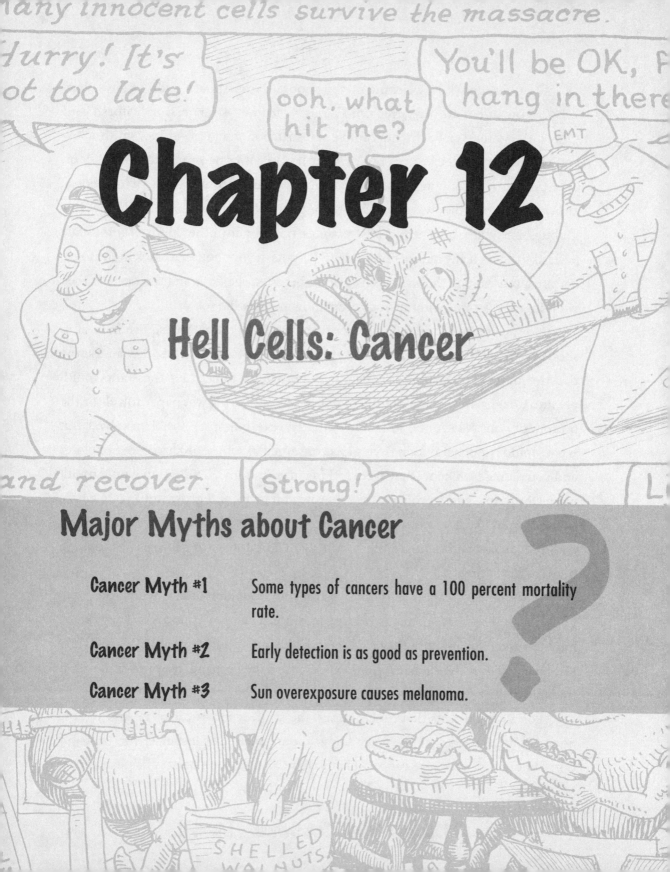

Chapter 12

Hell Cells: Cancer

Major Myths about Cancer

Cancer Myth #1	Some types of cancers have a 100 percent mortality rate.
Cancer Myth #2	Early detection is as good as prevention.
Cancer Myth #3	Sun overexposure causes melanoma.

You decide who's welcome in your house—your spouse, kids, in-laws, pets. You also have say over who's not welcome—strangers, solicitors, your daughter's ex-boyfriend. Simple construction and a good locksmith allow you to keep unwanted visitors out of your house with one simple tool—the door. One problem. As any ingenious teenager who wants to sneak out of the house knows, there are other ways in and out. For the teenager, it might be a window. But for bugs, ants, flies, spiders, roaches, termites, mice, or any other kinds of minuscule pests, it's through any number of vulnerable spots in your house: a crack in the foundation, a tiny hole in the wall, a silver of air between the door and the floor. If they want in, they get in—without your even knowing they did so.

Now, if it's an ant here or a spider there, it's no big deal. You squish it, swat it, shoo it, or flush it. But let's say the aforementioned ant decides to let other ants know that the joint at 201 Maple has got some sloppy eaters. In no time, these ants multiply into dozens, maybe hundreds. You wipe 'em out with a wet paper towel (or the bottom of your Nike) or poison them with a wave of bug spray. Problem solved. But what would happen if hundreds of pests converged in some obscure corner or closet and you didn't even know they were lurking in your home? The group would multiply faster than a math prodigy; they'd grow and grow and grow until your whole house looked like it was concocted by Stephen King or Alfred Hitchcock. Since you couldn't coexist with a house full of ants, you'd be forced to call a professional to help eradicate them.

In some ways, cancer cells can overrun your body the same way that pests can your house. They have no regard for the traditional rules of your body. They can be hard to catch, and, frankly, they frighten the hell out of a lot of people. As individuals, cancer cells aren't all that dangerous; yet when they expand, they prove to be formidable foes.

For all the threats that cancer poses, the truth is that most of us know more about 1970s sitcoms than we really know about cancer. For instance, you probably don't know that you have cancer. That's right. Every single person has had cancer cells in them. But in most cases, your body finds the cells, realizes that they're foreign, and kills them right away—without your even knowing that it happened.

Cancer cells are essentially normal cells that have something inside them that turns them bad. They're kind of like a gang of hooligans who have infiltrated your body. They may start out as good, but something inside them switches so they have total disregard for the rules that govern your body. Of course, your immune system serves as your own police force to bring down these bad cells. But cancer cells can be difficult to catch, because, like thugs who are used to committing and getting away with crimes, they are pretty smart about ways to beat the system.

Now, cancer is not a death sentence. In fact, there are no cancers that have a 100 percent mortality rate. Scientifically, this is where some really exciting cancer therapies lie—in studying people who have fought, beaten, and survived cancer: to find, identify, and replicate the mechanisms that helped each of them kill cancer cells. While, yes, some cancers like pancreatic cancer have lower survival rates, many cancers have extremely successful treatment rates—and many are even preventable. In some instances (like prostate cancer, which is more prevalent as you get older), it's even possible to coexist with cancer without it killing you or you killing it.

Myth Buster #1

Traditionally, we've viewed cancer as the body's dragon; it has no redeeming value whatsoever. But any doctor who studies, researches, and treats cancer gets an up-close look at how the body is supposed to work and how it responds when it doesn't. That's one of the great goals—and hopes—of oncologists: to find the mechanisms that kill cancer cells or prevent them from growing in the first place. To us, that's one of the important reasons why you should learn about cancer. By learning a little about the wonders of the human body and what happens when your body malfunctions, you can learn ways to make it work better. The bottom line in all of this discussion is this: Cancer doesn't always kill. But you can give yourself a hand with smart prevention strategies and early detection.

We should make it clear that this chapter isn't for people who have cancer; many resources exist to help you decide on treatment plans and courses of action. Instead, this is a guide for helping you understand the disease—so you can take steps now to increase your chances of preventing and detecting it.

Cancer: The Anatomy

It's a sign of the zodiac. It's a way sportswriters describe malcontent players on baseball teams. And ultimately, it's one of the scariest words anyone can hear. *Cancer.* We believe that the reason why cancer is so scary is not necessarily because of what it can do to our bodies but because many of us don't really understand what it is. Remember when you were a kid and you heard noises at night? In the dark of your room, you were convinced that a one-eyed, five-armed, hairy-nosed gremlin was rummaging around your bed, just waiting for the right time to pounce. It spooked you because you couldn't see it. Once you turned the light on—and realized that it was only the shadow of Raggedy Ann—things got a lot less scary. That's not to say cancer is only in your imagination. It does exist, and it's one SOB of a disease. But when we talk about it, we want your light to be turned on—so you can see the disease up close and understand how it operates. Knowing what you're confronting is the first step in fighting it.

While it's one word, cancer isn't one disease. It's hundreds of different diseases, all with different patterns of behavior and livelihood, and that makes it a complex affliction to understand. There's no one way to treat all cancers. Some cancers require surgery, while others are best treated with radiation, chemotherapy, or some combination of all of them. Unlike a heart attack, which is similar to a fire or lightning strike to your home, cancer is more of a slow-growing problem—termites, mold, a crack in the foundation—that can eventually destroy your home.

We think that understanding the way cancer grows can go a long way in understanding the disease. And it will ultimately help you take measures to detect it early enough so that it can be treated successfully—or perhaps even prevented altogether. So let's pull out our microscopes and take a look at one of the toughest cells in your body.

The Birth of Cancer Cells

Cancer is all about subtle mutations in your genes that are busy reproducing cells for the day's activities. This spectacular machinery, complete with accelerators for when you need more cells and inhibitors for when you need to slow down, occasionally loses a piece of a gene. Most are unimportant and no one notices. Then something in your normally functioning cell creates a genetic mutation that your immune system doesn't recognize and isn't able to react to. But this mutation process isn't something that happens in isolation every once in a while. It happens *all the time.* Every person has something like 70 million cell duplications a day (that's approximately the population of California, Texas, and Florida *combined*). What happens during duplication? A strand of DNA has four letters in its coding—A, G, C, T. When the cell duplicates, there are a certain number of duplications that have typographical errors in their coding, meaning that the cell doesn't recognize the code so it doesn't know what function it's supposed to perform. Imagine you're typing a hundred-page document; you're bound to make some mistakes when you're typing. But your cells don't have a backspace button to erase their errors. So if a letter gets mixed up in the cell duplication (a T becomes a U, for instance), it becomes an abnormal cell—a cell that your body doesn't recognize as normal (just as your spell-checker wouldn't know "fucniton" when you meant to type "function"). The majority of these typographical errors die—thanks to your immune system—but some of these errors can slip under the radar screen and can also lead to cancer.

To understand cell structure, it might help to think about your neighborhood (see Figure 12.1 [Acts 1–5]). You have all kinds of neighbors—friendly ones, quiet ones, benevolent ones who shovel the snow on your sidewalk before you even wake up, eccentric ones who mow their lawns wearing black socks and sneakers. But most of your neighbors fit into one category: They're socially responsible. That is, they respect your property, they fit in with everybody else, they're easy to get along with, and, darn it, when push comes to shove, their olive oil is your olive oil. It's the same with the normal cells in your body—they're very socially responsible. They get along with cells all around them, they live their own lives, and they even help each other out if necessary. Most important, they mind their own business and do their jobs without interfering with the well-being of neighboring cells. Liver cells let the spleen cells work, and abdominal muscle cells (even ones looking like tire treads) wouldn't dream of thinking they could do the work of your heart cells.

Now think of your bad neighbors—the neighbors who have no regard for anyone around them. They turf lawns, play loud music, let their Labrador drop digested Alpo bombs on other people's grass. They show total disrespect for everyone around them. Cancer cells are bad neighbors (see Figure 12.1 [Act 2]). They're not socially responsible; they're sociopathic. In essence, what they do is grow and divide and

FIGURE 12.1 (ACTS 1–5) Hell Cells and Recovery Cancer cells are sociopathic and do not respond to the normal messages to stop growing in crowded areas. Instead, surrounding healthy cells are crowded out and crushed. Sometimes the cancer outgrows its blood supply and starves to death. But the more dangerous cancers release chemicals that stimulate new blood vessels to grow into the tumor. The well-nourished cancer cells desire new fertile areas and can escape into blood tubes or follow the lymphatic channels. Accordingly, the metastases occur in tissues with lots of blood, like the lungs, liver, or brain or lymph nodes. Most chemotherapy works by killing the rapidly growing cancers as they try to grow, but this also hurts normal cells. Innovative ways to kill a cancer include stimulating immune systems to attack these invaders or preventing tumors from bringing in new blood supplies. Socialization, exercise, and the Owner's Manual Diet can help return cells to a more vital life and keep the sociopathic cells away.

Birth Of A Cancer
or, A Cell Goes Bad
ACT ONE

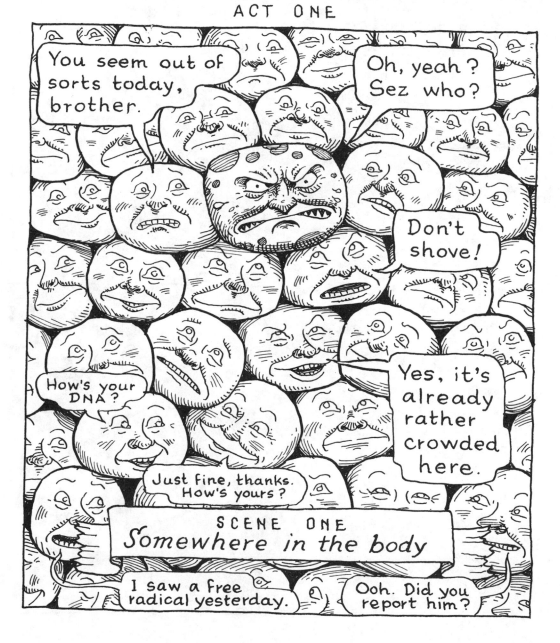

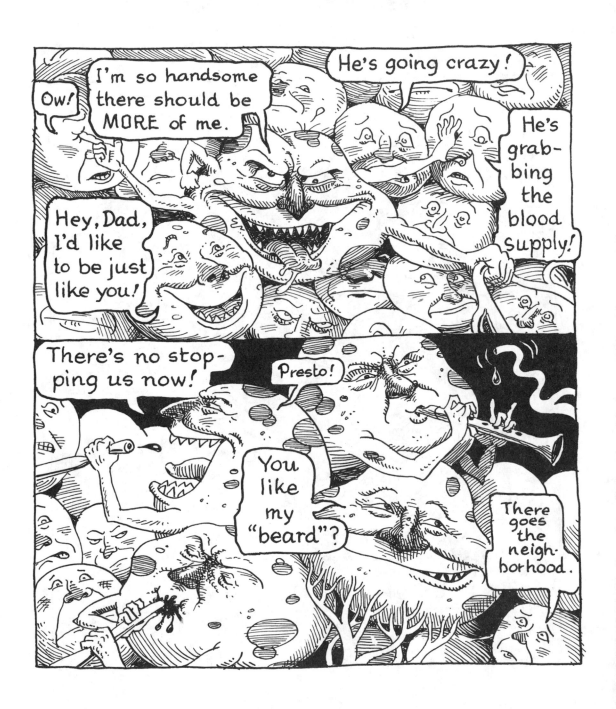

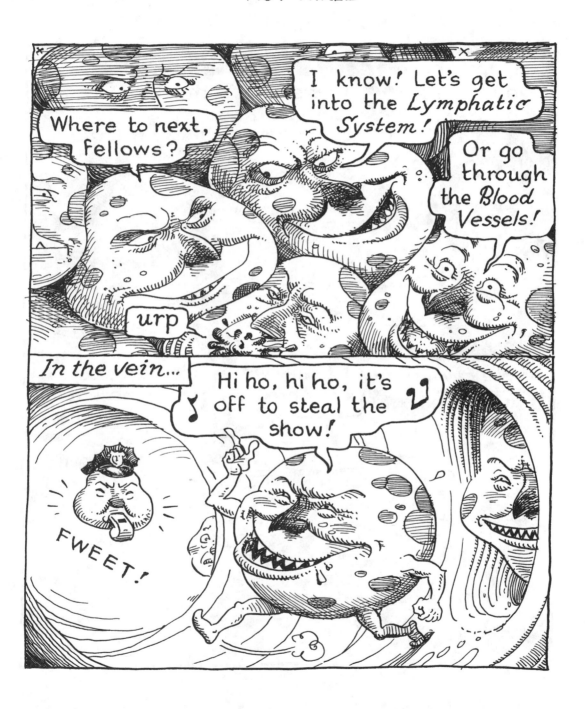

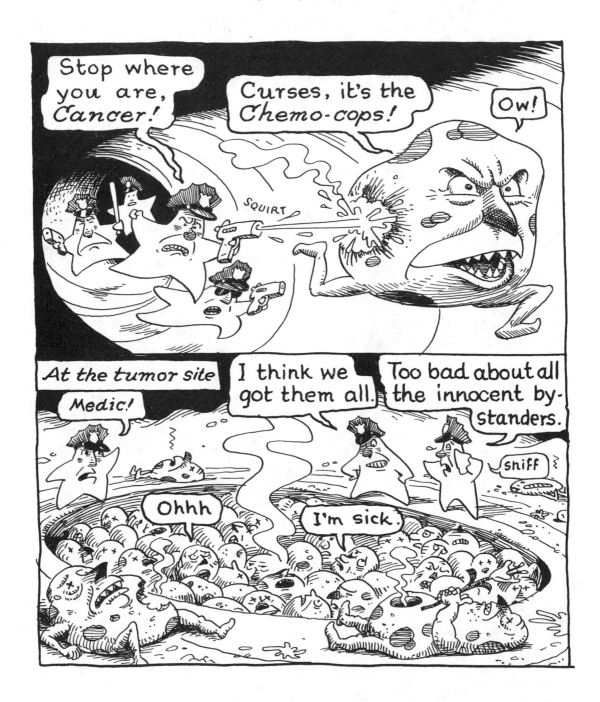

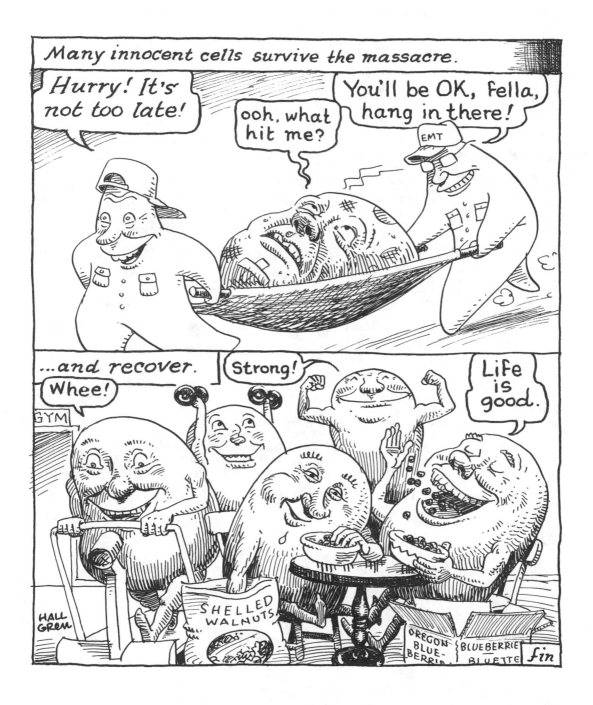

make life hell for the cells around them—just like that gang of thugs. They don't pay attention to the needs of other cells; they crush other cells; and then, in some circumstances, they can spread through the body and trash the whole neighborhood.

We get these bad neighbors—these mutations—in two ways. First, as indicated above, mutations come from mistakes in the cell-division process. Second, mutations can occur when the DNA in a cell is damaged by an irritant like radiation or free radicals (those are a charged atom or a group of atoms that can damage cells, proteins, and DNA by altering their chemical structure). The damage from free radicals can be prevented by binding the free radical with an antioxidant; perhaps the key function that antioxidants perform is to handcuff the free radicals, packaging them so that they can be washed out of the body through the kidneys and preventing them from damaging our cells and chromosomes. In both cases, these mutations—if they don't kill the cell or don't get fixed—get passed on when a cell divides.

Your second protection from cancer is your immune system; in the ideal situation, your immune system would be able to hunt down all these errors and impose the death penalty on all cells it doesn't recognize. Typically, your cells do that with a gene that's inside every cell in your body except red blood cells. That gene (called the P53 proofreader gene, if you're ever trying out for *Jeopardy!*) reads all the other genes to find the typos. Now, we know cancer is a dysfunctional neighbor—an evil neighbor, actually. So what it does is cut off the telephone lines so that you can't call your immune system cops to fight the thugs (remember, they're smart about ways to beat the system). In people with many forms of cancer, those cancer cells turn off the P53 gene.

While ordinarily the proofreader gene would stimulate the immune response to kill the weird cells, this mechanism doesn't work with people who have certain types of cancer cells—giving cancer a clear path to grow, develop, and damage your body. That's essentially how these hooligans are born—through mutation and the genetic coding that disarms the immune system's ability to rid the body of unwanted cells. You should note that the P53 gene requires vitamin D to function adequately, so one step in preventing cancer is getting adequate amounts of D (we'll discuss that more later). An interesting side note with potentially huge implications: In a study of rats with widespread metastatic cancer, when researchers found a way to turn the P53 proofreader genes back *on*, the cancer everywhere was killed.

It's also important to note how the oxidation process occurs. In many ways, oxidation is a good, naturally occurring process in your body. Your body needs oxidation for your immune system to work, for your body to protect itself. It helps kill off old cells to make room for new ones. So it's not a bad thing, but it has the potential to be bad. Cancer is part of the normal biological process that has gone a little awry. When oxidation turns bad, there's *too much* of it (your body's version of rusting); its products—free radicals—damage the DNA to cause malignant cells or inhibit the mechanism that can clear cancer cells from your body.

The Growth of Cancer Cells

Naturally, our immune system fights off most cancerous cells. So the logical first question is: Why wouldn't your body just call on the immune system to fight unwanted cells? Good question. In fact, your immune system does come in—and kills off many odd-looking cells, cells that have the potential to form cancer. That's why cancer-prevention measures like antioxidant-rich foods and vitamin D often work by strengthening your immune response. But your security network can be overwhelmed or even tricked. The challenge is that we don't quite know completely how our immune system works—why our immune system can fight some of these thug cells but not others. A rapidly growing area of research stems from the use of vaccines to prevent cancer, inasmuch as some cancers can be triggered by viral infections (hepatitis can lead to liver cancer, for example). It may turn out that viruses may play a more major role in the development and spread of cancer than anyone ever thought was possible.

In most cancerous mutations, these cells have some sort of genetic code that turns off your immune mechanisms, so they can grow quickly or avoid detection. But cancer cells can also have a mechanism that makes them replicate very efficiently—making cancer cells stronger and faster than the normal cells in your body. While they grow quickly, they can't grow by themselves. Just as a plant needs water or a child needs vitamins, cancer cells need nutrients to grow. The one thing that cancer cells want more than anything else is energy. If the cells don't get it, then they actually kill themselves off because they'd outgrow their energy supply. So the most successful cancers—the ones that grow large enough to be detected and to be harmful—often find ways to establish supply lines, such as attracting blood vessels to them. Once they create those supply lines, it's like an oxygen tank to someone under water—they have the means necessary to sustain themselves. And in cancer, that's what gives them a lifeline to live and grow. Since they're belligerent cells, cancer cells decide which blood vessels they want to take to other organs. They can surround regular tissue and dominate the organ they've invaded, and as they cluster together, they can form tumors—clumped masses

FACTOID

Some tumors don't have cancer cells; they're benign, but can still be dangerous. That's because tumors can grow to block off the pathway of important nutrients, or put pressure on critical organs. For example, even though many brain tumors will never spread, they are still removed.

of cancer cells—to block the normal functioning of that organ.

The Kinds of Cancer

The hundreds of types of cancers differ in the way they live, grow, and react to medication. But many cancers have similar characteristics. In some types of cancer, there are very clear causes. Lung cancer—the most common lethal cancer in both men and women—is overwhelmingly caused by cigarette smoke (though not all lung cancer is). More than 95 percent of people with lung cancer have smoked or been exposed to heavy doses of secondhand smoke, radon, or asbestos. What happens is, normal cells are repeatedly damaged by a toxin (in this case, hydrocarbons from the tobacco leaf that are formed with or without burning), so your lungs make new cells to repair and replace the damaged ones. The faster they need to work to replace and repair, the higher the likelihood that one of those typographical errors of duplication will take place—turning a normal cell into a bad one.

Though we don't know the primary causes of some cancers, like breast cancer, we do know that there's a large hereditary component involved and that an increased level of saturated and trans fat in your diet and obesity itself may influence cancer growth. Focus for these kinds of cancer needs to revolve around detection—by both self-exam as well as more sophisticated diagnostic testing (though prevention through getting more physical activity and taking folate and aspirin seem clear). Mammograms and PET scans are valuable tools for showing small tumors (though they don't prove cancer; only a biopsy can do that). And new tools for detection are constantly being developed. The routine operative breast endoscopy (ROBE), for instance, uses a viewing scope to magnify breast tissue up to sixty times its normal size

Myth or Fact? You can get heart cancer.

You never hear of heart cancer. That's because cancer rarely starts there. But the fact is, in end-stage cancer, there are actually cancer cells embedded in the heart quite frequently, which should not surprise us since cancers love energy-carrying blood.

and identify tumors 1/100th the size of what can be picked up on mammograms. With early detection of breast cancer, the treatment can usually be handled by a lumpectomy—the removal of the lump.

But not all cancers are tumors or lumps—making them even more difficult to diagnose. Blood-borne cancers such as leukemia are not like tumors in the usual sense. Instead, abnormal white blood cells accumulate in bone marrow and crowd or starve out healthy white and red blood cells—making your body unable to protect itself against infection and unable to deliver as much oxygen as you need. These blood-type cancers can destroy blood marrow and lymph nodes, and they destroy other cells that you need to live—up until the point that your blood marrow no longer contains healthy cells but consists completely of cancerous cells. A radical solution, which works for some cancers but not others, is to kill all the cells in your bone marrow and repopulate the remaining, barren terrain with bone marrow transplanted from a suitable donor.

The Spreading of Cancer

Cancer cells have a stealth quality to them. They don't possess the "sticky" quality that other cells have, so they can slip through their newly created blood vessels and spread to other parts of the body—very often to the liver, lungs, and brain—where metastases frequently occur. So, typically, cancer will escape to and grow in areas with lots of blood, which is why it's common for cancer from one area to jump and grow in another organ. And cancer loves traveling through the lymphatic system (the body's waste-disposal program) to the closest lymph nodes, which is why doctors always examine these areas carefully.

Cancer: The Live Younger Action Plan

Some of the most exciting research when it comes to cancer is in the world of genetics—that is, finding what cancer you're most prone to, given your family history and genetic makeup, and then having you make adjustments to your lifestyle to protect yourself against cancer growth. And maybe sometime in the future, we'll even be able to develop vaccines or other medications that can erase cancers by helping our immune system pick up their trail or by turning on defense mechanisms like the proofreader gene. But we're not there yet, which is why the most important thing you can do is to take your health into your own hands—and make decisions and choices about living in ways that will help prevent cancer. For example, sitting in the sun for long periods without sunscreen is the equivalent of sending an engraved invitation to cancer. And smoking? There is *such* a direct correlation between smoking and cancer you might as well take a syringe and shoot cancer cells right into your body. Tobacco doesn't just increase *lung* cancer, it's also been shown to increase the incidence of bladder, prostate, and breast cancers. And we know that some infectious diseases cause cancer, presumably because something in the interruption of the immune system promotes cancer growth.

With other cancers, we don't know their causes directly, but we do have some strong ideas about what can help prevent cancer. Most important: By following guidelines for keeping your heart and arteries young, you're also following a good prescription for preventing cancer. Obesity and inactivity have been linked to cancer, so eating a reasonable-calorie diet with the right kinds of foods and maintaining a physical activity program like the one we outline in this book are paramount for keeping your whole body young. You should also do these things to make sure your anatomical neighborhood is filled with good neighbors, not sinister ones.

Action 1: Fight with Nutrients

Some of the clearest evidence we have about preventing cancer comes in the form of food and nutrients. That is, in cases where avoidance isn't the first defense (like skin and lung cancer), nutrition is. Exterminators have their own set of chemicals, potions, and poisons they use to keep critters out of your house, but your cancer-fighting potions come in the form of a variety of nutrients and vitamins. For the ultimate cancer-preventing regimen, make sure to eat and supplement your diet with these ingredients.

VITAMIN D₃ Every proofreader needs a good dictionary and pair of eyes. Consider vitamin D to be the main tool in your proofreader's briefcase, because it appears to decrease immune aging and the incidence of cancer by strengthening the functioning of that proofreader gene. Though we're not sure this is the way it works, research has shown that vitamin D₃ does decrease the risk of cancer—in both epidemiological and test-tube studies. One theory is that a form of the vitamin actually kills cell mutations—meaning that D might be toxic to potentially cancerous cells. The second theory is that D bolsters the ability of the proofreader to spot cancerous cells and cause them to die—sort of acting like a magnifying glass for the proofreader gene. One form of vitamin D—D₃—helps make building blocks critical for healthy functioning of the P53 gene, which helps regulate proteins that have been shown to cause cancer when mutated. Most American adults don't get enough vitamin D (in fact, 30 to 40 percent may be deficient). We recommend getting 1,000 IU of vitamin D a day if you are sixty or younger and 1,200 IU if you're over sixty. You can take it in supplement form—or by drinking ten glasses of nonfat milk or fortified orange juice a day. (In addition, you can get some vitamin D through sunlight, as we discussed in Chapter 9. Spending ten to twenty minutes outside should give you proper levels in addition to the supplement, but we strongly believe in advising you to get your vitamin D through food and supplement and to wear SPF 45 and 4-star UVA protection every time you go out—even if the sun isn't shining.)

FOLATE Folate or folic acid, which is part of the B complex of vitamins, is often prescribed for pregnant women because it's essential for the normal development of the brain and spinal cord of the fetus. But when mothers started taking folate to prevent spina bifida (a specific birth defect), we also saw a 60 percent reduction in childhood cancers. A famous scientist, Bruce Ames, first hypothesized that folate helps prevent typographical errors when you duplicate your genes—by having enough folate, you supply enough T that the body doesn't miscopy it as a U. But folate is important for adults, too. If you don't get enough folate as an adult, that deficiency can lead to cancer. In four studies, folate supplementation decreased colon cancer rates by 20 to 50 percent, but more than 50 percent of Americans don't even get the recommended amount—and 90 percent don't get the amount that seems best to reduce colon cancer (800 micrograms a day).

Lots of foods—like spinach, tomatoes, and orange juice—contain folate, and many foods—like bread and cereal—are supplemented with it. But folate from food is absorbed less well than folic acid from supplements. When you consider that an eight-ounce glass of orange juice has only 43 micrograms of folate, that would mean you'd have to drink about twenty-five eight-ounce glasses of OJ a day to get the recommended amount. And when you consider that a slice of unsupplemented bread has only 6 micrograms of folate and spinach has only 2 micrograms, it's clear that you need to supplement. The average intake of folate through food is 275 to 375 micrograms, so you need a supplement of about 525 micrograms—to make cancer less likely. Unfortunately, there may be a downside. While folate prevents duplications and cancer, once you have the cancer, those bad cells need folate to grow fast. So at that point, supplemental folate may not be the best choice.

TOMATO PRODUCTS   Studies have shown that the risk of developing certain cancers decreases when you eat ten or more tablespoons a week of tomato or spaghetti sauce. The risk of developing prostate cancer is as much as one-third lower among men who frequently eat foods containing tomatoes or tomato paste. And studies have also shown that the risk of developing clinical breast cancer is 30 to 50 percent lower among women who frequently eat similar kinds of foods. Many believe that the active ingredient—the ingredient responsible for such astounding numbers—is lycopene, a carotenoid known for its antioxidant properties. Carotenoids work by attaching to free radicals (which can be cancer-causing) and packaging them so they can be washed out of the body so they don't damage cells or chromosomes. They may work in other ways, too. But they work, even if it seems magical. Tomato products all contain lots of lycopene, but it is more available to your body when it's cooked, and it's much better absorbed by your body when it's consumed with some fat. So it's important to eat tomato products with a little bit of olive oil or some nuts (not pepperoni) so you'll get some of the benefits. Eating more than ten servings of lycopene-rich products weekly can make your RealAge more than one year younger. One caution: We don't know for sure that it's the lycopene that gives cooked tomato products and sauces their cancer-preventing qualities, just that tomatoes reduce the risk of cancer. It could be another ingredient found in the tomato products.

SELENIUM   One of the trace minerals needed by our bodies, selenium largely comes from foods like garlic that absorb selenium from the soil. (Many fish, such as cod, herring, mackerel, and sardines, and Brazil nuts also have it.) One study showed a 50 percent reduction in cancer deaths among individuals who took 100 micrograms of selenium twice a day. Though there's still more work to be done, it does appear that taking selenium supplements may help reduce the incidence of cancer (but don't exceed 1,000 micrograms a day; you'll put yourself at risk of selenium toxicity). We wish we knew how it works, but the speculation centers around selenium helping power one of the main sanitation systems in your body that remove or detoxify harmful chemicals.

CRUCIFEROUS VEGETABLES LIKE BROCCOLI, BRUSSELS SPROUTS, CABBAGE, AND CAULIFLOWER These veggies have a chemical in them that prevents cancer. It's unclear whether they decrease cancer rates by turning on your immune system, by attacking the cancer, or by hindering the cancer cells from obtaining specialized nutrients. But it might be linked to two compounds found in these vegetables (for you *ER* junkies, they're indole-3 carbinol and sulforaphane). Whatever the mechanism, studies of patients with bladder cancer and gut cancer indicate it's likely that those eating seven or more nonfried servings (handfuls) of these veggies a week can prevent the growth of cancer by 50 percent.

OTHER VITAMINS Antioxidant vitamins in general quench the free radicals that can lead to miscopying of DNA and premature death of cells that force faster creation of new ones (and thus more chances for cancer-creating errors). Take 100 to 500 milligrams of vitamin C twice daily for boosting your immune system. Besides citrus fruits, vitamin C is also in berries, green vegetables, and tomatoes. And you can also take 400 IU of vitamin E daily (take it with vitamin C), because it helps reduce the risk of certain cancers. You can find E in wheat germ, nuts, and vegetable oils.

Action 2: Get Tested

It's safe to say that by now you know one of our main mottos: Organized medicine isn't responsible for your health; you are. *You're* responsible for your own healthy destiny. You make decisions regarding your health every day (fries or baked? stairs or elevator?), and you can influence how long and how well you live. But just because we've hammered home that message as if it's a box of carpenter nails, don't discount the important advances in medicine and the importance of having your health monitored by a professional. That's because cancer prevention isn't the same as cancer detection. Preventing the onset of the disease is our ultimate goal, but there's no guarantee you will. Bad luck and genes are important determinants in our lives—and our bodies as well. This is important because we don't want you to carry guilt with disease, but rather move on and fix the problem. That said, the next best goal is early detection. Early detection exponentially increases your chance of survival when diagnosed with cancer. We don't expect your garage to be filled with MRI scanners, syringes, or rubber gloves (unless you have a *serious* eBay problem), so it's important to know the best courses for early screening different types of cancer. One important note: Our screening guidelines are for people who have average risk factors. If you have a family history—especially if you have two first-degree relatives with certain kinds of cancer—it's crucial that you be screened at a much earlier age (twenty-five, in some cases).

Myth Buster #2

SKIN CANCER   The three main kinds of skin cancer (basal cell, squamous cell, and melanoma) originate from different cell types and therefore have very different behaviors. The one that really jumps around is melanoma, which is a peripatetic cell anyway. The basal and squamous cells are limited to the outer skin, so they invade locally; these are linked to sun exposure, while melanoma—the one most associated with risk of death—is not. Basal and squamous cell are very curable cancers that are usually treated by removal of the cancerous growth. Each kind of cancer has different physical characteristics, so keep a skin journal. That is, check your skin (and have a partner do the tough-to-see spots). If you notice any changes, that's the red flag that you need to have the blemish checked. We recommend that you get a skin screening by a dermatologist every year after age thirty. (If you're looking for a new project for your digital camera, you could even take photographs of any marks on your skin, upload the pictures, and then repeat the process every year. That's a good way to compare physical characteristics over time.) Plus, going to your doctor with a little ammunition like serial pictures of a mole will make the physician's decision easier, as he or she might not feel compelled to cut out every new skin change.

Myth Buster #3

Myth or Fact? If you're diagnosed with cancer, you need treatment right away.

While some cancer spreads quickly, it's always smart to get a second opinion. Although only 10 percent of patients get second opinions (even for serious diagnoses), 30 percent of second opinions change diagnosis or treatment. Good doctors will encourage you to get one—to confirm that the diagnosis is correct. The best second opinion comes from a doctor at a different institution from where your first doctor practices and one that is well regarded in cancer treatment. Even e–second opinions are available. After that, it's always best to see a specialist in the type of cancer you have because he or she will have a better handle on the different courses of treatment available.

BREAST CANCER   This is one case where family history is especially important. If you have two close relatives who've had either breast cancer or ovarian cancer, especially if it's before age forty, we recommend you start screening at age twenty-five.

But if you don't have a previous history, you should get a mammogram starting at age forty. And you should have one every year after that. Early mammograms don't prevent cancer, but if they detect it, and if it is caught early enough, breast cancer can be treated with the most conservative means—a lumpectomy and maybe some prophylactic treatment to lessen the chance of recurrence. While a self-exam is a very preliminary test without much reliability, it's a first step that can be taught to you by your gynecologist. Even now, new technologies are emerging to make early detection even more reliable.

PROSTATE CANCER   There's a reason why many men avoid physicals. It has nothing to do with disrobing in front of nurses or even the old turn-and-cough routine. It's about the rubber glove. The reason doctors insert a well-lubed and gloved finger into a man's rectum during a physical is to detect abnormal growths on the prostate—the gland that helps control the functions associated with urination and ejaculation. But there's a problem with the finger exam; doctors can't feel the whole prostate from that angle of insertion. So it's very possible that you could have a tumor on your prostate even if your doctor can't feel one during a manual exam. That's why it's important to have a PSA test (prostate-specific antigen test), which will help flag prostate cancer. Note: An elevated PSA doesn't mean you have cancer; an elevated level can also be associated with other conditions, like benign inflammation of the prostate. Only a biopsy can determine whether it's cancer or not. It is the change from your baseline value rather than the absolute number that interests the doctors; the trend can predict early cancer, which most responds to treatment. Get one at age fifty and every year after.

COLON CANCER   Most men and women should start having a Hemoccult test after age forty to screen for hidden blood in the stool (the tests are available in pharmacies). After fifty, you should have a colonoscopy every ten years to rule out

Food for Thought: Pop the Pill or Eat the Food?

Your car keys and the birthdays of all your nieces and nephews aren't the only things that are hard to keep track of. Advice is, too. We've given you a lot of information about foods and nutrients, so when do you get them from food and when do you visit the health store? Orange juice or vitamin C supplement? The easy answer is to take the pill, right? In some cases, that's right—it's been shown that the supplement form of a nutrient is powerful and is better absorbed than what's present in foods. But don't be misled into thinking that it's always better to down pills than to down vegetables. Orange juice has more in it than just vitamin C. And foods don't just have a biochemical importance; they create a kind of energy force in your body. For example, it may be quite possible that it's not one nutrient that helps prevent cancer or reduce heart disease but rather the combination of several ingredients that does it—and that's the kind of nutritional power you find only in the way nature makes food.

colon cancer and to detect polyps that could potentially turn into colon cancer. We know it's an invasive process—but newer virtual colonoscopies are improving dramatically—and if Katie Couric can do it in front of a national audience, you can do it on your own.

Action 3: Take the Almighty Aspirin

By now, you know that we think aspirin should have an airport—or at the very least, a long building—named after it, for all the good it can do. Just look at the stats: Taking 162 milligrams of aspirin a day can decrease the risk of getting colon cancer by 40 percent, the risk of breast cancer by 40 percent, and the risk of prostate cancer by 40 percent. And it's been shown to increase the risk of pancreatic cancer from two incidents in every hundred thousand people to only four incidents per hundred thousand. Though we don't know how aspirin decreases the incidence of cancer, we know that it does. Those benefits do not include its ability to prevent or reverse arterial aging. Just taking that half of a regular aspirin (or two baby aspirins) can make the RealAge average of a fifty-five-year-old 2.2 years younger. Take aspirin with a glass of warm water; it'll help dissolve the aspirin faster and decrease the risk of gastric side effects that occur when the aspirin lands directly on the stomach lining.

Chapter 13

The Owner's Manual Diet

So far, you've traveled all throughout the body—darting among neurons, streaking through arteries, and wading through intestines. Now that you've had an owner's view, we hope you realize the importance of everything that goes inside by understanding all the powerful effects food can have on preventing disease, on maintaining proper organ function, on helping you live a healthy life, and on keeping you feeling your best.

The Owner's Manual Diet will help you do that: this ten-day trial of delicious foods will not only satisfy your taste buds but also please all of your body's factories. It has more than thirty great-tasting recipes with all the right foods to fuel your body. After these ten days, you'll have a sense of how great healthy food can taste and how little effort eating this way takes. You'll also see how your body responds when you substitute nutrient-rich foods for the villainous ones.

Most diets, of course, focus on

one number: pounds lost. Why? Because so many people are obsessed about being overweight, about fitting into jeans, about impressing the casting director. But in the Owner's Manual Diet, we're not as concerned about the number of pounds lost. We're concerned about making you feel better, helping you live younger, and slowing the effects of aging. We feel it's more important to regulate other numbers and feelings in your life—things like your blood pressure, your waist size, your cholesterol and inflammation numbers, and your energy level. It is even possible to be overweight *and* fit if you make choices to control those things. Just to emphasize how important exercise is to health, we've included a Diet Activity Plan Crib Sheet (Table 13.1) that is just as easy to follow as the diet.

Now, it just so happens that one of the great side effects of this diet is that you

TABLE 13.1 The Owner's Manual Diet Activity Plan: Crib Sheet

Walking	30 minutes every day (or other general physical activity like swimming, if you cannot walk)
Stamina training (biking, swimming)	3 times a week, at a rate at which you are sweating for 20 minutes or are out of breath by the end
Resistance training	3 times a week, 10 minutes a day
Stretching or yoga	Every day, after walking
Deep breathing	Take 10 deep breaths every morning and night using the abdominal technique outlined in Chapter 5
Sleep	Plan time for 7 to 8 hours daily, and try our plan in Chapter 5 if you cannot sleep well

will lose weight on it, because these foods contain all the ingredients important to controlling weight. Of course, it's important to control obesity and make strides to living a healthy and active life, but we don't want you to panic if you don't lose fifty-three pounds in the next six hours. Even a ten-pound weight loss will have dramatic effects on your heart and blood pressure, your bones, your sex organs, and every other part of your body. And that's what makes this diet doable for the rest of your life. Some physicians even argue that obsessing over diets, pounds, and waist sizes is bad for your health, especially when you consider the inevitable cycle of fad diets—starve, binge, starve, binge. And the stress!

What we want is for you to relax about your weight. Enjoy and celebrate good, healthy foods described in our diet, and stop obsessing over points, pounds, and unfulfilled promises. Eat to feel good. Eat to live younger.

Try the Owner's Manual Diet for ten days. See how you feel. See how your body adjusts when it's fueled with the right balance of good food. And then make decisions about your long-term eating habits based on the guidelines we have outlined. We want you to develop an awareness of what you eat and the power of food so you can make your own choices. The way many of us eat today, it's as if our diets had been designed by the same people who designed the usual hospital gown. To us, changing your diet is like updating your home—whether it's modernizing an out-of-date kitchen, patching a hole in the roof, or even rearranging your furniture. You constantly update, upgrade, maintain, fix, and beautify your home, and you make those changes because you know they'll make your home function and feel better.

Don't you want the same for *you*?

The Owner's Manual Diet

If you learn nothing else about this diet (yes, we know we're repeating), understand this: The Owner's Manual Diet shouldn't be measured in pounds lost, but in the years younger you live and in the increased energy that you feel. The Owner's Manual Diet is designed so that you never feel hungry—and so that you have a right balance of nutrients for your long-term health. The Crib Sheet (Table 13.2) reminds you of the easy-to-follow rules for your diet (imagine all the basics on only one page). The diet tastes great and provides about 1,600 calories a day if you eat two of the breakfast choices, one lunch choice, one dinner choice, and two snacks, plus wine every day. This number is ideal for the medium body type. Keep in mind that the ideal daily calorie count for losing a pound a month is about nine times your ideal weight in pounds plus the calories you consume a day in physical activity. Here's a rough way to estimate your ideal weight: The preferable weight for a five-foot-tall person is roughly 100 pounds. You can add approximately five pounds per inch to calculate your ideal weight, so a six-foot person would have an ideal body weight of around 160 pounds. So, if your ideal weight is less than this, you can design a basic diet to provide around 1,600 calories a day using the selection formula above. You can even choose desserts intermittently as indicated. If your ideal body weight is 150 to 225 pounds, you can select an extra breakfast and/or lunch option depending on your daily physical activity.

Of course, there's also a more scientific way to calculate how much energy you burn per day (and thus how many calories you would need to consume in order to lose or maintain your weight). What you want to do is find your basal metabolic rate—your daily requirement of calories. Here's how:

Men
BMR = 66 + (13.7 × weight in kilograms) + (5 × height in centimeters)—
(6.8 × age in years)

Women
BMR = 655 + (9.6 × weight in kilograms) + (1.8 × height in centimeters)—
(4.7 × age in years)

TABLE 13.2 The Owner's Manual Diet Basics: Crib Sheet

Meal schedule	Eat when hungry, not famished, and make your last meal at least three hours before bed
Plate size	9 inches, not the usual 11- or 13-inch variety
Foods to eat daily	9 handfuls of fruits and vegetables; at least 1 ounce of nuts; whole-grain breads and cereals that contain fiber
Foods to eat at least three times a week	Fish (like line-caught salmon, mahi mahi, tilapia, catfish, and flounder)
Foods to eat weekly	10 tablespoons of cooked tomato products
Foods to avoid	(1) Processed foods that contain trans and saturated fats; (2) White foods like cream sauces, white bread, white rice, and simple sugar; (3) Products containing high-fructose corn syrup
To drink daily	64 ounces of water, 2 glasses skim or low-fat milk, 1 glass of wine (red or your other favorite choice, optional)
To take daily	(1) Multivitamin (taken with a little fat) that contains at least 400 micrograms of folate, 1,000 IU of vitamin D, 1200 milligrams of calcium, 400 milligrams of magnesium, and a daily value (DV) of all others; it's actually best for optimal body levels and absorption to take half of the total twice a day. (Reduce doses of vitamins C and E if you are taking a statin.) (2) Aspirin (taken with half a glass of warm water before and after); this dose can be two baby aspirin or half a regular-strength aspirin (162 milligrams), after age 40. (3) Omega-3 fatty acids (2 grams) or can be obtained by consuming 12 walnuts a day and fish as above, or 600 milligrams DHA capsules or fortified food.

★ To convert pounds to kilograms, divide by 2.2. To convert inches to centimeters, multiply by 2.54.

You should also factor in your activity level. Multiply your BMR by the following numbers:

Activity Level	Men	Women
Inactive: little or no activity	1.4	1.4
Light: some light daily exercise	1.5	1.5
Moderate: regular aerobic exercise	1.78	1.64
Heavy: energy-intensive job or serious athlete	2.1	1.82

Now you have the amount of calories you burn every day. Consume fewer calories than that, and you'll lose weight; consume more, and you'll gain it.

In the Owner's Manual Diet, you can pick breakfast, lunch, dinner, and snack recipes from our chart so you can design your diet around your own lifestyle—depending on how much time you have to prepare meals. For breakfast and lunch, at least one suggestion in each category requires either no or fewer than three minutes of preparation time. If you like to follow a stricter schedule, we also provide a ten-day sample diet with suggestions for what to eat every day. In the recipes that follow, you'll see the recipe's main benefit to a particular part of the body, but, of course, there's a lot of overlap: what's good for the heart, for example, can be good for your brain, for your senses, and for fighting cancer. And all the recipes follow the standards of being low in sodium, sugar, and saturated and trans fat—and high in taste.

BREAKFAST (Choose one or two)

★ Maple Oatmeal with Prunes and Plums   (PAGE 381)

★ Double Apple Cinnamon Smoothie   (PAGE 386)

★ Tunisian Egg Scramble   (PAGE 387)

★ Cheese Blintzes with Blueberry Lime Sauce   (PAGE 382)

★ Creamy Goat Cheese Omelet with Chives and Corn   (PAGE 385)

★ Huevos Rancheros Burritos with Chipotle, Chili Beans, and Corn   (PAGE 388)

★ Shiitake Mushroom and Asparagus Frittata with Smoked Salmon   (PAGE 384)

★ Raspberry-Orange Smoothie   (PAGE 383)

★ Double Strawberry Blender Blast   (PAGE 380)

★ Pineapple-Banana Frappé   (PAGE 379)

★ 1 slice toasted whole-wheat bread with 1 teaspoon peanut butter

★ 1 slice whole-wheat bread with 1 teaspoon apple or walnut butter

★ 2 to 3 hard-boiled eggs, no yolk

★ 2 pieces lean turkey, lean turkey sausage, tofu sausage, or veggie burgers

★ 1 cup Kashi High Fiber or cold oat cereal or 1 cup cooked oat cereal with 4 ounces of skim or low-fat soy milk

★ an egg-white omelet (3 egg whites) with ½ cup of sautéed vegetables

★ a 7-ounce Light 'n Fit smoothie with ¼ cup of fresh or frozen berries of your choice or 100 percent orange juice with pulp

SNACKS (one midmorning, one late afternoon)

★ Cacik   (PAGE 412)

★ Apple, plum, banana, or pear

★ Whole-grain cereal, dry, serving to be about 100 calories

★ Cut veggies

- ★ Sautéed veggies (sauté a week's worth of veggies in olive oil and season with salt, pepper, or garlic; store in refrigerator for snacks, as side dishes, or to use as part of recipes)
- ★ Low-fat yogurt covered with ½ cup canned unsweetened tangerines and some raisins
- ★ Nuts: 6 walnuts, or 12 almonds, or 12 cashews or pecans, or 20 peanuts, or ½ ounce unsalted roasted nuts; or ½ ounce real cocoa-based chocolate (before lunch; combine with any option)
- ★ ½ ounce nuts or real cocoa-based chocolate (before dinner)

And with all of the above choices: cup of coffee or tea and/or water

BEVERAGES

- ★ Cup of coffee, tea, or skim milk
- ★ Glass of water (or 100 percent orange juice with pulp with breakfast)
- ★ Glass of wine (with dinner)

LUNCH (Choose one)

- ★ *Tomato Bruschetta*   (PAGE 401)
- ★ *Grilled Vegetable Sandwich with Fresh Goat Cheese*   (PAGE 390)
- ★ *Persian Kidney Beans*   (PAGE 404)
- ★ *Pasta e Fagioli Soup*   (PAGE 394)
- ★ *Portuguese Bean Soup*   (PAGE 397)
- ★ *The Ultimate Chicken Soup*   (PAGE 392)
- ★ *Non-Caesar Caesar Salad (no egg)*   (PAGE 396)
- ★ *Grilled Tilapia with Asian Red Lentils and Kale*   (PAGE 405)
- ★ *Ginger, Carrot, and Orange Cappuccino Cup Soup*   (PAGE 398)
- ★ *Bowl of Edamame with Asian Salad*   (PAGE 391)
- ★ *Texas Slaw*   (PAGE 407)

- ★ *The Reds and Greens Parade*   (PAGE 408)
- ★ *Power Quesadillas*   (PAGE 409)
- ★ *Warm Teriyaki Beef with Pea Shoots*   (PAGE 399)
- ★ *Roasted Red Pepper and Kalamata Olive Sicilian Salad*   (PAGE 395)
- ★ *Dijon Chicken*   (PAGE 406)
- ★ *Guacamole*   (PAGE 400) and either *Roasted Tomato Basil Soup*   (PAGE 403) *or* ½ *Avocado Stuffed with Canned Salmon*   (PAGE 389)
- ★ *Broccoli Sandwich*   (PAGE 402) (or serve with an arugula and shaved fresh Parmesan salad, olive oil, lemon, pepper, and salt)
- ★ *Hearty Hummus Sandwich*   (PAGE 393) (can use 3 tablespoons per sandwich of store-bought hummus if you do not want to make your own)
- ★ *The Un-Bagel:* 1 piece whole-wheat toast, 1 ounce low-fat cream cheese, 2 ounces sliced or canned salmon, one onion slice, one tomato slice, capers
- ★ 3 cups (cut-up and colorful noniceberg) salad mixed with ¼ cup drained and washed garbanzo beans or chickpeas or four-bean salad with 1 or 2 tablespoons of balsamic vinegar / olive oil mix (2 parts vinegar to 1 part oil)
- ★ 3 cups (cut-up and colorful noniceberg) salad with ¼ cup canned salmon or ¼ cup cut-up grilled chicken added
- ★ Grilled veggie burger on toasted whole-grain English muffin with sliced tomato, red onion, ketchup, and romaine lettuce

DINNER (Choose one)

- ★ *Succulent Salmon and Salsa*   (PAGE 411)
- ★ *Salmon with Spinach and Mustard*   (PAGE 414)
- ★ *Grilled Chicken or Fish with Wasabi Mashed Potatoes with Caramelized Sweet Onions*   (PAGE 415)
- ★ *Warm Spinach Salad with Chicken, Apples, and Toasted Almonds*   (PAGE 413)
- ★ *Barbecued Red Snapper with Spicy Red Beans and Rice*   (PAGE 416)

- ★ Grilled Tuna Niçoise   (PAGE 417)
- ★ Smoked Mozzarella and Veggie–Stuffed Pizza   (PAGE 418)
- ★ Mandarin Chicken   (PAGE 419)
- ★ Roasted Chicken with Pesto Gemelli   (PAGE 420)
- ★ Tuscan Tuna with Grilled Tomato   (PAGE 421)
- ★ Teriyaki Tofu with Red Bell Pepper and Shiitakes over Whole-Grain Jasmine Rice   (PAGE 422)
- ★ Rainbow Shrimp Moo Shu Roll-ups   (PAGE 423)
- ★ Grill 4 ounces of your favorite fish or chicken breast, and add 1 cup of sautéed vegetables; serve with dinner salad with 2 tablespoons of balsamic vinegar/olive oil dressing (2 parts vinegar to 1 part oil)
- ★ Just for the Halibut   (PAGE 424)
- ★ Pasta with Heart   (PAGE 425)
- ★ Lovely Lamb   (PAGE 426)
- ★ Stir-fry Friday Favorite   (PAGE 427)
- ★ Raisin Curry Chicken   (PAGE 428)

DESSERT (one every three days)

- ★ Chocolate Soy Sundae Smoothie   (PAGE 429)
- ★ Chocolate Strawberry Sundae   (PAGE 430)
- ★ Maple-Cranberry–Topped Frozen Yogurt   (PAGE 431)

Suggested Ten-Day Schedule

Note: Two options are given for breakfast and lunch, because, depending on your ideal weight and calories consumed with physical activity, you may be eating two options in those categories. See next page.

	Day 1	Day 2
Breakfast	1 slice toasted whole-wheat bread with 1 teaspoon peanut butter **Pineapple-Banana Frappé** (page 379)	2 pieces lean turkey, lean turkey sausage, tofu sausage, or veggie burgers 1 cup Kashi High Fiber or cold oat cereal or 1 cup cooked oat cereal with 4 ounces of skim or low-fat soy milk
Midmorning snack	6 walnuts	Apple, plum, pear, or banana
Lunch	**Grilled Vegetable Sandwich with Fresh Goat Cheese** (page 390) 3 cups (cut-up and colorful noniceberg) salad with ¼ cup canned salmon or ¼ cup cut-up grilled chicken (page 371)	**Grilled Tilapia with Asian Red Lentils and Kale** (page 405) **The Un-Bagel** (page 371)
Midafternoon snack	Apple, plum, banana, or pear	**Cacik** (page 412) with cut veggies
Dinner	**Succulent Salmon and Salsa** (page 411) **Chocolate Soy Sundae Smoothie** (page 429)	**Warm Spinach Salad with Chicken, Apples, and Toasted Almonds** (page 413)

	Day 3	Day 4
Breakfast	**Maple Oatmeal with Prunes and Plums** (page 381) 2 to 3 hard-boiled eggs, no yolk	**Cheese Blintzes with Blueberry Lime Sauce** (page 382) 7-ounce Light 'n Fit smoothie with ¼ cup fresh or frozen berries of your choice or 100 percent orange juice with pulp
Midmorning snack	Banana	Orange
Lunch	**Hearty Hummus Sandwich** (page 393) 3 cups (cut-up and colorful noniceberg) salad mixed with ¼ cup drained and washed garbanzo beans (chickpeas) or four-bean salad with 1 or 2 tablespoons of balsamic vinegar/olive oil mix (2 parts balsamic to 1 part oil) (page 371)	**Pasta e Fagioli Soup** (page 394) 3 cups (cut-up and colorful noniceberg) salad with ¼ cup grilled, smoked, or canned salmon or ¼ cup cut-up grilled chicken (page 371)
Midafternoon snack	Whole-grain cereal, dry, serving to be about 100 calories	Pear, peach, apple, or banana
Dinner	**Barbecued Red Snapper with Spicy Red Beans and Rice** (page 416)	**Grilled Tuna Niçoise** (page 417) **Chocolate Strawberry Sundae** (page 430)

	Day 5	Day 6
Breakfast	1 slice toasted whole-wheat bread with 1 teaspoon apple or almond butter **Raspberry-Orange Smoothie** (page 383)	2 pieces lean turkey, lean turkey sausage, tofu sausage, or veggie burgers **Shiitake Mushroom and Asparagus Frittata with Smoked Salmon** (page 384)
Midmorning snack	6 walnuts	**Cacik** (page 412) with cut veggies
Lunch	**Roasted Red Pepper and Kalamata Olive Sicilian Salad** (page 395) **Dijon Chicken** (page 406)	**Non-Caesar Caesar Salad (no egg)** (page 396) **or Portuguese Bean Soup** (page 397) **The Un-Bagel** (page 371)
Midafternoon snack	Apple or cut veggies	6 walnuts, or 12 cashews or pecans, or 20 peanuts, or ½ ounce unsalted roasted nuts; or ½ ounce real cocoa-based chocolate
Dinner	**Smoked Mozzarella and Veggie–Stuffed Pizza** (use sautéed vegetables) (page 418) *or* Grill 4 ounces of your favorite fish or chicken breast, and add 1 cup of sautéed vegetables (page 371)	**Mandarin Chicken** (page 419)

	Day 7	Day 8
Breakfast	**Huevos Rancheros Burritos with Chipotle, Chili Beans, and Corn** (page 388) *or* 2 to 3 hard-boiled eggs, no yolk	**Creamy Goat Cheese Omelet with Chives and Corn** (page 385) 1 cup Kashi High Fiber or cold oat cereal or 1 cup cooked oat cereal with 4 ounces of skim or low-fat soy milk
Midmorning snack	6 walnuts	Low-fat yogurt covered with ½ cup of canned unsweetened tangerines and some raisins
Lunch	**Bowl of Edamame with Asian Salad** (page 391) *or* **Warm Teriyaki Beef with Pea Shoots** (page 399)	**Guacamole** (page 400) Grilled veggie burger on toasted whole-grain English muffin with sliced tomato, red onion, ketchup, romaine lettuce (page 371)
Midafternoon snack	1 cup whole-grain cereal	Apple, plum, pear, or banana
Dinner	**Roasted Chicken with Pesto Gemelli** (page 420) *or* Grill 4 ounces of your favorite fish or chicken breast, and add 1 cup of sautéed vegetables (page 371)	**Tuscan Tuna with Grilled Tomato** (page 421) *or* Grill 4 ounces of your favorite fish or chicken breast, and add 1 cup of sautéed vegetables (page 371)

	Day 9	Day 10
Breakfast	2 pieces lean turkey, lean turkey sausage, tofu sausage, or veggie burgers **Double Apple Cinnamon Smoothie** (page 386)	**Tunisian Egg Scramble** (page 387) Egg-white omelet (3 egg whites) with ½ cup of sautéed vegetables
Midmorning snack	Sautéed veggies	6 walnuts, or 12 cashews or pecans, or 20 peanuts or ½ ounce roasted unsalted nuts
Lunch	**Tomato Bruschetta** (page 401) **Broccoli Sandwich** (page 402) or serve with arugula and shaved fresh Parmesan salad; olive oil, lemon, pepper, and salt	Either **Roasted Tomato Basil Soup** (page 403) or ½ **Avocado Stuffed with Canned Salmon** (page 389) **Persian Kidney Beans** (page 404)
Midafternoon snack	**Cacik** (page 412) with cut veggies	6 walnuts, or 12 cashews or pecans, or 20 peanuts; or ½ ounce unsalted roasted nuts
Dinner	**Teriyaki Tofu with Red Bell Pepper and Shiitakes over Whole-Grain Jasmine Rice** (page 422) *or* Grill 4 ounces of your favorite fish or chicken breast, and add 1 cup of sautéed vegetables (page 371)	**Rainbow Shrimp Moo Shu Roll-ups** (page 423) *or* Grill 4 ounces of your favorite fish or chicken breast, and add 1 cup of sautéed vegetables (page 371) **Maple-Cranberry–Topped Frozen Yogurt** (page 431)

The Owner's Manual Diet: The Recipes

Taste Note: Every recipe was selected for both its appeal to taste buds and its ease of preparation (less than thirty minutes, and by twenty naive-about-cooking medical students, nonetheless). All recipes were tested repeatedly by amateurs and professional chefs—in at least five groups of eight to twelve people. Each recipe was tested on a rating scale (see below) and scored at least an 8. These are the top-rated recipes from more than 350 tested—made only from ingredients that make your RealAge younger. Special thanks to Dr. John La Puma and the chefs he worked with at the Frontera Grill and Kendall College of Nutrition in Chicago. For more recipes, go to www.RealAge.com.

The Rating Scale

Based on Taste, Color, and Texture:	Rating
I wouldn't feed this to my neighbor's dog—even the one that keeps me up all night.	0
I wouldn't send this back at a restaurant, but I wouldn't order it again either.	6
I'd order this again at a restaurant.	8
This is almost as good as great sex. We said *almost*.	10

Breakfast

PINEAPPLE-BANANA FRAPPÉ

1 large ripe banana

½ cup low-fat (1 percent) soy milk or skim cow's milk with a touch of vanilla flavoring

½ can (4 ounces) crushed pineapple in juice, undrained

½ cup pineapple passion sorbet

Peel banana; break into chunks. Combine all ingredients in blender container. Cover; blend until fairly smooth.

2 SERVINGS

MODIFICATIONS You can modify the frappé and decrease the simple carbohydrate load by adding a scoop of soy protein powder and 1 tablespoon of flaxseed oil; you can also add 1 cup of pineapple chunks (packed in water) straight from a can or 1 cup of frozen mango chunks as a substitute for the sorbet.

HORMONES Potassium in bananas has been shown to help regulate blood pressure, which plays a key role in many hormonal functions.

NUTRITIONAL INFORMATION, PER SERVING	
CALORIES:	175
FAT:	0.8 GRAM
AGING FATS:	0.5 GRAM
FIBER:	12.1 GRAMS
CARBOHYDRATES:	38 GRAMS
PROTEIN:	3 GRAMS
SODIUM:	31 MILLIGRAMS
POTASSIUM:	428 MILLIGRAMS

Body Benefit

DOUBLE STRAWBERRY BLENDER BLAST

1½ cups (6 ounces) hulled, halved fresh strawberries
½ cup fat-free or light soy milk or skim cow's milk with a touch of vanilla
    flavoring
½ cup (3 ounces) strawberry sorbet

Combine strawberries and milk in blender container. Cover and blend until fairly smooth. Add sorbet; cover and blend until smooth and thick.

2 SERVINGS

MODIFICATIONS You can decrease simple carbohydrate load by adding a scoop of soy protein powder and 1 tablespoon of flaxseed oil; or you can add 1 cup of pineapple chunks (packed in water) straight from a can or 1 cup of frozen mango chunks as a substitute for the sorbet.

NUTRITIONAL INFORMATION, PER SERVING	
CALORIES:	103
FAT:	0.5 GRAM
AGING FATS:	0.2 GRAM
FIBER:	5.3 GRAMS
CARBOHYDRATES:	35.3 GRAMS
PROTEIN:	5.4 GRAMS
SODIUM:	18 MILLIGRAMS
POTASSIUM:	374 MILLIGRAMS

HORMONES Potassium and antioxidants in strawberries have been shown to help regulate blood pressure, which plays a key role in many hormonal functions.

Body Benefit

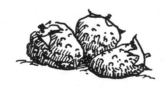

MAPLE OATMEAL WITH PRUNES AND PLUMS

1½ cups fat-free milk
1½ cups old-fashioned oats, uncooked
¼ cup apple cider or juice
2 small plums, seeded and diced
½ cup dried prunes, diced
⅛ ounce sliced almonds
1½ tablespoons pure maple syrup
⅛ teaspoon ground cinnamon

Bring milk to a simmer in a medium saucepan; mix in oats and simmer 5 to 8 minutes or until thickened, stirring once or twice. Stir in apple cider, then plums, prunes, almonds, syrup, and cinnamon; heat through. Serve in bowls.

2 SERVINGS

DIGESTIVE SYSTEM
Oatmeal and fruit contain fiber to keep your digestive system running smoothly.

Body Benefit

NUTRITIONAL INFORMATION, PER SERVING	
CALORIES:	519
FAT:	9.1 GRAMS
AGING FATS:	2.4 GRAMS
FIBER:	10.5 GRAMS
CARBOHYDRATES:	96.9 GRAMS
PROTEIN:	18.3 GRAMS
SODIUM:	1,011 MILLIGRAMS
POTASSIUM:	1,069 MILLIGRAMS

CHEESE BLINTZES WITH BLUEBERRY LIME SAUCE

¾ cup light ricotta cheese

½ package (5 ounces) light silken tofu

⅛ teaspoon salt

½ pint (6 ounces, about 1 cup) fresh blueberries

2½ tablespoons whole-fruit blueberry preserves

4 prepared crepes

Cooking oil spray

½ lime

Heat oven to 400 degrees. In a medium bowl, whisk together ricotta cheese, tofu, and salt. Stir ¼ cup blueberries into cheese mixture; set aside remaining ¾ cup blueberries for sauce. Spread 1½ tablespoons of the preserves (about 1 teaspoon per crepe) thinly over bottom half of crepes. Spread the cheese mixture over preserves. Fold both sides of crepe in 1 inch over filling, then roll up completely to enclose filling. Coat a 9-×-13-inch baking or casserole dish with cooking spray. Arrange blintzes in dish, seam side down. Cover dish with foil; bake 10 minutes or until warm.

Meanwhile, finely grate or zest 1 teaspoon lime peel from the lime; set aside. Squeeze enough lime juice from lime to measure 1 tablespoon. Combine reserved blueberries, lime juice, and remaining 1 tablespoon preserves in medium saucepan. Bring to a simmer; simmer gently 3 to 4 minutes or until berries pop and mixture is slightly thickened, stirring occasionally. Transfer blintzes to 2 serving plates; top with blueberry sauce and sprinkle with lime zest.

2 SERVINGS

BONES Calcium in cheese helps build bones.

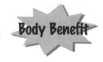
Body Benefit

NUTRITIONAL INFORMATION, PER SERVING	
CALORIES:	352
FAT:	5.6 GRAMS
AGING FATS:	2.9 GRAMS
FIBER:	4.7 GRAMS
CARBOHYDRATES:	63.3 GRAMS
PROTEIN:	26.6 GRAMS
SODIUM:	401 MILLIGRAMS
POTASSIUM:	446 MILLIGRAMS

RASPBERRY-ORANGE SMOOTHIE

1 cup nonfat or 1 percent vanilla soy milk

1 medium ripe banana

1 cup frozen raspberries

1 tablespoon frozen orange juice concentrate or ½ cup 100 percent orange
    juice with 1 ice cube

Combine all ingredients in blender. Cover; blend until smooth.

2 SERVINGS

IMMUNE SYSTEM

Vitamin C, antioxidants, and
flavonoids help boost your
immune system.

Body Benefit

NUTRITIONAL INFORMATION, PER SERVING	
CALORIES:	253
FAT:	0.2 GRAM
AGING FATS:	0.1 GRAM
FIBER:	5.3 GRAMS
CARBOHYDRATES:	28 GRAMS
PROTEIN:	4.8 GRAMS
SODIUM:	15 MILLIGRAMS
POTASSIUM:	584 MILLIGRAMS

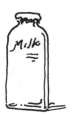

SHIITAKE MUSHROOM AND ASPARAGUS FRITTATA WITH SMOKED SALMON

Butter-flavored cooking oil spray or olive oil in a mister

3 ounces shiitake mushrooms, stems discarded, caps sliced

3 ounces asparagus spears, trimmed and cut into 1-inch pieces

2 large egg whites

½ large egg

1½ tablespoons fat-free soy milk or skim cow's milk

1 tablespoon plus 1 teaspoon chopped fresh dill

⅛ teaspoon salt

⅛ teaspoon freshly ground pepper

2 ounces smoked salmon, coarsely chopped

1 tablespoon reduced-fat sour cream

Heat an ovenproof, slope-slided, 10-inch nonstick skillet coated with cooking oil spray, over medium heat. Add mushrooms and asparagus; cook 5 minutes, stirring occasionally. Preheat broiler. In a medium bowl beat together egg whites, egg, milk, 1 tablespoon dill, salt, and pepper. Stir in smoked salmon; pour mixture into skillet over vegetables; mix well. Press vegetables down into an even layer under the egg mixture. Cook without stirring until eggs are set on bottom, about 4 minutes (center will be wet). Transfer to broiler; broil 4 to 5 inches from heat for 2 minutes or until eggs are set. Cut into wedges. Drop spoonfuls of sour cream on wedges, and sprinkle remaining dill over frittata before serving.

2 SERVINGS

BRAIN Omega-3 fatty acids found in salmon have been shown to increase brain function.

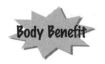
Body Benefit

NUTRITIONAL INFORMATION, PER SERVING	
CALORIES:	108
FAT:	3.9 GRAMS
AGING FATS:	1.8 GRAMS
FIBER:	1.3 GRAMS
CARBOHYDRATES:	5 GRAMS
PROTEIN:	13.7 GRAMS
SODIUM:	805 MILLIGRAMS
POTASSIUM:	439 MILLIGRAMS

CREAMY GOAT CHEESE OMELET WITH CHIVES AND CORN

Cooking oil spray, or olive oil in a mister
¼ cup fresh or thawed frozen corn kernels
3 large egg whites
1 large egg
2 tablespoons nonfat soy milk or skim milk
¼ teaspoon salt
¼ teaspoon freshly ground pepper
4 tablespoons (1 ounce) crumbled goat or herbed goat cheese
1 tablespoon plus 1 teaspoon chopped fresh chives

Heat a large nonstick skillet over medium heat, coated lightly with cooking oil spray, until hot. Add corn; cook 2 to 3 minutes or until corn begins to brown, stirring occasionally. In a medium bowl, beat together egg whites, egg, milk, salt, and pepper. Add to skillet and cook for 2 minutes or until eggs begin to set on bottom. Gently lift edges with spatula to allow uncooked portion of eggs to flow to edges and set. Continue cooking for 2 minutes or until center is almost set. Scatter 3 tablespoons of cheese and 1 tablespoon chives over the egg mixture. Reserve remaining 1 tablespoon cheese and 1 teaspoon chives for garnish. Using a large spatula, fold one half of omelet over the filling; cook 1 minute or until cheese is melted. Cut in half; transfer to serving dishes and garnish with remaining cheese and chives.

2 SERVINGS

BONES Calcium in cheese and calcium, vitamin D, and magnesium in milk help build bones.

Body Benefit

NUTRITIONAL INFORMATION, PER SERVING

CALORIES:	140
FAT:	5.6 GRAMS
AGING FATS:	3.6 GRAMS
FIBER:	0.9 GRAM
CARBOHYDRATES:	10.6 GRAMS
PROTEIN:	12.2 GRAMS
SODIUM:	462 MILLIGRAMS
POTASSIUM:	198 MILLIGRAMS

DOUBLE APPLE CINNAMON SMOOTHIE

¼ cup frozen apple juice concentrate, not thawed

½ cup cinnamon applesauce

¾ cup vanilla or plain fat-free or light soy milk

¾ cup low-fat vanilla frozen yogurt

⅛ teaspoon apple pie spice

Combine all ingredients in blender container. Cover; blend at high speed for 1 minute. Pour into frosty mugs, if desired.

2 SERVINGS

HORMONES   Cinnamon increases insulin receptivity.

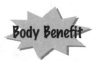

Body Benefit

NUTRITIONAL INFORMATION, PER SERVING	
CALORIES:	204
FAT:	3.4 GRAMS
AGING FATS:	1.3 GRAMS
FIBER:	2.7 GRAMS
CARBOHYDRATES:	34.9 GRAMS
PROTEIN:	9.1 GRAMS
SODIUM:	266 MILLIGRAMS
POTASSIUM:	566 MILLIGRAMS

TUNISIAN EGG SCRAMBLE

1 medium poblano chili
1 teaspoon olive oil
¼ cup chopped onion
2½ large egg whites
1 large egg
¼ teaspoon salt
¼ teaspoon ground cumin
⅛ teaspoon paprika
⅛ cup chopped pitted Kalamata olives
⅛ cup golden raisins
⅛ cup flat-leaf parsley
2 whole-wheat pitas

Heat broiler. Split chili in half; discard stems and seeds. Place cut side down on foil-lined baking sheet. Broil 3 to 4 inches from heat source until skin blackens, about 8 minutes. Wrap chili in foil; let cool 5 minutes. Unwrap chili; discard blackened skin and cut into strips. Meanwhile, heat a large nonstick skillet over medium-high heat. Add oil, then onion; cook 4 minutes, stirring occasionally. Beat together egg whites, egg, salt, cumin, and paprika; add to skillet and cook 1 minute, stirring constantly. Stir into egg mixture slices of chili, olives, raisins, and parsley. Continue cooking until eggs reach desired doneness. Serve in pita bread.

2 SERVINGS

HEART AND ARTERIES

The B vitamins help lower homocysteine levels, and olive oil helps keep arteries clear.

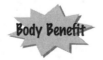
Body Benefit

NUTRITIONAL INFORMATION, PER SERVING	
CALORIES:	246
FAT:	8.1 GRAMS
AGING FATS:	3 GRAMS
FIBER:	2.1 GRAMS
CARBOHYDRATES:	32 GRAMS
PROTEIN:	13.5 GRAMS
SODIUM:	752 MILLIGRAMS
POTASSIUM:	286 MILLIGRAMS

HUEVOS RANCHEROS BURRITOS WITH CHIPOTLE, CHILI BEANS, AND CORN

8 ounces chili beans in spicy sauce, undrained

½ cup frozen whole kernel corn

⅛ cup salsa, preferably chipotle

1½ large egg whites

1 large egg

1 tablespoon low-fat sour cream

Cooking spray

2 large (10-inch) flour tortillas (even better made with corn or whole-wheat tortillas)

⅛ cup chopped cilantro

In a medium saucepan, combine beans, corn, and salsa. Bring to a boil over high heat; reduce heat and simmer uncovered for 5 minutes. Beat together egg whites, egg, and sour cream. Heat a large nonstick skillet, coated with cooking spray, over medium-high heat until hot. Add egg mixture; cook, stirring occasionally, until eggs are set. Break into chunks and stir in bean mixture. Stack tortillas on clean kitchen towels. Sprinkle a few drops of water on the top of tortillas. Fold tortillas up into the towel; heat in microwave oven for 20 seconds. Place tortillas on 2 serving plates and divide egg mixture between them. Top with cilantro, and roll tortillas, burrito-style.

2 SERVINGS

DIGESTIVE SYSTEM

Beans are important sources of digestive-friendly fiber. Remember the Beano.

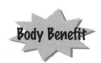
Body Benefit

NUTRITIONAL INFORMATION, PER SERVING	
CALORIES:	446
FAT:	11.3 GRAMS
AGING FATS:	3.5 GRAMS
FIBER:	8.6 GRAMS
CARBOHYDRATES:	68.3 GRAMS
PROTEIN:	19.1 GRAMS
SODIUM:	928 MILLIGRAMS
POTASSIUM:	279 MILLIGRAMS

Lunch

AVOCADO STUFFED WITH CANNED SALMON

1 tablespoon canola oil mayonnaise
1 medium ripe avocado
½ cup canned salmon
Pinch of dried oregano
¼ small onion, chopped fine
Splash of wine vinegar
Salt and pepper to taste

Drain salmon, and mix with canola oil mayonnaise. Add oregano, onion, vinegar, and spices, and blend lightly. Slice and seed avocado, removing half of pulp for guacamole, and stuff remainder of avocado "shell" with salmon mixture.

2 SERVINGS

IMMUNE SYSTEM
Avocados provide healthy
anti-inflammatory fat.

Body Benefit

NUTRITIONAL INFORMATION,
PER SERVING

Calories:	210
Fat:	17.2 grams
Aging Fats:	1.8 grams
Fiber:	3.4 grams
Sugar:	0.8 grams
Carbohydrates:	4.3 grams
Protein:	10.9 grams
Sodium:	280 milligrams
Potassium:	407 milligrams

GRILLED VEGETABLE SANDWICH WITH FRESH GOAT CHEESE

½ large yellow summer squash

½ large zucchini

½ small eggplant or white eggplant

½ large red or orange bell pepper

¾ tablespoon garlic-infused olive oil

½ teaspoon dried thyme leaves

⅛ teaspoon salt

⅛ teaspoon freshly ground black pepper

4 slices dark rye or pumpernickel bread

Cooking oil spray or olive oil in a mister

½ cup (3½ ounces) crumbled feta or other soft goat cheese

1 teaspoon chopped fresh thyme (optional)

Trim ends and cut yellow and zucchini squash lengthwise into ¼-inch-thick slices. Trim end and cut eggplant lengthwise into four ½-inch-thich slices (reserve any remaining eggplant for another use). Cut bell pepper lengthwise into quarters; discard stem and seeds. Combine oil and dried thyme leaves; brush lightly over both sides of the vegetables and sprinkle with salt and pepper. Grill vegetables over medium-hot coals or in a ridged grill pan (in batches) over medium-high heat 4 to 5 minutes per side, or until vegetables are tender. During last 2 minutes of cooking, coat bread lightly with cooking oil spray and place around outer edges of grill to toast (or grill in the ridged grill pan after the vegetables cook). Top 2 slices of the bread with the vegetables; sprinkle with cheese and thyme. Close sandwiches.

2 SERVINGS

NUTRITIONAL INFORMATION, PER SERVING	
CALORIES:	245
FAT:	9 GRAMS
AGING FATS:	4.3 GRAMS
FIBER:	5.3 GRAMS
CARBOHYDRATES:	35 GRAMS
PROTEIN:	7.7 GRAMS
SODIUM:	427 MILLIGRAMS
POTASSIUM:	464 MILLIGRAMS

HEART AND ARTERIES   Garlic, folic acid, and monounsaturated fat in the olive oil help keep arteries clear, while the vegetables have many disease-preventing characteristics.

EDAMAME WITH ASIAN SALAD

1 cup frozen edamame
1 cup chopped lettuce
1 cup shredded cabbage
1 tablespoon sesame seeds
1 large carrot, shredded
1 scallion, chopped

Dressing:
½ cup rice vinegar
¼ teaspoon sesame oil
1 teaspoon ponzu sauce
1 tablespoon canola oil
1 teaspoon grated fresh ginger
½ teaspoon sugar

Boil edamame until tender and salt to taste. Combine salad ingredients and add the dressing.

2 SERVINGS

DIGESTIVE SYSTEM
Soybeans and fiber in salad facilitate gut health.

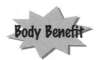

NUTRITIONAL INFORMATION, PER SERVING	
Calories:	275
Fat:	16.7 grams
Aging fats:	1.8 grams
Fiber:	7.3 grams
Carbohydrates:	22.7 grams
Protein:	14 grams
Sodium:	24 milligrams
Potassium:	807 milligrams

THE ULTIMATE CHICKEN SOUP

1 whole chicken (3 to 3½ pounds), skinned, with visible fat removed
Sea salt to taste
Freshly cracked black pepper to taste
1 large carrot, peeled
1½ stalks celery
1½ small onions, peeled but left whole
2 or 3 Yukon Gold potatoes
½ medium turnip
½ bunch of fresh thyme

Place the chicken in large soup pot (one big enough to later hold chicken plus all other ingredients, with at least 4 inches left at the top) and cover it with water. Bring to a light boil over medium-high heat. Reduce the heat to a gentle simmer. Cook, skimming occasionally, for 1 hour, or until the chicken is tender enough to pull easily from the bone. Use a pair of large tongs and a large ladle to remove the chicken from the pot, holding it over the pot for a few seconds to allow chicken cavity to drain. Remove bones and skin, discard, then set chicken meat aside. Season the chicken broth with salt and pepper, then place the chicken meat back in the pot with the vegetables; add water to cover everything by an inch or two. Bring to a simmer and cook, skimming occasionally, for 1 hour. Add the fresh thyme during the last 10 minutes of cooking. Cut up vegetables with ladle while cooking in pot, if you prefer; or wait until soup has cooled, then cut and reheat before serving.

2 SERVINGS

IMMUNE SYSTEM Chicken soup has been found to be one of the three things that decrease the length of the common cold.

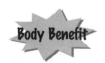
Body Benefit

NUTRITIONAL INFORMATION, PER SERVING	
CALORIES:	343
FAT:	3.4 GRAMS
AGING FATS:	1.3 GRAMS
FIBER:	6.4 GRAMS
CARBOHYDRATES:	48 GRAMS
PROTEIN:	29.9 GRAMS
SODIUM:	80 MILLIGRAMS
POTASSIUM:	1,500 MILLIGRAMS

HEARTY HUMMUS SANDWICHES

½ large garlic clove, peeled

½ can (8 ounces) chickpeas (garbanzo beans), rinsed and drained

1 tablespoon lemon juice

½ tablespoon extra-virgin olive oil

½ teaspoon dark sesame oil

¼ teaspoon ground cumin

⅛ teaspoon salt

¼ cup (2 ounces) low-fat silken tofu

1½ tablespoons chopped fresh mint

2 (6-inch) whole-wheat pita pockets

1 cup mesclun

¼ cup thinly sliced radishes

With motor running, drop garlic clove through tube of food processor and process until minced. Add chickpeas; process until finely chopped. Add lemon juice, olive oil, sesame oil, cumin, and salt; process 30 seconds. Add tofu; process until smooth. Stir in mint.

Cut each pita in half; open pockets. Stuff pockets with half the mesclun and radishes; top with hummus, then add remaining mesclun and radishes.

2 SERVINGS

BONES Tofu contains calcium for stronger bones.

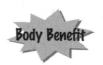
Body Benefit

NUTRITIONAL INFORMATION, PER SERVING	
CALORIES:	353
FAT:	8.6 GRAMS
AGING FATS:	2.3 GRAMS
FIBER:	3.9 GRAMS
CARBOHYDRATES:	82.4 GRAMS
PROTEIN:	30.6 GRAMS
SODIUM:	526 MILLIGRAMS
POTASSIUM:	1,093 MILLIGRAMS

PASTA E FAGIOLI SOUP

½ teaspoon olive oil

1 carrot, thinly sliced

2 garlic cloves, minced

⅛ teaspoon crushed red pepper flakes

1½ cups low-salt vegetable or chicken broth

¼ cup uncooked whole-wheat gemelli (small twisted pasta)

½ can (8 ounces) seasoned diced tomatoes, undrained

½ can (8 ounces) kidney or red beans, rinsed and drained

¼ cup frozen baby peas, thawed

⅛ cup chopped fresh basil

⅛ cup grated Romano or Asiago cheese

Heat a large saucepan over medium heat. Add olive oil and carrot slices; cook 2 minutes. Stir in garlic and red pepper flakes; cook 1 minute. Add broth and pasta; bring to a boil over high heat. Reduce heat; simmer 10 minutes. Stir in tomatoes and beans; return to a simmer and cook 5 minutes or until pasta is tender. Stir in peas; heat through. Ladle into shallow bowls; top with basil and cheese.

2 SERVINGS

SEX ORGANS Lycopene, folate, and perhaps selenium, found in tomato products and garlic, help protect the sex organs.

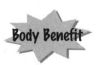
Body Benefit

NUTRITIONAL INFORMATION, PER SERVING

CALORIES:	268
FAT:	3.5 GRAMS
AGING FATS:	0.7 GRAM
FIBER:	8.9 GRAMS
CARBOHYDRATES:	40.9 GRAMS
PROTEIN:	19.3 GRAMS
SODIUM:	684 MILLIGRAMS
POTASSIUM:	888 MILLIGRAMS

ROASTED RED PEPPER AND KALAMATA OLIVE SICILIAN SALAD

1½ cups packed romaine lettuce

1½ cups escarole or curly endive

½ jar (3½ ounces) roasted red bell peppers, drained, cut into short, thin strips

½ cup yellow tomatoes

4 pitted Kalamata olives, halved

⅛ cup golden raisins

1½ tablespoons white balsamic vinegar

¾ tablespoon extra-virgin olive oil

Salt to taste

Freshly ground black pepper to taste

1 tablespoon crumbled feta or other soft goat cheese (optional)

In a large bowl, combine lettuce, escarole, bell peppers, tomatoes, olives, and raisins. Combine vinegar and oil; add to lettuce mixture. Toss well and season with salt and pepper to taste. Transfer to 2 plates. Top with cheese, if desired.

2 SERVINGS

HEART AND ARTERIES

Olives contain high amounts of monounsaturated fats, which help keep arteries clear. The flavonoids from many ingredients also help the arteries stay young.

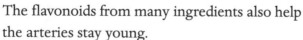

Body Benefit

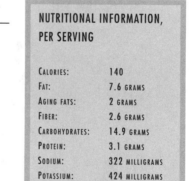

NUTRITIONAL INFORMATION, PER SERVING	
CALORIES:	140
FAT:	7.6 GRAMS
AGING FATS:	2 GRAMS
FIBER:	2.6 GRAMS
CARBOHYDRATES:	14.9 GRAMS
PROTEIN:	3.1 GRAMS
SODIUM:	322 MILLIGRAMS
POTASSIUM:	424 MILLIGRAMS

NON-CAESAR CAESAR SALAD (NO EGG)

1 cup romaine lettuce
Juice of ½ lemon (roll the lemon first)
2 tablespoons olive oil
½ teaspoon Dijon mustard
Dash Worcestershire sauce
1 garlic clove (pressed or minced)
Pinch of sugar
Salt and pepper to taste
Anchovies (optional)

Place lettuce in a large bowl. Combine lemon juice, olive oil, mustard, Worcestershire garlic, and sugar in a cup; add to lettuce. Toss well and season with salt and pepper to taste. Transfer to 2 plates.

2 SERVINGS

IMMUNE SYSTEM Olive oil contains anti-inflammatory monounsaturated fats.

Body Benefit

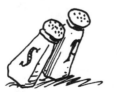

NUTRITIONAL INFORMATION, PER SERVING	
CALORIES:	130
FAT:	13.6 GRAMS
AGING FATS:	1.8 GRAMS
FIBER:	0.5 GRAMS
CARBOHYDRATES:	20 GRAMS
SUGAR:	1.1 GRAMS
PROTEIN:	0.6 GRAM
SODIUM:	3 MILLIGRAMS
POTASSIUM:	87 MILLIGRAMS

PORTUGUESE BEAN SOUP

½ teaspoon olive oil

½ cup coarsely chopped white onion

1½ cups reduced-sodium chicken broth

½ cup diced (½-inch pieces) unpeeled sweet potatoes

1½ to 2 teaspoons chili garlic sauce

½ can (7 ounces) diced tomatoes, undrained

½ can (8 ounces) cannelloni beans, drained and rinsed

2 cups packed sliced Swiss chard or collard greens

2 teaspoons balsamic vinegar (optional)

Heat a large saucepan over medium-high heat. Add oil, then onion; cook 3 minutes, stirring occasionally. Add broth, sweet potato, and chili garlic sauce; bring to a boil over high heat. Reduce heat and simmer uncovered 5 minutes. Stir in tomatoes and beans; return to simmer. Stir in Swiss chard. Simmer 5 more minutes or until sweet potatoes and chard are tender. Stir in vinegar and ladle into bowls.

2 SERVINGS

LUNGS Spices like chili and garlic help open up airways.

Body Benefit

NUTRITIONAL INFORMATION, PER SERVING

CALORIES:	270
FAT:	3.7 GRAMS
AGING FATS:	1.3 GRAMS
FIBER:	8.2 GRAMS
CARBOHYDRATES:	30 GRAMS
SUGAR:	7.3 GRAMS
PROTEIN:	9.9 GRAMS
SODIUM:	899 MILLIGRAMS
POTASSIUM:	801 MILLIGRAMS

GINGER, CARROT, AND ORANGE CAPPUCCINO CUP SOUP

Cooking oil spray

¼ cup thinly sliced yellow onion

½ rib celery (½ cup), thinly sliced

¼ pound carrots, very thinly sliced

1½ cups low-salt vegetable broth or stock

¾ teaspoon finely grated ginger

¼ cup orange juice

¼ teaspoon salt

1 teaspoon extra-virgin olive oil

Heat a large nonstick saucepan or Dutch oven, coated with cooking oil spray, over medium heat. Add onion and celery; cook 5 minutes, stirring occasionally. Add carrots; continue to cook another 5 minutes. Add broth and ginger; bring to a boil. Add orange juice and salt. Reduce heat; cover and simmer until vegetables are very tender, about 20 minutes. Transfer mixture (in batches, if necessary) to a blender or food processor; blend until smooth. Reheat, if necessary; ladle into bowls. Drizzle oil over soup.

2 SERVINGS

SENSES Lots of vitamins and nutrients from orange juice, celery, onions, and carrots to help improve your eyes and other sensory organs.

Body Benefit

NUTRITIONAL INFORMATION, PER SERVING

CALORIES:	83
FAT:	2.5 GRAMS
AGING FATS:	0.4 GRAM
FIBER:	3.5 GRAMS
CARBOHYDRATES:	14.9 GRAMS
PROTEIN:	5.2 GRAMS
SODIUM:	568 MILLIGRAMS
POTASSIUM:	573 MILLIGRAMS

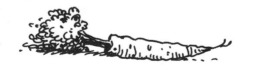

WARM TERIYAKI BEEF WITH PEA SHOOTS

2 tablespoons plus 2 teaspoons light teriyaki sauce, such as Kikkoman brand
1 teaspoon dark sesame oil
½ pound well-trimmed boneless top sirloin steak, cut 1 inch thick
½ tablespoon rice wine or cider vinegar
3 cups packed mesclun salad mix or torn salad greens
½ cup pea shoots
½ can (4 ounces) whole baby corn, such as Dynasty brand, drained
¼ cup corn nuts

Combine teriyaki sauce and sesame oil. Spoon 1 tablespoon of the mixture over both sides of steak; let stand 5 minutes. Combine remaining teriyaki mixture and vinegar; set aside. Prepare a charcoal or gas grill or heat a ridged grill pan over medium-high heat until hot. Add steak; grill or pan-sear 2 to 3 minutes per side for rare steak or longer until desired doneness is reached. Transfer to a carving board; let stand 5 minutes. Toss mesclun with 1½ tablespoons of reserved teriyaki mixture; transfer to serving plates and top with pea shoots. Cut steak crosswise into ⅛-inch-thick slices; arrange over salad. Arrange corn around edges of salad, forming a "box." Sprinkle corn nuts over beef and drizzle remaining teriyaki mixture over all.

2 SERVINGS

HORMONES Potassium in this dish keeps your blood pressure normal and glands happy.

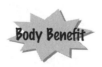

Body Benefit

NUTRITIONAL INFORMATION, PER SERVING	
CALORIES:	452
FAT:	21.4 GRAMS
AGING FATS:	5.6 GRAMS
FIBER:	4.4 GRAMS
CARBOHYDRATES:	25.5 GRAMS
PROTEIN:	42.4 GRAMS
SODIUM:	1,169 MILLIGRAMS
POTASSIUM:	1,025 MILLIGRAMS

GUACAMOLE

    1 medium ripe avocado
    ½ large plum tomato, diced
    ½ tablespoon minced white or yellow onion
    ½ tablespoon lime or lemon juice
    1 teaspoon minced, seeded Serrano or jalapeño chili
    ½ small garlic clove, minced
    ¼ teaspoon salt

Peel and seed avocado. Scoop available avocado flesh into medium bowl; coarsely mash with a fork. Add remaining ingredients; mix well. Serve immediately with fresh vegetable dippers, baked tortilla chips, or fresh corn tortillas.

2 SERVINGS

LUNGS Spicy ingredients, like chili peppers, help open airways, and avocados provide healthy anti-inflammatory fat.

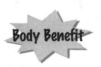
Body Benefit

NUTRITIONAL INFORMATION, PER SERVING	
CALORIES:	178
FAT:	13.6 GRAMS
AGING FATS:	3.9 GRAMS
FIBER:	4.5 GRAMS
CARBOHYDRATES:	15.5 GRAMS
PROTEIN:	2.7 GRAMS
SODIUM:	10 MILLIGRAMS
POTASSIUM:	805 MILLIGRAMS

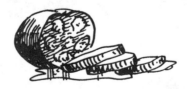

TOMATO BRUSCHETTA

½ small whole-wheat or French bread baguette

Olive oil cooking spray

½ tablespoon extra-virgin olive oil

1½ large garlic cloves, unpeeled

1 medium tomato (about 12 ounces or 1 cup), chopped

½ tablespoon chopped basil

⅛ teaspoon salt

Dash freshly ground black pepper

Heat oven to 450 degrees. Cut bread crosswise into sixteen ½-inch-thick slices. Spray cooking oil spray lightly over both sides of each slice and arrange on baking sheet. Bake 6 to 8 minutes or until lightly toasted. Cool at room temperature. Meanwhile, heat olive oil in a small nonstick skillet over medium heat until hot. Add garlic cloves; cook until the skin is slightly charred, about 5 minutes, turning occasionally. Cool, peel, and chop garlic. Use the back of a large knife to mash garlic to a paste. Combine tomatoes, garlic, basil, salt, and pepper. Spoon mixture over toasted bread.

2 SERVINGS

ANTICANCER Lycopene, folate, and perhaps selenium, found in tomato products and garlic, have anticancer properties.

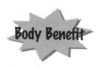
Body Benefit

NUTRITIONAL INFORMATION, PER SERVING	
CALORIES:	210
FAT:	5.9 GRAMS
AGING FATS:	1.6 GRAMS
FIBER:	2.5 GRAMS
CARBOHYDRATES:	33 GRAMS
PROTEIN:	6.3 GRAMS
SODIUM:	321 MILLIGRAMS
POTASSIUM:	247 MILLIGRAMS

BROCCOLI SANDWICH

½ cup (3 ounces) extra-firm light silken tofu, such as Mori-Nu brand

1 tablespoon chopped flat-leaf parsley

¾ tablespoon lemon juice

½ tablespoon water

½ teaspoon salt, divided

½ tablespoon olive oil

½ cup thinly sliced red onion

1½ cups chopped broccoli florets

⅛ teaspoon freshly ground black pepper

2 tablespoons barbecue sauce

2 whole-wheat or whole-grain English muffins, split, toasted

Combine tofu, parsley, lemon juice, water, and ¼ teaspoon salt in a blender container or food processor. Blend until smooth; set aside.

Heat a large nonstick skillet over medium-high heat. Add oil, then onion; cook 4 minutes, stirring occasionally. Add broccoli, remaining ¼ teaspoon salt, and pepper; cook 4 minutes, stirring occasionally. Add barbecue sauce; continue cooking 2 minutes or until thickened. Spoon broccoli mixture evenly over bottom halves of muffins. Add tofu dressing and replace muffin tops.

2 SERVINGS

ANTICANCER   Nutrients in broccoli are great at warding off cancer.

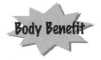
Body Benefit

NUTRITIONAL INFORMATION, PER SERVING	
CALORIES:	224
FAT:	5.6 GRAMS
AGING FATS:	0.9 GRAM
FIBER:	10.1 GRAMS
CARBOHYDRATES:	37 GRAMS
PROTEIN:	9 GRAMS
SODIUM:	902 MILLIGRAMS
POTASSIUM:	500 MILLIGRAMS

ROASTED TOMATO BASIL SOUP

1 white onion, diced
2 large garlic cloves, finely minced
1 tablespoon olive oil
1 bay leaf
Pinch of thyme
½ tablespoon sugar
Pinch of salt
Pinch of freshly ground pepper
2 cups canned tomatoes, diced or whole plum
Chopped fresh basil leaves

In a heavy-bottomed pan, combine the onion, minced garlic, olive oil, bay leaf, thyme, sugar, salt, and freshly ground pepper. Cook for 15 minutes over medium heat until soft and sweet, stirring occasionally. Next, add the tomatoes and chopped basil leaves. (If you want, puree the ingredients to make them smooth.) Bake in 450-degree oven for 30 minutes. Stir in any black parts that accumulate. Taste for basil flavor; a little more can be added for secondary flavor. Remove bay leaf. Serve or reheat for later.

2 SERVINGS

ANTICANCER The stuff in tomatoes seems to be a great way to prevent breast and prostate cancer cells from growing.

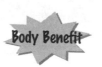

Body Benefit

NUTRITIONAL INFORMATION, PER SERVING

CALORIES:	140
FAT:	7.1 GRAMS
AGING FATS:	1 GRAM
FIBER:	2.8 GRAMS
CARBOHYDRATES:	18.6 GRAMS
PROTEIN:	3 GRAMS
SODIUM:	393 MILLIGRAMS
POTASSIUM:	624 MILLIGRAMS

PERSIAN KIDNEY BEANS

¾ teaspoon olive oil

½ cup finely chopped white or yellow onion

1½ garlic cloves, minced

½ teaspoon salt

½ teaspoon ground cumin

⅛ teaspoon cinnamon

½ cup fresh orange juice

1 tablespoon fresh lime juice

1 tablespoon tomato paste

½ teaspoon bottled or fresh seeded, minced red jalapeño chili

1½ cans (24 ounces total) red kidney beans, rinsed and drained

¼ teaspoon finely shredded lime peel

¼ teaspoon finely shredded orange peel

2 tablespoons freshly grated Romano cheese (optional)

Heat a large saucepan over medium heat. Add oil, then onion. Cook 5 minutes, stirring occasionally. Add garlic, salt, cumin, and cinnamon; cook 3 minutes. Add orange and lime juices, tomato paste, and chili; simmer uncovered 5 minutes. Add beans; bring to a boil. Reduce heat; simmer uncovered 5 minutes, stirring occasionally. Ladle into shallow bowls; top with lime and orange zests and cheese.

2 SERVINGS

DIGESTIVE SYSTEM

Beans are important sources of digestive-friendly fiber.

Body Benefit

NUTRITIONAL INFORMATION, PER SERVING

CALORIES:	311
FAT:	2.4 GRAMS
AGING FATS:	0.6 GRAM
FIBER:	7.1 GRAMS
CARBOHYDRATES:	31.6 GRAMS
PROTEIN:	8.1 GRAMS
SODIUM:	1,098 MILLIGRAMS
POTASSIUM:	582 MILLIGRAMS

GRILLED TILAPIA WITH ASIAN RED LENTILS AND KALE

½ pound fresh tilapia fillet, cut about ½ inch thick

1 tablespoon soy sauce

½ tablespoon mirin

1 clove garlic, minced

½ teaspoon finely grated fresh ginger

½ teaspoon dark sesame oil

½ cup red lentils

1 cup low-salt chicken broth

2 cups (4 ounces) packed, sliced kale

1 tablespoon water

1 teaspoon sesame seeds, toasted (optional)

Prepare a charcoal or gas grill. Place fish on a shallow plate. Combine soy sauce, mirin, garlic, ginger, and sesame oil; mix well. Pour over fish, turning to coat. Let stand 10 minutes. Meanwhile, combine lentils and broth in a large, deep skillet. Bring to a boil over high heat. Reduce heat; simmer uncovered 10 minutes, stirring occasionally. Add kale; cover and simmer 5 more minutes or until lentils and kale are tender, stirring once. Drain fish, reserving marinade. Grill fish over medium-high heat 3 to 4 minutes per side or until fish is opaque in center. Transfer marinade to a small saucepan; add 1 tablespoon water. Bring to a boil; boil gently 30 seconds. Spoon lentil mixture onto 2 warmed serving plates; top with fish. Sprinkle with sesame seeds, if desired. Drizzle boiled marinade over fish and lentil mixture.

2 SERVINGS

DIGESTIVE SYSTEM The lentils provide fiber to aid digestion.

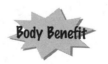

Body Benefit

NUTRITIONAL INFORMATION, PER SERVING	
CALORIES:	294
FAT:	36 GRAMS
AGING FATS:	1 GRAM
FIBER:	8.9 GRAMS
CARBOHYDRATES:	25 GRAMS
PROTEIN:	36.7 GRAMS
SODIUM:	657 MILLIGRAMS
POTASSIUM:	908 MILLIGRAMS

DIJON CHICKEN

¼ cup Dijon mustard, divided
1 tablespoon white wine (such as a chardonnay or sauvignon blanc)
⅛ teaspoon Worcestershire sauce
Freshly ground black pepper to taste
1 tablespoon finely minced shallot, divided
1½ tablespoons real maple syrup, divided
2 (4-ounce) boneless and skinless chicken breast halves or fillets, trimmed of
   all visible fat

Combine ⅛ cup mustard, wine, Worcestershire sauce, pepper, ½ tablespoon shallots, and ½ tablespoon maple syrup in a shallow dish. Add chicken and turn to coat thoroughly; let stand for 5 minutes. Preheat charcoal or gas grill or heat a ridged grill pan. Remove chicken from marinade; discard marinade. Grill or pan-grill chicken 3 to 5 minutes per side or until chicken is no longer pink in the center.

Meanwhile, in a small bowl, combine the remaining mustard, shallots, and maple syrup. Mix well and serve as a dipping sauce for the chicken.

2 SERVINGS

IMMUNE SYSTEM The chicken and onions provide nutrients that help your immune cells keep fighting for you.

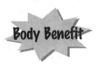
Body Benefit

NUTRITIONAL INFORMATION, PER SERVING	
CALORIES:	174
FAT:	3.2 GRAMS
AGING FATS:	0.5 GRAM
FIBER:	0.2 GRAM
CARBOHYDRATES:	6.9 GRAMS
PROTEIN:	35 GRAMS
SODIUM:	582 MILLIGRAMS
POTASSIUM:	314 MILLIGRAMS

TEXAS SLAW

4 cups green cabbage, shredded
1 cup red cabbage, shredded
¼ cup red onion, chopped
2 jalapeño chili peppers, finely chopped
2 tablespoons fresh cilantro, chopped
1 can (11 ounces) Mexicorn, drained and rinsed (lowers sodium content)
¼ cup cheddar cheese, finely shredded
¾ cup low-fat, low-sodium wine vinegar salad dressing
1 tablespoon fresh lime juice
1 teaspoon ground cumin
Cilantro sprigs

In a large bowl, combine green and red cabbage, onion, chilies, cilantro, corn, and cheese. Mix together dressing, lime juice, and cumin, and pour over vegetables. Toss to coat. Serve immediately or cover and chill up to 24 hours before serving. Garnish with cilantro sprigs. You can substitute frozen corn and diced red, green, orange, and yellow bell peppers for the Mexicorn.

4 SERVINGS

GI SYSTEM   Fiber helps maintain health of digestive system.

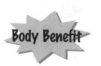
Body Benefit

NUTRITIONAL INFORMATION, PER SERVING	
CALORIES:	151
FAT:	4.7 GRAMS
AGING FATS:	1.8 GRAMS
FIBER:	4.8 GRAMS
CARBOHYDRATES:	30 GRAMS
SUGAR:	10 GRAMS
PROTEIN:	5.3 GRAMS
SODIUM:	803 MILLIGRAMS
POTASSIUM:	212 MILLIGRAMS

THE REDS AND GREENS PARADE

1 tablespoon extra-virgin olive oil

1 small onion, finely chopped

1 small carrot, finely chopped

½ teaspoon crushed red pepper flakes

4 cloves garlic, minced

1 can (14½ ounces) diced red tomatoes, drained, skin on

1 tablespoon sun-dried tomato bits

8 ounces mustard greens, torn

Freshly ground black pepper (optional)

Onion salt (optional)

¾ cup (4 ounces) cooked chickpeas (garbanzo beans)

Heat oil in a large, deep nonstick skillet over medium heat. Add onion, carrot, pepper flakes, and garlic. Cook 3 minutes, stirring occasionally. Add tomatoes and tomato bits and simmer for 3 minutes. Stir in mustard greens, and, if desired, pepper and onion salt to taste. Cover and cook 15 to 20 minutes or until greens are tender. Add chickpeas and heat through.

2 SERVINGS

HEART Olive oil promotes good arterial health.

Body Benefit

NUTRITIONAL INFORMATION, PER SERVING

CALORIES:	241
FAT:	8 GRAMS
AGING FATS:	1 GRAM
FIBER:	9.7 GRAMS
CARBOHYDRATES:	33.4 GRAMS
SUGAR:	10.4 GRAMS
PROTEIN:	9.7 GRAMS
SODIUM:	380 MILLIGRAMS
CALCIUM:	173 MILLIGRAMS
POTASSIUM:	675 MILLIGRAMS

POWER QUESADILLAS

1 tablespoon olive oil

1 small onion, chopped

1 carrot, thinly sliced

¼ cup red cabbage, chopped

1 cup packed spinach leaves, chopped

1 tablespoon fresh parsley, chopped

½ teaspoon ground cumin

¼ teaspoon chili powder

6 pitted black olives, rinsed (reduces salt) and finely chopped (2 tablespoons)

1 cup canned black beans, rinsed and drained

2 (6- to 8-inch) 100% whole-wheat flour or corn tortillas

2 tablespoons finely crumbled feta cheese

2 tablespoons prepared salsa

Heat oil in a large nonstick skillet over medium heat. Add onion and cook 3 minutes. Add carrot and red cabbage and continue cooking 3 minutes. Add spinach, parsley, cumin, chili powder, olives, and beans. Cook 3 minutes. Coat a nonstick skillet with cooking spray and place over medium-high heat. Add 1 tortilla and cook until golden brown on bottom. Turn and fill with half of vegetable mixture, 1 tablespoon of cheese on each, and 1 tablespoon of salsa. Use a large spatula to fold tortilla over filling. Cook 2 minutes or until heated through. Transfer to a serving plate and repeat with remaining ingredients to prepare second quesadilla.

NUTRITIONAL INFORMATION, PER SERVING	
CALORIES:	393
FAT:	14.8 GRAMS
AGING FATS:	2.4 GRAMS
FIBER:	9.6 GRAMS
CARBOHYDRATES:	51 GRAMS
SUGAR:	9.3 GRAMS
PROTEIN:	12.7 GRAMS
SODIUM:	568 MILLIGRAMS
POTASSIUM:	270 MILLIGRAMS

2 SERVINGS

GI SYSTEM Beans provide fiber to promote healthy intestines.

Body Benefit

CURRIED CHICKEN WITH SAUCE

1¼ cups low-salt chicken broth, divided
½ cup red lentils
1 teaspoon curry powder
½ teaspoon ground cumin
¼ teaspoon salt
⅛ teaspoon cayenne pepper
2 large or 4 small bone-in chicken thighs, skin removed (about 12 ounces)
2 teaspoons olive oil
¼ cup low-fat Greek-style thick yogurt
1 tablespoon fresh mint leaves, chopped

Combine 1 cup of the broth and lentils in a medium saucepan. Bring to a boil over high heat. Reduce heat to low; cover and simmer 20 to 25 minutes or until liquid is absorbed and lentils are tender. Meanwhile, combine curry powder, cumin, salt, and cayenne pepper. Rub mixture over both sides of chicken. Heat oil in a large nonstick skillet over medium-high heat. Add chicken and cook 3 minutes per side. Add remaining ¼ cup broth to skillet, cover, and cook over medium-low heat 8 to 10 minutes or until chicken is no longer pink in center. Transfer chicken to serving plates. Increase heat to high and cook juices in skillet 1 minute or until reduced and thickened. Stir in yogurt and mint; simmer 1 minute longer, stirring constantly. Transfer lentils to serving plates and top with chicken. Spoon sauce over chicken and lentils.

2 SERVINGS

BRAIN Curry helps clear the memory clogging amyloid from your brain. And fiber, healthy fat, and potassium keeps the arteries in your brain younger.

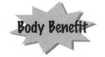
Body Benefit

NUTRITIONAL INFORMATION, PER SERVING	
CALORIES:	410
FAT:	14.9 GRAMS
AGING FATS:	3.6 GRAMS
FIBER:	7.4 GRAMS
CARBOHYDRATES:	31.5 GRAMS
SUGAR:	3.8 GRAMS
PROTEIN:	37 GRAMS
SODIUM:	472 MILLIGRAMS
POTASSIUM:	704 MILLIGRAMS

SUCCULENT SALMON AND SALSA

¼ teaspoon salt

⅛ teaspoon freshly ground black pepper

2 (4 to 5 ounce) skinless wild salmon fillets

1 teaspoon olive oil

1 clove garlic, minced

1 cup ripe tomato (1 medium), chopped

2 tablespoons Kalamata olives (6 olives), chopped, pitted

2 tablespoons port wine

2 tablespoons fresh basil, chopped

Sprinkle salt and pepper over salmon. Heat oil in a large nonstick skillet over medium heat until hot. Add salmon and cook 4 to 5 minutes per side or until salmon is opaque in center. Transfer to serving plates and keep warm. Add garlic to skillet and cook 30 seconds. Stir in tomato, olives, and wine. Simmer 2 to 3 minutes or until thickened. Spoon salsa over salmon and top with basil.

2 SERVINGS

SKIN Omega-3 fatty acids in fish have been shown to help improve skin health.

Body Benefit

NUTRITIONAL INFORMATION, PER SERVING	
CALORIES:	279
FAT:	13.7 GRAMS
AGING FATS:	2 GRAMS
FIBER:	1.3 GRAMS
CARBOHYDRATES:	7.3 GRAMS
SUGAR:	3.5 GRAMS
PROTEIN:	26.9 GRAMS
SODIUM:	537 MILLIGRAMS
POTASSIUM:	879 MILLIGRAMS

Snack

CACIK

½ cucumber, chopped finely or grated
½ pint low-fat plain yogurt
1 clove garlic
Salt to taste
Pepper to taste
4 cups cut raw cauliflower

Mix all ingredients except cauliflower together. Use as a dip for cauliflower, and enjoy.

2 SERVINGS

IMMUNE SYSTEM Yogurt promotes growth of healthy bacteria in the intestines.

Body Benefit

NUTRITIONAL INFORMATION, PER SERVING	
CALORIES:	130
FAT:	2 GRAMS
AGING FATS:	1.2 GRAMS
FIBER:	5.7 GRAMS
CARBOHYDRATES:	20.5 GRAMS
PROTEIN:	10.5 GRAMS
SODIUM:	141 MILLIGRAMS
POTASSIUM:	933 MILLIGRAMS

Dinner

WARM SPINACH SALAD WITH CHICKEN, APPLES, AND TOASTED ALMONDS

2 tablespoons sliced almonds

1 cup plus 3 tablespoons apple juice, preferably unfiltered, divided

6 ounces (about 1½ cups) shredded or chopped, cooked skinless chicken breast

½ teaspoon canola or olive oil

2 tablespoons plus 2 teaspoons sliced shallots or chopped sweet onion

½ tablespoon brown sugar

⅛ teaspoon cinnamon

⅛ teaspoon salt

3 cups (5 ounces) packed, torn spinach leaves

½ apple, preferably Fuji or Gala, unpeeled and cut into ½-inch cubes

Place almonds on a baking sheet and bake in a 350-degree oven until lightly browned and fragrant, 6 to 8 minutes; set aside. In a very large bowl, combine 3 tablespoons apple juice and the chicken; toss well and set aside. Heat a large skillet over medium heat. Add oil, then shallots; sauté 5 minutes. Add remaining 1 cup apple juice, brown sugar, cinnamon, and salt. Simmer 5 minutes, stirring occasionally. Add spinach, apple, and almonds to chicken mixture. Add hot shallot mixture; toss well and transfer to 2 serving plates. Serve with freshly ground black pepper, if desired.

Tip: Toasting doubles the flavor, enabling you to eat just half of what you would otherwise. Thinly sliced almonds go further and have more flavor than whole or slivered ones.

NUTRITIONAL INFORMATION, PER SERVING	
CALORIES:	327
FAT:	12 GRAMS
AGING FATS:	2.5 GRAMS
FIBER:	3.8 GRAMS
CARBOHYDRATES:	26.7 GRAMS
SUGAR:	19.6 GRAMS
PROTEIN:	29.7 GRAMS
SODIUM:	136 MILLIGRAMS
POTASSIUM:	926 MILLIGRAMS

2 SERVINGS

HEART AND ARTERIES   Nuts are a terrific source of healthy protein, unsaturated fat, and, of course, great flavor.

Body Benefit

SALMON WITH SPINACH AND MUSTARD

   2 (4- to 5-ounce skinless salmon fillets)
   1 tablespoon soy sauce
   ½ tablespoon dry white wine
   ½ tablespoon lemon juice
   ½ tablespoon Dijon mustard
   ½ tablespoon olive oil
   ½ package (5 ounces) fresh spinach, coarsely chopped
   1 teaspoon finely shredded lemon peel (optional)

Rinse salmon in cold water; pat dry with paper towels. Place salmon on a shallow plate; top with soy sauce and let stand for 10 minutes. Combine wine, lemon juice, mustard, and oil; set aside. Roast salmon in a 450-degree oven for 16 minutes (it should be a little pink inside). Move salmon to serving plate, and heat spinach in nonstick skillet. Cook until wilted. Pour spinach and sauce over salmon.

2 SERVINGS

BONES   Omega-9 fatty acids help lubricate joints, and the spinach contains bone-boosting calcium.

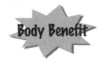

Body Benefit

NUTRITIONAL INFORMATION, PER SERVING	
Calories:	409
Fat:	12.4 grams
Aging Fats:	3 grams
Fiber:	3.2 grams
Carbohydrates:	24.2 grams
Protein:	22.7 grams
Sodium:	667 milligrams
Potassium:	538 milligrams

GRILLED CHICKEN OR FISH WITH WASABI MASHED POTATOES WITH CARAMELIZED SWEET ONIONS

1 pound red potatoes
¾ tablespoon extra-virgin olive oil
1 cup chopped sweet or yellow onions
½ cup low-fat (1 percent) buttermilk
½ tablespoon wasabi powder

Bring a large pot of water to a simmer. Cut potatoes into 1-inch chunks. Add to water; return to simmer. Simmer uncovered until potatoes are tender when pierced with a tip of a knife, about 14 minutes. Meanwhile, heat a medium saucepan over medium-high heat. Add oil, then onions. Cook 8 to 10 minutes or until onions begin to brown, stirring occasionally. Remove from heat. Drain potatoes. Sprinkle salt (if desired) over potatoes and heat over medium heat for 30 seconds to dry them. Add buttermilk and wasabi powder; turn off heat. Mash with a potato masher until desired consistency. Stir in onions. Serve with grilled chicken or fish and add a vegetable of your choice.

2 SERVINGS

LUNGS Wasabi, onions, and olive oil help open the airways for better breathing.

Body Benefit

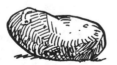

NUTRITIONAL INFORMATION, PER SERVING OF MASHED POTATOES	
CALORIES:	305
FAT:	6.4 GRAMS
AGING FATS:	1.6 GRAMS
FIBER:	4.7 GRAMS
CARBOHYDRATES:	56.1 GRAMS
SUGAR:	9.5 GRAMS
PROTEIN:	7.6 GRAMS
SODIUM:	822 MILLIGRAMS
POTASSIUM:	1,005 MILLIGRAMS

BARBECUED RED SNAPPER WITH SPICY RED BEANS AND RICE

2 tablespoons plus 2 teaspoons hickory barbecue sauce

1 teaspoon Caribbean jerk seasoning mix

2 (4- to 5-ounce) skinless red snapper fish fillets

¾ cup spicy vegetable juice

1 cup water

1 cup quick-cooking brown rice

1½ cups packed, sliced kale or collard greens

½ can (8 ounces) red beans, rinsed and drained

1 tablespoon light sour cream

Combine the barbecue sauce and jerk seasoning. Mix well. Brush 3 tablespoons of the mixture onto fillets; set aside fillets and remaining mixture. In a small bowl, reserve 1 tablespoon of the vegetable juice. Combine the remaining barbecue sauce, vegetable juice, and 1 cup of water in a large skillet. Bring to a simmer. Stir in rice; cover and simmer 8 minutes. Meanwhile, grill fish on medium-hot coals for 3 to 4 minutes per side, or until fish is opaque and firm to touch. Stir kale and beans into rice mixture. Cover and simmer for 3 to 4 minutes more until kale is wilted and liquid is absorbed. Add sour cream to the reserved vegetable juice; mix well. Serve fish over rice; drizzle some cream sauce over fish.

2 SERVINGS

BRAIN Omega-3 fatty acids, healthy protein, potassium, and folate found in fish and green leafy vegetables help improve brain function.

Body Benefit

NUTRITIONAL INFORMATION, PER SERVING	
CALORIES:	642
FAT:	6.5 GRAMS
AGING FATS:	1.1 GRAMS
FIBER:	15 GRAMS
CARBOHYDRATES:	101.4 GRAMS
SUGAR:	9.5 GRAMS
PROTEIN:	42.4 GRAMS
SODIUM:	921 MILLIGRAMS
POTASSIUM:	1,475 MILLIGRAMS

GRILLED TUNA NIÇOISE

1 tablespoon olive oil

½ tablespoon coarse-grained mustard

1½ tablespoons tarragon white wine vinegar

½ teaspoon dried tarragon

⅜ teaspoon salt

¼ teaspoon freshly ground black pepper

2 (4-ounce) fresh tuna steaks, cut about ½ inch thick

½ pound small red boiling waxy potatoes

4 ounces whole fresh green beans

4 cups (5 ounces) mesclun or torn salad greens

8 grape, teardrop, or cherry tomatoes

In a small bowl, combine oil, mustard, vinegar, tarragon, salt, and pepper; mix well. Brush 1½ tablespoons of the mixture over tuna; set tuna and remaining dressing aside. Rinse potatoes and green beans but do not dry. Place potatoes in an 8-inch-square baking dish or microwave-safe casserole. Cover; cook at high power for 3 minutes. Add green beans; cover and continue to cook at high power 4 minutes more or until vegetables are tender. Transfer to a colander and rinse with cold water to stop the cooking and cool the vegetables. Meanwhile, heat a ridged grill pan over medium-high heat. Add tuna; cook 2 minutes per side or until seared and still very pink in center.

Arrange greens on 2 serving plates. Quarter the potatoes and cut green beans in half if large; arrange over greens. Top with tuna and reserved dressing. Garnish with tomatoes.

---

2 SERVINGS

HEART AND ARTERIES

Olive and fish oils help keep your arteries clear.

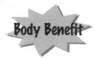

Body Benefit

NUTRITIONAL INFORMATION, PER SERVING	
Calories:	291
Fat:	8.1 grams
Aging fats:	1.6 grams
Fiber:	5.3 grams
Carbohydrates:	32.5 grams
Protein:	30.6 grams
Sodium:	556 milligrams
Potassium:	1,268 milligrams

SMOKED MOZZARELLA AND VEGGIE–STUFFED PIZZA

Cooking oil spray

1 pound fresh, cut stir-fry vegetables, like broccoli, zucchini, mushrooms, bell pepper, red onion

Salt to taste

Freshly ground pepper to taste

¼ cup tomato paste

2 tablespoons olive relish

2 tablespoons sun-dried tomato bits

1 (12-inch or 10-ounce) prepared thin pizza crust

¼ cup chopped mixed green herbs such as chives, thyme, parsley, basil

½ cup (2 ounces) finely shredded smoked mozzarella cheese

Heat oven to 425 degrees. Heat a large nonstick skillet over medium-high heat until hot. Coat with cooking spray; add vegetables. Stir-fry 3 to 4 minutes or until vegetables are crisp-tender. Add salt and pepper to taste. Combine tomato paste, olive relish, and sun-dried tomato bits. Spread over pizza crust; top with cooked vegetables, herbs, and cheese, in that order. Bake the pizza directly on oven rack for about 10 to 15 minutes, or until crust is golden brown and cheese melts.

4 SERVINGS

ANTICANCER The vegetables work as antioxidants, and contain phytonutrients that have cancer-preventing properties.

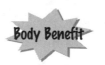
Body Benefit

NUTRITIONAL INFORMATION, PER SERVING	
CALORIES:	297
FAT:	9.5 GRAMS
AGING FATS:	4.1 GRAMS
FIBER:	5.3 GRAMS
CARBOHYDRATES:	42.7 GRAMS
PROTEIN:	12.2 GRAMS
SODIUM:	682 MILLIGRAMS
POTASSIUM:	481 MILLIGRAMS

MANDARIN CHICKEN

2 tablespoons rice wine vinegar

1 teaspoon dark sesame oil

½ tablespoon minced garlic

½ tablespoon julienned pickled ginger

1 tablespoon low-sodium soy sauce

¼ pound cooked boneless, skinless chicken breast, chopped

¾ cup drained canned mandarin orange segments

¼ cup blanched snow peas

¼ cup drained canned bamboo shoots

¼ cup drained canned water chestnuts

2 cups shredded lettuce

1 teaspoon toasted sesame seeds

Mix the vinegar, sesame oil, garlic, ginger, and soy sauce thoroughly. Add chicken and orange segments; marinate for about 10 minutes. Add snow peas, bamboo shoots, and water chestnuts. Distribute lettuce on 2 serving plates. Top with chicken mixture, sprinkle with sesame seeds, and serve.

2 SERVINGS

ANTICANCER The flavonoids and vitamins found in the vegetables have cancer-preventing properties.

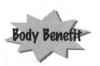
Body Benefit

NUTRITIONAL INFORMATION, PER SERVING	
CALORIES:	184
FAT:	5.7 GRAMS
AGING FATS:	1.6 GRAMS
FIBER:	4.1 GRAMS
CARBOHYDRATES:	26.3 GRAMS
PROTEIN:	23 GRAMS
SODIUM:	485 MILLIGRAMS
POTASSIUM:	850 MILLIGRAMS

ROASTED CHICKEN WITH PESTO GEMELLI

4 ounces whole-grain pesto gemelli pasta

6 ounces boneless, skinless chicken thighs

½ tablespoon olive oil

1 teaspoon dried herbes de Provence

½ bunch (about 7 ounces) asparagus spears, cut into 1-inch pieces

¼ cup low-salt chicken broth

2 tablespoons prepared reduced-fat basil pesto

½ teaspoon salt

¼ teaspoon freshly ground pepper

Optional: fresh basil, parsley, grated Asiago cheese, toasted pine nuts

Heat broiler. Cook pasta according to package directions. Cut chicken into 1-inch chunks; toss with oil and dried herbs and spread out on nonstick jelly-roll pan. Broil 5 to 6 inches from heat for 6 minutes. Add asparagus to chicken, stirring to coat lightly with oil. Continue broiling 4 minutes or until chicken is cooked through and asparagus is crisp-tender. Transfer cooked pasta to colander to drain. Add broth, pesto, salt, and pepper to pot; top with optional ingredients, if using.

2 SERVINGS

HEART AND ARTERIES

Olive oil, whole-grain pasta, and asparagus decrease the inflammatory gremlins that age your arteries.

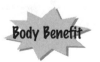

Body Benefit

NUTRITIONAL INFORMATION, PER SERVING	
CALORIES:	439
FAT:	12.5 GRAMS
AGING FATS:	4.9 GRAMS
FIBER:	1.8 GRAMS
CARBOHYDRATES:	18.7 GRAMS
PROTEIN:	29 GRAMS
SODIUM:	808 MILLIGRAMS
POTASSIUM:	84 MILLIGRAMS

TUSCAN TUNA WITH GRILLED TOMATO

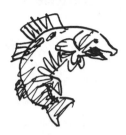

1½ tablespoons high-quality balsamic vinegar

¾ tablespoon extra-virgin olive oil

1 teaspoon chopped fresh rosemary

¼ teaspoon salt

¼ teaspoon fresh ground pepper

2 (4-ounce) tuna steaks (½ inch thick)

2 plum tomatoes, halved lengthwise

2 slices red or sweet onion

½ can (8 ounces) cannelloni beans, rinsed

½ cup packed arugula leaves

Prepare a charcoal or gas grill. In a small bowl, combine vinegar, oil, rosemary, salt, and pepper; mix well. In a small bowl, reserve 1 tablespoon of vinegar mixture. Brush remaining mixture over both sides of tuna, tomatoes, and onion slices. Grill the tomatoes and onion slices 4 minutes per side or until tender. Grill the tuna 2 to 3 minutes per side (for medium-rare). In large bowl, combine beans and arugula. Cut the grilled tomatoes into chunks and separate the onions into rings; add to bean mixture. Add reserved vinegar mixture; toss well. On each plate, top bean mixture with tuna; sprinkle with pepper.

2 SERVINGS

SEX ORGANS Fish oils keep arteries clear, and cooked tomato products protect the prostate and breasts.

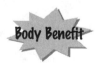

Body Benefit

NUTRITIONAL INFORMATION, PER SERVING	
CALORIES:	314 CALORIES
FAT:	7.2 GRAMS
AGING FATS:	1.2 GRAMS
FIBER:	8.8 GRAMS
CARBOHYDRATES:	46.6 GRAMS
PROTEIN:	44.7 GRAMS
SODIUM:	347 MILLIGRAMS
POTASSIUM:	142 MILLIGRAMS

TERIYAKI TOFU WITH RED BELL PEPPER AND SHIITAKES OVER WHOLE-GRAIN JASMINE RICE

1½ tablespoons dark sesame oil

1 tablespoon light teriyaki sauce

2 garlic cloves, minced

¼ teaspoon five-spice powder

6 ounces baked teriyaki-flavored tofu, cut into 1-inch squares

2 cups broccoli florets (cut into 2-inch pieces)

2 cups asparagus spears (cut into 2-inch pieces)

1 cup sliced shiitake mushrooms

1 cup diced red bell pepper

½ cup vegetable broth or stock

1 teaspoon Chinese hot chili sauce (optional)

1½ cups hot cooked jasmine rice

In a large bowl, combine 1 tablespoon of the oil, teriyaki sauce, garlic, and five-spice powder; mix well. Add tofu, tossing to coat. Heat a Dutch oven over medium-high heat. Add remaining ½ tablespoon of oil, then tofu mixture. Stir-fry 1 minute. Add broccoli, asparagus, mushrooms and bell peppers; stir-fry 2 minutes. Add broth; stir-fry 2 minutes. Stir in hot chili sauce, if desired. Transfer to 2 shallow bowls; serve with rice.

2 SERVINGS

IMMUNE SYSTEM   Garlic has properties to protect against various fungal conditions, and healthy fats and folate strengthen immune function.

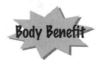
Body Benefit

NUTRITIONAL INFORMATION, PER SERVING

CALORIES:	514
FAT:	14.9 GRAMS
AGING FATS:	1.7 GRAMS
FIBER:	6.1 GRAMS
CARBOHYDRATES:	127 GRAMS
PROTEIN:	29.1 GRAMS
SODIUM:	1,087 MILLIGRAMS
POTASSIUM:	952 MILLIGRAMS

RAINBOW SHRIMP MOO SHU ROLL-UPS

6 ounces uncooked, peeled, and deveined small, medium, or halved large
    shrimp, thawed if frozen
1 tablespoon chili sauce
Garlic-flavored cooking oil spray
½ red bell pepper, cut into short, thin strips
½ yellow bell pepper, cut into short, thin strips
2 cups coleslaw mix (shredded cabbage and carrots)
4 green onions, cut into ½-inch-thick slices
⅛ cup oyster sauce
½ tablespoon cornstarch
4 (10-inch) whole-wheat or honey whole-wheat flour tortillas, warmed
1 teaspoon coriander seeds (optional)

In a medium bowl, combine shrimp and chili sauce, tossing to coat. Heat a
Dutch oven or large saucepan over medium heat; coat with cooking oil spray.
Add shrimp; stir-fry 1 minute. Add bell peppers, coleslaw mix, and green
onions; stir-fry 1 minute. Add oyster sauce; stir-fry 2 minutes or until shrimp
are opaque and vegetables are crisp-tender. In a small bowl, combine cornstarch with 1 tablespoon cold water; mix well. Add to shrimp mixture; cook 1
minute or until thickened, stirring constantly. Spoon mixture down center of
tortillas; sprinkle coriander seeds over mixture, if
desired. Fold one end of tortilla over filling; roll up
burrito-style.

2 SERVINGS

HORMONES Complex
carbohydrates and reduced
intake of sugar help decrease
risk of diabetes.

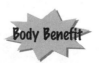
Body Benefit

NUTRITIONAL INFORMATION, PER SERVING	
CALORIES:	270
FAT:	1.9 GRAMS
AGING FATS:	0.3 GRAM
FIBER:	7.2 GRAMS
CARBOHYDRATES:	57.4 GRAMS
PROTEIN:	25.3 GRAMS
SODIUM:	968 MILLIGRAMS
POTASSIUM:	569 MILLIGRAMS

JUST FOR THE HALIBUT

3 tablespoons fresh lime juice

4 (4-ounce) halibut fillets

1 teaspoon olive oil

2 cups onion, thinly sliced

3 cups ripe tomato, diced, seeded

¼ cup bottled diced pimiento, divided

2 tablespoons capers, drained

1 tablespoon jalapeño chili pepper, finely chopped, seeded

¼ teaspoon sea salt

¼ cup water

3 cups hot cooked brown rice (1 cup dry)

2 tablespoons fresh parsley, chopped

4 lime wedges

Combine lime juice and fish in a zip-top plastic bag. Seal bag, turning to coat. Marinate in refrigerator at least 30 minutes or up to 2 hours, turning once. Heat oil in a large nonstick skillet over medium heat. Add onion and cook 8 minutes or until tender, stirring frequently. Stir in tomato, 2 tablespoons pimiento, capers, jalapeño, and salt. Cover and cook 5 minutes. Stir in water. Add fish, discarding remaining lime juice. Cover and cook 6 minutes, turning fish after 3 minutes. Uncover and cook 3 minutes or until fish flakes easily when tested with a fork. Transfer rice to serving plates and top with fish and sauce. Garnish with remaining pimiento, parsley, and lime wedges.

4 SERVINGS

IMMUNE SYSTEM

Tomatoes, chili peppers, and onions spice up your immune system.

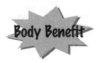
Body Benefit

NUTRITIONAL INFORMATION, PER SERVING	
CALORIES:	353
FAT:	5.5 GRAMS
AGING FATS:	0.9 GRAM
FIBER:	5.5 GRAMS
CARBOHYDRATES:	46 GRAMS
SUGAR:	6.7 GRAMS
PROTEIN:	29.6 GRAMS
SODIUM:	397 MILLIGRAMS
POTASSIUM:	998 MILLIGRAMS

PASTA WITH HEART

8 ounces whole-wheat rotini

1 teaspoon extra-virgin olive oil

2 shallots, minced

2 garlic cloves, minced

1 tablespoon fresh oregano, chopped

¼ cup dry white wine

3 tablespoons fresh lemon juice

1 can (14 ounces) quartered artichoke hearts, drained

6 ounces baby spinach leaves

½ cup part-skim ricotta cheese

2 teaspoons grated lemon zest

Freshly ground black pepper

3 tablespoons prepared basil pesto sauce

Cook pasta according to package directions. Heat oil in a large nonstick skillet. Add shallots and garlic, and sauté over medium heat until soft, about 5 minutes. Add oregano, wine, lemon juice, and artichoke hearts. Cook, stirring frequently, until artichokes are heated through. Add spinach and turn with tongs until the spinach is wilted, about 2 minutes. Remove from heat and stir in ricotta cheese, lemon zest, and pepper to taste. Drain pasta and return to same pot. Add pesto sauce and toss well. Serve immediately.

4 SERVINGS

BONES Minerals in spinach help strengthen bones.

Body Benefit

NUTRITIONAL INFORMATION, PER SERVING	
CALORIES:	387
FAT:	12.4 GRAMS
AGING FATS:	3.1 GRAMS
FIBER:	10.6 GRAMS
CARBOHYDRATES:	51.9 GRAMS
SUGAR:	4.7 GRAMS
PROTEIN:	17.1 GRAMS
SODIUM:	379 MILLIGRAMS
POTASSIUM:	65.5 MILLIGRAMS

LOVELY LAMB

1 tablespoon extra-virgin olive oil

8 ounces boneless leg of lamb cut into ½-inch cubes

1 tablespoon curry powder

½ large onion, chopped

½ green bell pepper, cut into short, thin strips

½ red or orange bell pepper, cut into short, thin strips

1 clove garlic, minced

¾ cup low-salt chicken broth

½ cup unfiltered apple juice

Freshly ground pepper

1 medium red apple such as Gala, diced

1½ cups hot cooked brown rice (½ cup dry)

2 tablespoons fresh parsley, chopped

Heat oil in a large nonstick skillet over medium heat. Add lamb and curry powder. Cook just until lamb is no longer pink on the outside, about 6 minutes, stirring often. (Lamb will be rare but will be returned to sauce to cook further.) Use a slotted spoon to transfer lamb to a plate and set aside. Add onion to same skillet; cook 5 minutes, stirring occasionally. Add the bell peppers and garlic; cook 5 minutes. Add broth, apple juice, and pepper to taste. Simmer 10 minutes. Add apple and cook 3 minutes. Return lamb to skillet and cook 3 minutes or until lamb is barely pink in center or longer to desired doneness. Serve over rice; garnish with parsley.

2 SERVINGS

BRAIN Curry and peppers boost brain cell communication.

Body Benefit

NUTRITIONAL INFORMATION, PER SERVING	
Calories:	516
Fat:	15.4 grams
Aging Fats:	3.8 grams
Fiber:	8.4 grams
Carbohydrates:	65 grams
Sugar:	21 grams
Protein:	30.6 grams
Sodium:	146 milligrams
Potassium:	881 milligrams

STIR-FRY FRIDAY FAVORITE

1 tablespoon canola oil
½ large onion, sliced
1 clove garlic, minced
½ teaspoon fresh ginger, minced
1 orange or yellow bell pepper, cut into short, thin strips
1 green bell pepper, cut into short, thin strips
⅛ teaspoon cayenne pepper
⅛ teaspoon onion salt
8 ounces firm tofu, cut into cubes*
1½ cups hot cooked brown rice (½ cup dry)

Heat oil in a large nonstick skillet over medium-high heat. Add onion, garlic, and ginger. Cook 5 minutes, stirring occasionally. Add bell peppers, cayenne, and onion salt, and cook 5 minutes, stirring occasionally. Stir in tofu and heat through. Serve over rice.

2 SERVINGS

IMMUNE Onions, garlic, ginger, and peppers rev your immune system to beat back your invaders.

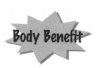
Body Benefit

NUTRITIONAL INFORMATION, PER SERVING

Calories:	376
Fat:	14.5 grams
Aging Fats:	1.6 grams
Fiber:	6.4 grams
Carbohydrates:	48.3 grams
Sugar:	6.8 grams
Protein:	15.7 grams
Sodium:	57 milligrams
Potassium:	405 milligrams

*8 ounces cooked whitefish or chopped cooked chicken breast may be substituted.

RAISIN CURRY CHICKEN

1 tablespoon olive oil

1 medium onion, sliced

8 ounces skinless, boneless chicken breast, cut crosswise into
    ½-inch thick slices

2 teaspoons curry powder

½ teaspoon ground cinnamon

1 clove garlic, minced

1 cup low-salt chicken broth

⅓ cup orange juice

3 tablespoons raisins

4 orange wedges, peeled

1½ cups cooked brown rice (½ cup dry)

Freshly ground black pepper to taste

Heat oil in a large nonstick skillet over medium heat. Add onion and cook 8 to 10 minutes or until tender, stirring occasionally. Toss chicken with curry powder and cinnamon. Add chicken and garlic to skillet and cook, stirring frequently, until chicken is no longer pink, 2 to 3 minutes. Add broth and orange juice. Simmer uncovered 8 minutes or until chicken is cooked through. Stir in raisins, orange wedges, and brown rice; heat through.

2 SERVINGS

ARTERIES   Healthy fat, fiber, and potassium keep the inner layer of your arteries young.

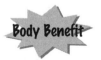

Body Benefit

NUTRITIONAL INFORMATION, PER SERVING

CALORIES:	462
FAT:	10.4 GRAMS
AGING FATS:	2.0 GRAMS
FIBER:	5.4 GRAMS
CARBOHYDRATES:	57 GRAMS
SUGAR:	17 GRAMS
PROTEIN:	33.6 GRAMS
SODIUM:	159 MILLIGRAMS
POTASSIUM:	671 MILLIGRAMS

Dessert

CHOCOLATE SOY SUNDAE SMOOTHIE

1 cup low-fat (1 percent) chocolate soy milk
½ cup frozen chocolate nondairy soy dessert
12 frozen medium strawberries
½ medium banana, broken into chunks
⅛ cup chocolate syrup
Sprinkles (optional)

Combine all ingredients except sprinkles in blender container. Cover and blend at high speed until thick and smooth. Pour into frosted mugs; garnish with sprinkles, if desired.

2 SERVINGS

BRAIN   Chocolate helps raise levels of the feel-good hormone, dopamine, in the brain.

Body Benefit

NUTRITIONAL INFORMATION, PER SERVING

CALORIES:	145
FAT:	4 GRAMS
AGING FATS:	1.7 GRAMS
FIBER:	4.5 GRAMS
CARBOHYDRATES:	25 GRAMS
PROTEIN:	6 GRAMS
SODIUM:	32 MILLIGRAMS
POTASSIUM:	523 MILLIGRAMS

CHOCOLATE STRAWBERRY SUNDAE

2 (½-cup) scoops nonfat or low-fat chocolate frozen yogurt
¾ cup sliced strawberries
½ cup low-fat granola cereal
1 teaspoon confectioners' sugar

Scoop yogurt into 2 serving bowls; top with strawberries and granola. Place sugar in strainer and shake over sundaes.

2 SERVINGS

ANTICANCER
Strawberries contain powerful antioxidants, which can help prevent cancer.

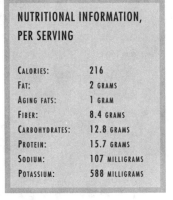

NUTRITIONAL INFORMATION, PER SERVING	
CALORIES:	216
FAT:	2 GRAMS
AGING FATS:	1 GRAM
FIBER:	8.4 GRAMS
CARBOHYDRATES:	12.8 GRAMS
PROTEIN:	15.7 GRAMS
SODIUM:	107 MILLIGRAMS
POTASSIUM:	588 MILLIGRAMS

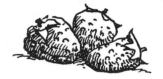

MAPLE-CRANBERRY–TOPPED FROZEN YOGURT

½ cup fresh or frozen cranberries
½ cup orange juice
¼ cup dried cranberries
1½ tablespoons pure maple syrup
¾ cup low-fat frozen vanilla yogurt
½ teaspoon finely shredded orange peel

Combine fresh or frozen cranberries, orange juice, and dried cranberries in a medium saucepan. Bring to a boil over high heat. Reduce heat; simmer uncovered 7 to 8 minutes or until cranberries pop and sauce thickens slightly. Remove from heat; stir in syrup. Serve warm, at room temperature, or chilled over frozen yogurt. Garnish with orange peel.

2 SERVINGS

IMMUNE SYSTEM Foods such as berries and orange juice that contain vitamin C, folate, and flavonoids help raise immunity levels.

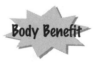
Body Benefit

NUTRITIONAL INFORMATION,
PER SERVING

CALORIES:	193
FAT:	1.1 GRAMS
AGING FATS:	0.7 GRAM
FIBER:	1.7 GRAMS
CARBOHYDRATES:	30.1 GRAMS
PROTEIN:	4.4 GRAMS
POTASSIUM:	332 MILLIGRAMS

To calculate nutrient changes to these recipes, you can go to the USDA calculator at www.nal.usda.gov/fnic/foodcomp/.

Note: If you want the dishes delivered to your cafeteria or local grocery, check our Web site—www.YOUtheownersmanual.com—we may have a helpful national distribution source for you.

Chapter 14

The Owner's Manual Workout

A good workout should be one that works all your major muscles by strengthening and stretching them. The benefit: more muscle tone, a higher metabolism, stronger bones, and a healthier and more flexible body that allows you to handle the rigors of life. Below you'll find the Owner's Manual Workout, (designed by Joel Harper, www.fitpackdvd.com), which does indeed work your entire body.

To build muscle, you have to tire within your thirteenth repetition or two minutes. Most women want to tone and tighten muscles. To do that, use light weights and the number of reps recommended here, and do them quickly. Most men want to strengthen and bulk. To do that, use a weight that you cannot lift more than twelve times with each exercise and do them slowly.

Before starting any exercise, always look down and make sure that your toes are lined up. Most people have a tendency to favor one side; you can prevent this imbalance with proper foot position and it will also help prevent over-stressing your knees. Imagine a string pulling from the top of your head to elongate your spine, and lift your chest in order to keep your shoulders from rolling forward. Proper breathing is also imperative. If you catch yourself holding your breath, count your repetitions out loud to normalize your breathing.

#1 Swimming
(Warms up shoulders)

Put your feet together with the weights in your hands, and your arms and shoulders relaxed. "Swim" your shoulders backward ten times and forward ten times. When your right shoulder is up, your left shoulder is down; when your right shoulder is forward, your left shoulder is back. Get a full range of motion to open and warm up your shoulders. Resist bending your elbows, and relax your arms so that you isolate the rotation in your shoulder. Do ten times in each direction.

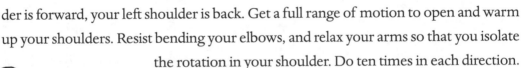

#2 Shrugs
(Strengthens trapezoid muscles and shoulders)

With weights in your hands, let your relaxed arms hang down throughout the entire movement. Lift your shoulders up toward your ears as high as you can and slowly lower them back down. Focus on having your shoulders doing the only movement (don't jut your chin out). Lift forty times.

Advanced variation: Do it while balancing on your toes.

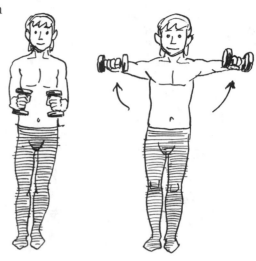

#3 Lateral Raises

(Strengthens shoulders and arms)

With your elbows at your sides, lift your hands up with your knuckles facing forward to make a 90-degree angle. While maintaining this position throughout the entire exercise, lift your elbows out to your sides at shoulder height and then lower them back down. Lift twenty times.

Advanced variation: Balance on one foot, switch sides, and do another set.

#4 Field Goal

(Strengthens rotator cuff muscles, arms, and shoulders)

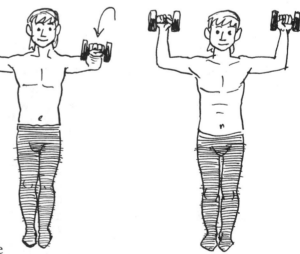

With your arms in the up position of lateral raises, lift your arm from elbows to hands and bring your hands palm-side forward above your elbows. During the entire movement, your elbows remain in line with your shoulders. Do twenty times. Don't let your shoulders scrunch up toward your ears.

Advanced variation: Bring your knee out in line with your hip, do twenty times, and then switch knees and do another twenty.

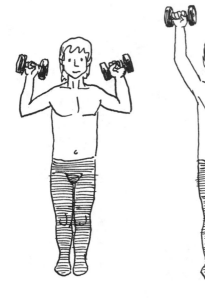

#5 Shoulder Press

(Strengthens shoulders)

With your arms in the up position of field goal, straighten your arms above your head and lower them back down. Keep your palms facing forward and your belly pulled taut to prevent from arching your back. Exhale on the way up and inhale on the way down. Do twenty times.

Advanced variation: After twenty times, hold in the up position for thirty seconds.

#6 Hug Yourself

(Stretches shoulders, arms, and upper back)

Take your right hand below your left and reach back as far as you can toward your shoulder blades. Relax your elbows down and take deep breaths into the upper part of your back; expand the back muscles as much as possible. To increase the stretch, reach your hands closer to each other. Release and shake your arms out, and switch your left hand below your right.

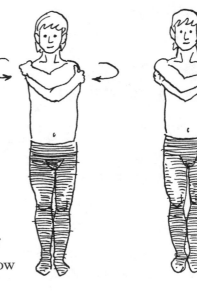

#7 One-Arm Row

(Strengthens upper back and arms)

Put your left foot forward and your left arm supporting yourself on your left leg or a sturdy chair if you need additional support. While keeping a straight line from the top of your head to your tailbone, use your back muscles to lift up your right elbow. Barely rub against your side when lifting toward the ceiling and stretch all the way back down. Resist rocking from side to side and isolate by only using your right arm. Do fifty times.

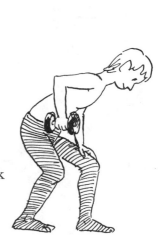

Advanced variation: Do one hundred times each side.

#8 Kickbacks

(Strengthens triceps muscles)

Stay in same body position as for one-arm row. Leaving your elbow in the up position, kick the weight backward and twist your palm toward the ceiling. Breathe normally. Maintain the up position (don't drop the elbow). Do fifty times each side.

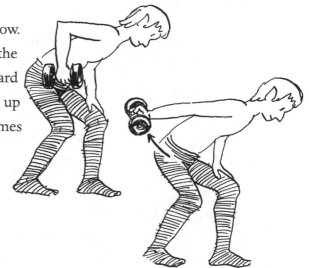

Advanced variation: Do one hundred times each side.

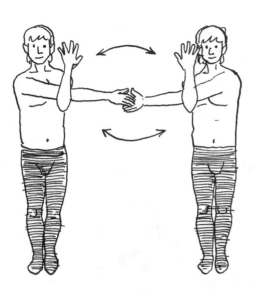

#9 Vogue

(Stretches triceps, shoulders, and upper back)

Take your left hand and reach it across your chest, palm facing backward. Take your opposite hand, with the fingers pointing to the ceiling, and hook your left arm with your right, then pull your left hand backward. Take deep breaths throughout entire stretch. Resist raising your shoulder up toward your ear. If you were looking in a mirror, your shoulders would be level with each other. Hold for fifteen seconds and switch sides.

Advanced variation: Look in the direction of your left hand and twist your entire body from your heel to your left fingertips.

#10 Obliques

(Strengthens and stretches oblique muscles)

With your feet together and weights in hands, lift the right weight as high as you can toward your right armpit by bending your elbow toward the ceiling, simultaneously lowering the left weight with your straight arm toward your left ankle. Then switch by lowering the right and lifting the left. During the entire movement, keep your chest lifted and look straight ahead. Curve your

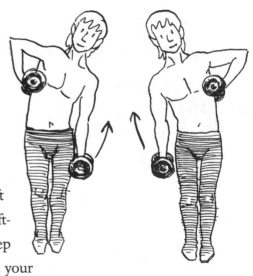

spine from side to side to increase movement. Do twenty times each side.

Advanced variation: Do one hundred times each side.

#11 Ballet Stretch

(Stretches sides)

With legs apart and toes pointed at angles, put your right hand on your waist and your left hand above your head like a ballerina. Keep your knees slightly bent (don't lock). Press your hips slightly to the left with your right hand, and reach your left hand to the right, palm-side down. Take deep breaths and expand your rib cage. Hold for ten seconds and switch sides. Do twice each side.

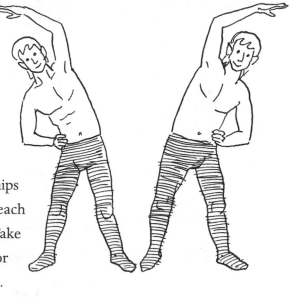

#12 Ballet Squat

(Strengthens entire leg and buttocks)

Open legs to second position in ballet, with feet pointed out to sides. To make sure you have correct leg positioning, your knees should always remain over your ankles when you lower yourself. Place weights in both hands below your chin, keep arms straight but relaxed, and lower yourself as far down as you can go comfortably, stopping with your thighs parallel to the ground. When straightening back up, make sure you keep your knees slightly bent. Don't lock them. Keep a straight line from the top of your

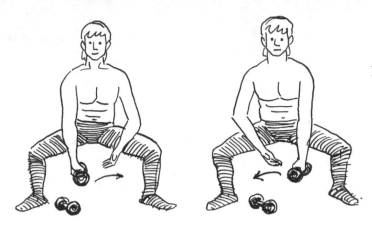

head to your tailbone so that you don't lean forward. Lower twenty-five times.

Advanced variation: Stay at the lowest point and swing weights between hands twenty times.

#13 Weeping Willow Stretch
(Stretches hamstrings, calves and back)

With your feet in the same position as the ballet squat, drop down toward your right ankle. Relax your upper body and let your head dangle down, releasing all the tension in your neck. It's more important to keep your legs straight than to bend your knee and touch your toe. Do for twenty seconds and switch sides.

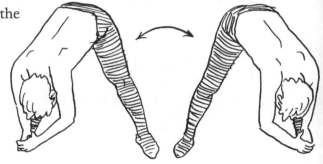

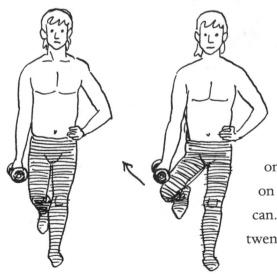

#14 Side Leg Lift
(Strengthens buttocks and legs)

With your feet together and toes pointed forward, place weight in your right hand and rest it on the side of your right leg. With your left hand on your waist, lift your right knee as high as you can. Lower back to the other knee and repeat. Do twenty-five times.

Advanced variation: Put both weights in your hand and do fifty times. If you have trouble balancing, use your opposite hand from the lifting knee and lean against a wall.

#15 Calf Stretch
(Stretches, uh, calves)

With your hands on your waist, lunge your right foot three feet forward. While keeping your left heel on the ground, bend your left knee toward your left toe to stretch out your left calf. Keep your chest lifted and look straight ahead toward your left shin. Hold for fifteen seconds and switch sides.

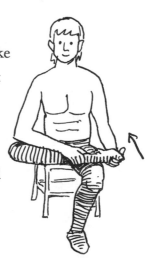

Advanced variation: Drop down with straight legs and pull your left toe up with your right hand and let your forehead relax down toward your right shin.

#16 Airplane Stretch
(Stretches hips and hamstring muscles)

While seated, cross your right leg on top of your left knee. Take your right elbow and set it on top of your right knee, and put your hand on your right ankle. Lean forward and press your lower back toward your right calf while keeping your back straight. Look straight ahead.

Advanced variation: Simultaneously take your left hand and pull your right foot toward the ceiling.

#17 French Curl
(Strengthens biceps muscles)

Put weight in your right hand, take your left hand, and put it palm-side down on your right quad, slightly above your knee. Put your right elbow over and on the outside of your left wrist. Straighten your right arm all the way down toward the ground and curl all the way up. Do twenty-five each side.

Advanced variation: Use both weights in your right hand and do twelve times each arm. No weight: Do fifty times each side.

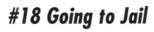

#18 Going to Jail
(Stretches arms and chest)

Interweave your hands behind your tailbone with your knuckles away from you, and lift your straight arms up as high as you can comfortably. Keep your chest lifted. Take deep breaths, expanding your rib cage. Hold for twenty seconds.

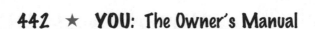

#19 Tree Hug

(Strengthens chest and arms)

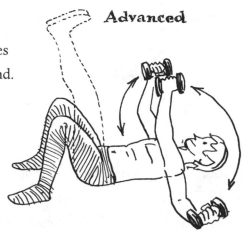

Lie flat on your back with your knees bent and your feet flat on the ground. Raise your arms out to side. Raise your arms toward the ceiling, keeping your hands above your shoulders. Lower the weights down to the ground, tap your elbows, and come back up. Pretend you're hugging a tree. Do fifty times.

Advanced variation: Lift your straight legs up in the air with your feet directly above your hips, while doing usual version.

#20 Tailbone Lift

(Strengthens lower abdominal muscles)

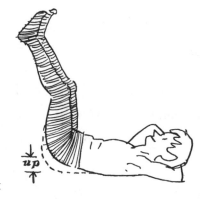

While lying on your back, and with your hands interwoven behind your head and used as a pillow, lift up your legs as straight as you can above your hips. While maintaining this position, lift your tailbone off the ground one inch and tap it slowly back down. Do twenty-five times. Don't allow your chin to compress down to your chest; leave a tennis ball's distance.

Advanced variation: Lift upper body simultaneously and use your hands to hold your head, so your neck is completely relaxed.

#21 One-Legged Crunch

(Strengthens core muscles)

While lying on your back, interweave your
hands behind your head and keep your
knees bent and feet flat on the ground.
Lift your right leg straight up toward the ceiling and flex this foot.
Using your abs, lift your upper body up
toward your right toe. Pretend there is a string in
your belly button, and it's pulling your stomach down toward the ground. Keep your
neck relaxed and hold your head as if it were an egg. Do twenty-five times and switch
legs.

Advanced variation: Keep the lower leg straight and one inch off the ground for
the entire set.

#22 Side Crunch

(Works entire core)

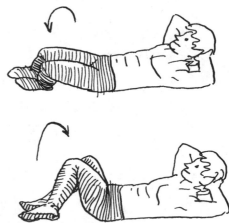

Lie on your back and rest your head in interwoven hands. Drop your bent knees down to
the left, resting your right leg on your left.
Crunch your upper body up, keeping your
chin a tennis ball's distance from your chest.
Focus on pulling your belly button toward
your spine. Do twenty-five times each side.

Advanced variation: Keep your legs one
inch off the ground and crunch your upper and lower
body up each rep.

#23 Sun's in Eyes
(Stretches abs and chest)

While on your knees, take your interwoven hands and place them knuckle-side back on your forehead. Lift your right elbow toward the ceiling as high as you can, away from your right knee, and press your right hip slightly forward. Hold for ten seconds, taking in deep breaths to release any tight muscles.

Advanced variation: Try to look up toward the ceiling.

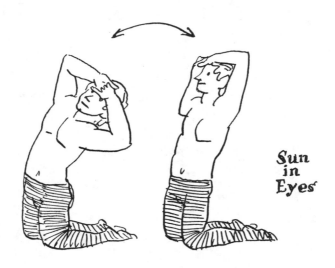

Sun in Eyes

The Owner's Manual Workout Crib Sheet

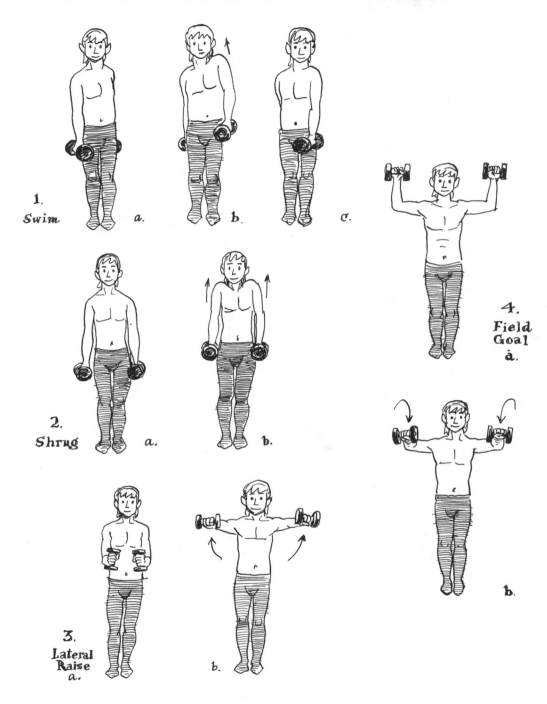

1. Swim   a.   b.   c.

2. Shrug   a.   b.

3. Lateral Raise a.   b.

4. Field Goal â.   b.

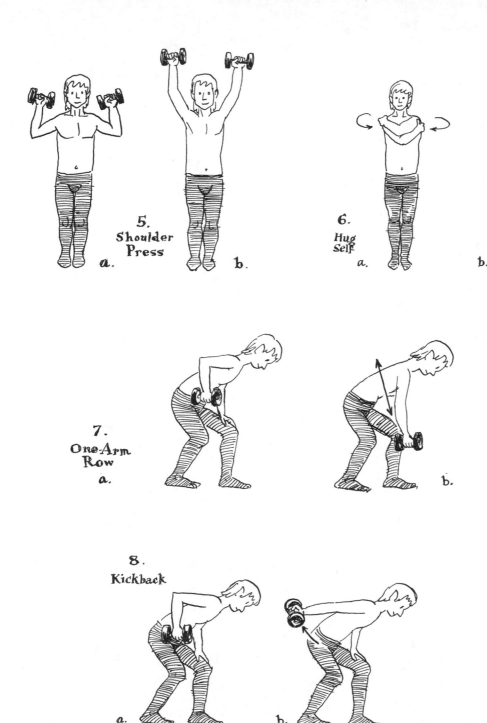

5.
Shoulder
Press
a.   b.

6.
Hug
Self
a.   b.

7.
One-Arm
Row
a.   b.

8.
Kickback
a.   b.

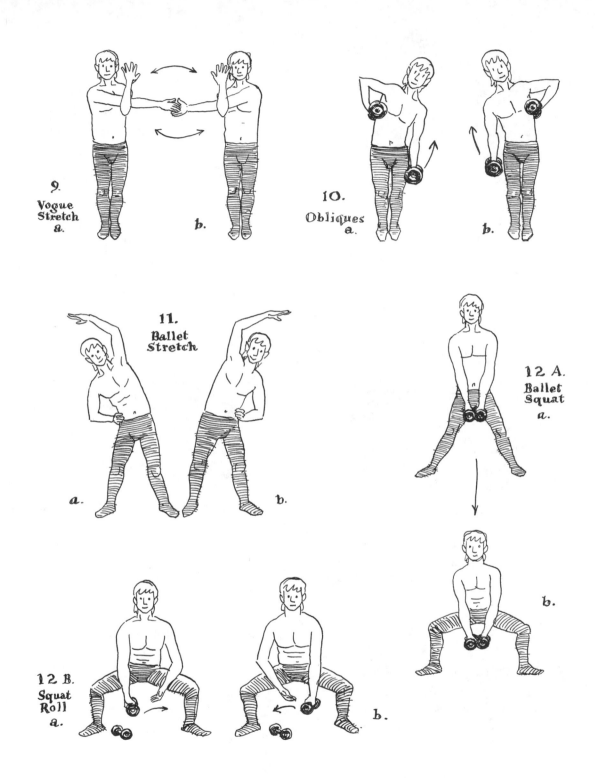

9.
Vogue
Stretch
a.

b.

10.

Obliques
a.

b.

11.
Ballet
Stretch

a.

b.

12 A.
Ballet
Squat
a.

b.

12 B.
Squat
Roll
a.

b.

13.
Weeping Willow Stretch

a.   b.

14.
Side Leg Lift
a.   b.

15.
Calf Stretch

16.
Airplane Stretch

17.
French Curl

18.
Going To Jail

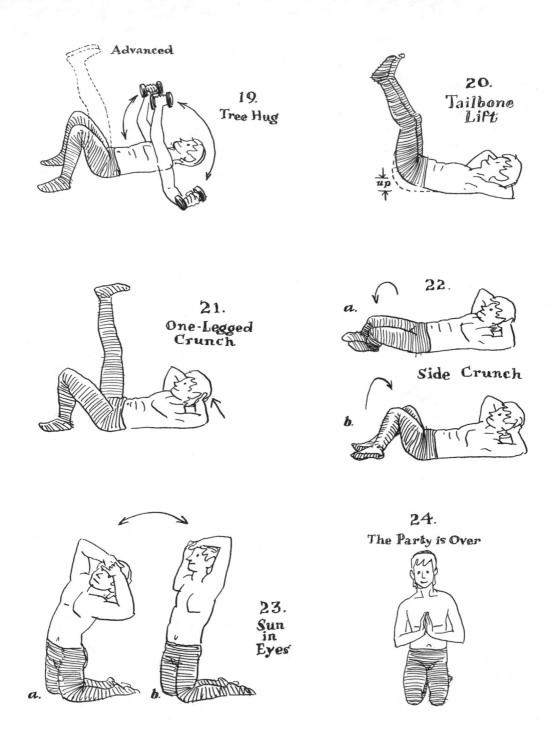

19. Tree Hug

Advanced

20. Tailbone Lift

up

21. One-Legged Crunch

22. a. b. Side Crunch

23. Sun in Eyes

a. b.

24. The Party is Over

More Strength-Training Moves

Want more options? The following strength-training moves are ones you can work into your strength routine or put all together for a workout. Follow these guidelines when performing them:

★ Do one set of each exercise (two if the exercise works only one side of the body at a time). You can increase to two (or four) sets of each exercise as you progress.

★ Train at threshold: Follow the eight/twelve rule. For each exercise, choose a weight light enough that you can lift it eight times in the given exercise but heavy enough that you can't lift it more than twelve times.

★ Start by doing only the exercises in part 1. Add those in part 2 after a month—or earlier if you're comfortable with the first workout.

★ Do not lock your legs or arms. Straight legs and straight arms do not mean that they should be locked.

★ Suck in your abdominals when doing all exercises. That will lead to a stronger midsection and better posture.

★ Breathe. Exhale when you're pushing or pulling the weight, and inhale when you're releasing it back to the starting position.

Strength-Training Moves, Part 1

Squats

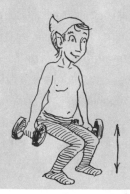

(Strengthens legs and butt)

Stand with your feet a little wider than shoulder width apart and with your hands by your side. Without curling your back, squat down to the point where your thighs are approximately parallel to the floor (or before that, if you have knee or lower-back pain). Pause, then rise up to the original standing position. Look forward throughout the movement. Breathe in on the way down; breathe out on the way up. When twelve repetitions feels too easy, you can add resistance by holding dumbbells or other low-weight objects at your sides.

Lunges

(Strengthens legs and butt)

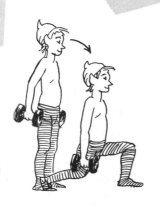

Stand with your feet shoulder width apart with your hands on your hips. Take a long step forward with your left foot. Bend your left knee so that your thigh is parallel to the floor (use the same rule as above if you have knee pain, and make sure that when you're lunging, your knee does not extend farther than your foot). Pause, then step back into the original standing position. Repeat by stepping forward with your right foot. Breathe in when you lunge forward; breathe out when you step back. When twelve reps feels easy, you can add resistance by holding dumbbells or other objects that have weight at your sides. Or do one entire leg at a time, then switch.

Bent-Over Back Rows

(Strengthens back)

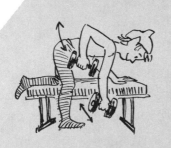

Stand next to a weight bench (or a chair or a piano bench). Put one knee on the bench and hold a dumbbell (or a can of soup or a book) in the opposite hand. With your other hand also resting on the bench, bend over so your back is approximately parallel to the ground. Keep your other arm straight down so the dumbbell dangles toward the floor. Using your back muscles, pull the dumbbell up while slightly skimming your elbow against your side and lifting the weight to your chest. Pause, then lower it. Breathe in when you pull up, out when you lower it. Resist overextending your neck by looking straight down.

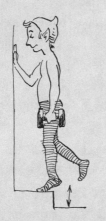

One-Leg Calf Lift

(Strengthens calves)

Stand with the ball of your left foot near the edge of a stair. Hold a weight in your left hand and hold on to a wall or railing with your right hand to balance yourself. Lift your right foot so it hangs relaxed near your left ankle. Lower your left heel off the edge of the stair as far as you comfortably can. Keeping your knee straight, use your left calf muscle to press yourself up on your toes as high as you can.

Push-ups

(Strengthens upper body)

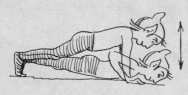

Get in a classic push-up position with your hands on the floor at shoulder width apart, your back straight, and your toes or knees on the floor. Lower yourself until your chest nearly touches the ground and push back up. You can also do modified push-ups on your knees (and with your hands on a stair step, if that's still too difficult). When they become too easy, you can increase the number of repetitions, as well as change the position of your hands, by moving them closer together or farther apart. Look three inches above your fingertips so you don't overextend your neck. Also, resist snapping your elbows in the up position; leave them slightly bent.

Crunch Variations

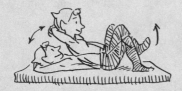

(Strengthens abdominals)

A strong abdominal section supports your back muscles and reduces your risk of injury, as well as speeds recovery if you do have a back strain. Abdominal exercises tend to be a little bit like ice-cream flavors. There are a couple of traditional favorites, but it seems as if somebody is always inventing a new variety to satisfy different tastes. To perform a traditional crunch, lie on your back with your knees bent and feet flat on the floor. Using your abdominal muscles, crunch up about 30 degrees from the floor. You can add variety and hit different parts of your midsection with crunch variations. At the same time you crunch your body up, curl your legs off the ground toward your head, and squeeze your belly button toward the floor. In this variation, you'll use all three pairs of muscles—the upper with the upper crunch, the lower with the leg pull, and the middle with the squeeze. Or try doing crunches with your back flat on an exercise ball. Or lie flat on the floor and lift your knees toward your chest. In this variation, you'll use more of the lower region of your abdominals.

Arm and Leg Lifts

(Strengthens abdominals)

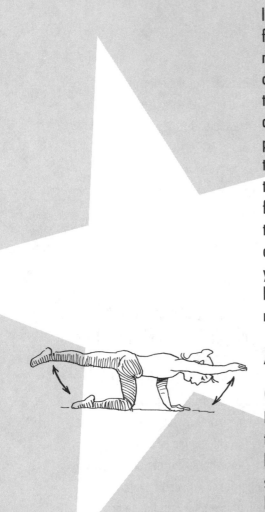

Place both hands and knees on the floor with your arms and thighs parallel to each other and perpendicular to the floor. Your knees should be directly under your hips, and your hands should be under your shoulders. Look to the floor, keeping your head in line with your spine. Keep your back straight. Lift your right arm and left leg slowly off the floor and extend them straight out so that your leg, back, and arm are roughly in one line. Slowly lower them to the starting position. After one set, switch positions—lifting your left arm and right leg.

Strength-Training Moves, Part 2

Chest Press

(Strengthens chest)

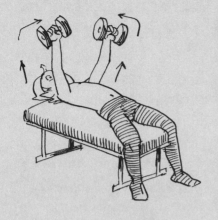

With a dumbbell (or other kind of weight) in each hand, lie on the floor, holding the weights close to your chest. Bend your knees and place your feet on the floor (you can also do this from a bench). Press the weights straight up from your shoulders with your palms facing each other or facing your toes, and bring the weights close together. Slowly lower the weights out to the sides until your elbows are even with your shoulders.

Biceps Curl

(Strengthens arms)

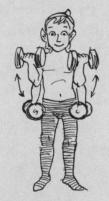

Stand or sit with your feet approximately shoulder width apart, your arms down at your sides and your palms facing forward. Hold a dumbbell (or other kind of weight) in each hand. Bend your elbows slowly, bringing your hands toward your shoulders, keeping your elbows down at your sides. Slowly return to the starting position. Resist rocking and dropping your chin, and keep your shoulders back.

Standing Side Lift

(Strengthens shoulders)

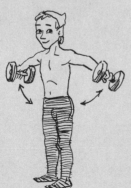

Stand with your feet shoulder width apart and your knees and hips slightly bent. Hold a dumbbell (or other kind of weight) in each hand. Lean forward slightly from the hips and let your arms hang straight down, with your elbows bent and your palms facing each other. Pull your arms up and out to your side, keeping your wrists straight and elbows slightly bent. Lift until your arms are almost parallel to the floor and your hands are slightly in front of you. Lead with your elbows, not your wrists. Slowly lower them back to the starting position.

Rotator-Cuff Rotation

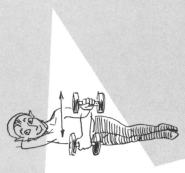

(Strengthens rotator cuff)

Lie on your side on a bench or on the floor with a weight in your top hand. Bend your elbow at a 90-degree angle and hold your upper arm against the side of your body with your forearm down across your body. Lift the weight by rotating the top shoulder outward while keeping your upper arm against the side of your body. Lift until your forearm is almost perpendicular to the floor. Resist sliding your elbows on your side. Try to stay locked in.

Overhead Press

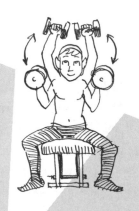

(Strengthens shoulders)

Sit on a bench or chair with back support. Hold one weight in each hand and lift the weights until your forearms are perpendicular to the floor, with the weights at shoulder level. With your palms facing forward, press the weights above you until they come together over your head, with your elbows bent ever so slightly.

Lateral Deltoid Lift

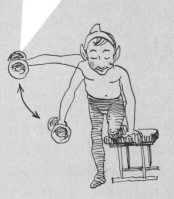

(Strengthens shoulders)

Place your left knee and left arm on a bench; your right foot remains on the floor. Pick up a weight with your right hand. Pull your arm up and out to the side until your elbows are slightly higher than the level of your torso and your hand has reached the level of your shoulders. Slowly return to the starting position. Resist locking your support arm; always keep it slightly bent.

Chapter 15

YOU: The Owner's Manual FAQs

The YOU Docs Answers Your Questions about Your Body and Your Health

We now know how Santa feels come December. After we published *YOU: The Owner's Manual* in 2005, we received more than one hundred thousand letters with questions about health. While this book is intended to serve as a health bible of sorts to help you understand your body, we also know that the body is a universe of its own—with limitless possibilities. That's why we're including an entire chapter in this edition on FAQs—frequently asked questions—to address your particular concerns about your particular body.

Your Heart and Arteries

Family Matters

Question: What percentage does my family history play as opposed to my lifestyle in my chances of having heart disease? I'm a female and live a very healthy life. I'm a vegetarian, eat no saturated or trans fats, and run and do weight training. But I also have a strong family history of heart disease.—Irene, fifty-five

Answer: About 25 percent of your risk of disease is the genes you inherit. You actually control your genes to a large part. All genes do is watch other genes or are protein factories, and which factories you turn on or off are under your control. Aging fats turn on a gene that makes your arteries become more stiff and age, while walking turns on a gene that decreases cancer growth.

Change of Heart

Question: I'm in my fifties, and I have been eating very unhealthily and fear it may be too late. Is it possible to reverse heart problems? I have never been told I had a heart problem, and my cholesterol has always been normal, but I do have high blood pressure (usually 130/90) and am very overweight. Is there any hope?—Lisa M., fifty-five

Answer: Of course there's hope. As long as the heart has a reason to keep beating, it's going to hang in there for you. Your job? To be a compassionate owner of your heart—so you give it reason to keep pumping out more blood than a low-budget horror flick. You get a do-over in life—you can literally pull plaque out of aged arteries. But you need to act now. Because of your waist and blood pressure, your heart is under a fair amount of stress, so it probably feels more overworked than a first-year law student. You can help out your heart by making some changes. If you lose the extra weight (especially around your stomach), I bet your blood pressure will start coming down. And since this is the single biggest factor in aging us, you'll get to live longer as well. So start walking thirty minutes a day and follow our guidelines in *YOU: On a Diet* as if your heart depended on it. Because it does.

More questions?

Send them to Oprah.com or RealAge.com. We'll answer as many as we can and post them on one of the Web sites.

Take a Pill

Question: Should I take aspirin, even if I take omega-3s daily?—Jackie, forty

Answer: Though some pairs seem to go great together (beer and nuts) and others don't (salami and sorbet), it's not always easy knowing what's best to mix in your mouth. These two pills? Well, they have more power than a Lamborghini, so we recommend that you talk to your doc about taking both. Aspirin and omega-3s both decrease inflammation in your arteries; that reduces the risk of heart disease, stroke, memory loss, and impotence. Omega-3s also decrease the risk of depression and arthritis, while aspirin drops the risks of colon cancer, breast cancer, and prostate cancer. And both seem to help keep your brain working like it did ten years ago. For typical men over thirty-five and women over forty, we recommend taking them both. We take 162 milligrams aspirin (that's two baby aspirin or half a regular aspirin). Take it with a large glass of water to help avoid potential gastrointestinal side effects. For omega-3s, you can gulp down 2 grams of distilled fish oil or 600 milligrams of DHA supplements (from algae—where the fish get their highest-quality and longest-chain omega-3s), or enjoy twelve walnuts a day. You can also get the same benefits by eating four ounces of nonfried fatty fish three times a week. Wild salmon, mahi-mahi, flounder, and tilapia are four that are neither overfished nor associated with toxins.

Take Two

Question: Why two baby aspirin for heart protection and not just one per day? —Ernestine, sixty

Answer: Like they say in Vegas, it's all about the odds. When you take 162 milligrams or greater of aspirin, you reduce your arterial aging by 36 percent. With 82 milligrams, the reduction is 13 percent. Since the side effects are just a little more pronounced with 162 milligrams, the benefit of taking 162 milligrams is far greater—with only a little increase in risk. Las Vegas won't give you such odds without your paying a much higher price. For aspirin, the bump is great for the increased risk. We'll take those odds every time.

Stroke Story

Question: Once a person has a stroke, what's the likelihood that they'll have another one if they control their blood pressure?—Andy W., forty-eight

Answer: It depends, because there are so many kinds of strokes. Certainly, many strokes are caused by high blood pressure. For those people, there's a 20 percent recurrence rate within two years if they control their BP, compared to a 50 percent rate if they don't. You can lower that 20 percent by about 70 percent more by avoiding smoke (even secondhand smoke), eating healthy fats (like 2 grams of distilled fish oil or an ounce of walnuts a day—see "Take a Pill," above), controlling stress and meditating daily, taking 162 milligrams of aspirin a day if your doc says it's okay, and taking 200 milligrams of coenzyme Q10 a day.

Your Weight

Worth the Weight

Question: I'm three weeks into the YOU Diet and have lost two inches and ten pounds. I have been stuck at the same exact weight for a week now, and I'm not sure why. I'm really frustrated because I started lifting weights on Monday, I've been walking every day, and I've really been trying to watch what/how much I'm eating. What now?—Anita, forty-seven

Answer: Don't worry about daily weight when you first start muscle building. You will accumulate water in these newly worked muscles, so the weight gain (or lack of loss) is water, which will go away with time. It is the opposite of the weight loss that occurs on an Atkins or South Beach type of diet—the majority of early weight loss on those low-carb diets is from ridding your muscles of water. That water loss in muscles will come back like an unwanted boyfriend when you eat carbs again. So your steady weight now is actually progress.

Mean Genes

Question: How common are genetics as a cause of diabetes or obesity? Is it possible to overcome your genetics?—Pat J., forty-five

Answer: Sure would be nice to blame Aunt Mabel for the shape of your thighs, but it doesn't quite work that way. For obesity and diabetes (we're talking type 2 diabetes, which makes up 95 percent of diabetes cases in the U.S.), your environment (that is, your lifestyle, your behaviors, and those Nutter Butters in your pantry) is a much more dominant trait than genetics. Diabetes ages you one and a half years for every year you live with it. For example, if you get it at age thirty and live to sixty, you're not really sixty—you have the energy and disability risks of a seventy-five-year-old.

Here's how it works: Type 2 diabetes is a genetic disease. That is, if you were an identical twin and your twin got type 2 diabetes, you'd have the genetics for it.

Type 2 diabetes makes sugar build up in your bloodstream rather than directly into your cells. That causes weakness in the seals between cells in your arteries, allowing cholesterol to seep in. It also causes sugar to attach to proteins and make them less effective. That causes a host of health problems. For example:

★ It increases your blood pressure.
★ It increases your risk of heart attacks, strokes, memory loss, kidney failure, eye problems, arthritis, and lung disease.
★ It decreases your ability to fight off infections.

But here's the thing: You can control your genes if you want to. To keep blood sugar levels down, you should avoid foods with simple sugar, syrups, any grain but 100% whole grain, and lousy aging fats (trans and saturated fats). About 2,000 calories' worth of activity a week—about thirty minutes of walking every day (no excuses) and thirty minutes of weight lifting a week—causes your muscles to be so much more sensitive to insulin, which allows sugar into your cells. Good foods to eat for diabetics (or anyone—it is the same goal) are featured on the RealAge.com Web site.

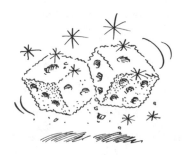

Your Brain

Memory Booster

Question: Several articles have listed pyroglutamate for memory. Have you heard of it?—Greta, thirty-nine

Answer: What was that again? Kidding. The primary claim made for the product is that it can help overcome memory defects induced by alcohol abuse and in those with some forms of dementia. Some people in Italy use the supplement to treat alcoholism, senility, and mental retardation. While such sweeping use is unwarranted based on current findings, there are some data suggesting a cognitive-enhancing role. In one double-blind study (the best kind of study) of older people, verbal memory was said to be improved in those taking arginine pyroglutamate compared with controls who received placebo. An even better bet for cognitive enhancement? Walking, coffee, omega-3s (especially DHA), curry and mustard, and mental games like bridge, chess, and crossword puzzles.

In the Mood

Question: Is depression more common in women?—Karen, thirty-nine

Answer: Most investigators report that depression is two to three times as common in women as in men. Hormonal changes around the times of pregnancy, menopause, and the premenstrual cycle can cause mood disturbances. Sexual or physical abuse may contribute to higher rates of depression. The last explanation: Our wives argue that a woman is bound to be depressed when she has to put up with a man who never listens, talks incessantly about sex, poop, and sports, and babbles on obsessively about some books he wrote.

Lasting Love

Question: Does falling in love really cause chemical changes in the brain?
—Renee, thirty-two

Answer: It's not just butterflies in your stomach or tingling in your private parts that you're feeling; when you're in love, you actually experience major chemical changes in your brain as well. Research shows that serotonin—a feel-good chemical—in lovesick subjects was just as low as the serotonin levels in people with obsessive-compulsive disorder. So if your heart hurts or you feel a little insane in the membrane, there's a solid scientific basis for losing your heart and your marbles! By the way, hugging increases the release of oxytocin (another feel-good chemical) throughout your body.

Positively Positive

Question: I'm sick and I'm tired of everyone telling me to have a positive attitude. Is there any truth to the idea that positive thinking and humor can heal?
—Lilly, fifty

Answer: Now, it's not like your doc can write up a prescription-strength, 500-milligram joke and send you on your healthy way. But don't dismiss positive thinking. Attitude and fun are as good for your body as water, sunscreen, and a six-hand massage. Besides the fact that humor has been shown to boost brainpower and improve immune-cell function (which can help ward off cancer), a positive attitude works wonders because that means you're more likely to do things such as walk, eat cruciferous vegetables, and avoid saturated fats—three choices that substantially help the chance of survival after heart attacks, strokes, and cancer. So instead of feeling bluer than our scrubs, take charge of your life. While you're at it, TiVo Letterman, Stewart, or Leno (because sleep is just as important for your health, bucko).

Remember, miracles do happen, and you can bet your sweet aspirin that they happen more often to people who are positively positive.

Speak Not So Easy

Question: I tend to freeze up whenever I have to talk to more than a couple people at a time. Why do we sometimes panic and feel like deer stuck in the headlights? —Patty I., forty-eight

Answer: This response is called tonic immobility, and it's not to be confused with the inability to walk out of a bar after a half-dozen cocktails. The response is common in animals that are avoiding other predators. See, most animals will not eat meat that they didn't kill, so if you're caught and play dead, the hunter will pass by. This same instinct is sometimes stimulated by our autopilot nervous system to make us feel like a Volkswagen in two feet of mud—completely stuck and paralyzed about spinning our wheels trying to get out of the situation. The solution: Focus by speaking to one person during group talks, then move to another. We do that too.

Brain Freeze

Question: What causes an ice-cream headache?—Larry, fifty

Answer: Ah, downed your triple-dipped chocolate a little too quickly, eh? There are two theories as to what causes the rush of pain that comes with frozen food. One, the rapid cooling of air in the frontal sinuses may trigger local pain receptors. Two, after the cold rush passes, the constricted blood vessels in the roof and rear of the mouth relax; as blood rushes into the area, it overloads local pain receptors and shoots the pain to the head. These are correlated with migraine headaches in some people, which makes sense, since the cause of these headaches is also dilation of arteries. To reduce the pain: Keep your tongue touching the roof of your mouth—and stop eating so much ice cream!

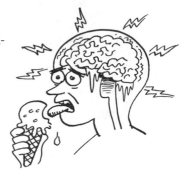

Nosing Around

Question: **The hairs in my nose grow fast, so I pull them out—like, six a day. I heard that may be bad for your brain. Is it?—David, forty-two**
Answer: Yes, pulling nose hairs can be bad for your brain. The danger is that you will break the skin somehow and give root to an infection, which could subsequently migrate inward into the base of the brain. Blood from your nose (to be precise, from a triangular region of the face centered on the nose) drains to the rear toward your brain, where it joins various other veins, including the ones that drain blood out of your brain. If a nasal infection were to travel downstream and block this junction point (a condition known as intracranial thrombophlebitis—say that three times fast), you'd have big problems. Some doctors call it "the triangle of death." Use a special nose-hair clipper; it's a great present and a clue to a loved one.

Your Bones, Joints, and Muscles

Bone Crusher

Question: I was recently diagnosed with osteoporosis of the spinal column. What are your recommendations?—Lila E., sixty-three
Answer: Some of us like to call osteoporosis the Rottweiler disease, because it can

chew up bones fast. Your job is to do what you can to build your bones and make sure they stay as dense as the third-grade class clown. For starters, do resistance exercises such as lunges, bent-over back rows, and squats with a weight in each hand, or the exercises in the Owner's Manual Workout on page 433. Strength training builds muscle *and* bone—and that can help slow the progression of osteoporosis. Also, take the following twice a day: 200 milligrams of magnesium, 300 milligrams of vitamin C, and 600 milligrams of calcium with 400 IU of vitamin D. And be sure to eat some spinach or another leafy green with vitamin K in it. Then take another DEXA scan in twelve months to gauge your levels.

Joint Lessons

Question: I have joint pain. I heard that people who are allergic to shellfish shouldn't take the glucosamine-chondroitin product for joint pain. Are there other options that don't contain shellfish products?—Patricia, forty-four

Answer: The most common form of joint pain isn't the kind felt by those running out of reefer at a reggae concert. It's osteoarthritis, and it can be so debilitating that it can make everything—from walking to getting up off the couch—more uncomfortable than a wet pair of jeans. To slow the progression of osteoarthritis, you should take these steps:

★ Exercise the muscles surrounding affected joints.
★ Take aspirin or other anti-inflammatories.
★ Take vitamin D (1,000 IU a day), vitamin C (300 milligrams twice a day, assuming you're not taking a statin drug such as Lipitor), calcium (600 milligrams twice a day), and DHA (600 mg a day) or fish or walnut oil (2 grams a day).

We don't know of any substitute for glucosamine and chondroitin sulfate except Avosoy Complete. Three smooth-coated tablets daily provide 300 milligrams of

ASU (that's avocado-soybean unsaponifiables, not Arizona State University), 1,500 milligrams of shellfish-free glucosamine, and 800 milligrams of "cow-free" chondroitin, plus vitamins C and E and the mineral manganese. See www.drtheo.com.

Fast Action

Question: I have five minutes every morning that I watch the news; I feel I should exercise in that time. What should I do?—Juanita H., thirty-five

Answer: You are smart. Just stretch that to ten minutes every day, and you could do all the resistance exercises you need. Start by learning how to do lunges, push-ups, crunches, and back rows. Then do lunges and push-ups one day, and crunches and back rows the next. You can do these using your own body as the weight to lift or graduate to milk containers filled with water or sand or real weights. You can find those described at www.Real Age.com, and you can do them while watching the news.

Your Lungs

Clean Air Action

Question: Do air filters work? I am in a newer home that was built three years ago, but I feel like there are pollutants in it. What can be done about this?—Lindsey, twenty-nine

Answer: Old air filters work about as well as remote controls without batteries. Make sure to clean or replace your filters every year and your air ducts every three years to keep air inside the home free of toxins. Also, don't store any toxin-containing substances within your home.

Pump Up Lungs?

Question: Do human growth hormone pills help strengthen my lungs and help me get more oxygen to my brain and lungs?—Phyllis, fifty

Answer: Oral—or over-the-counter—human growth hormone (HGH) is as worthless to your lungs as a car without a windshield and wheels. There's no research to show that the HGH pills are absorbed, and studies show that any effectiveness is from the placebo effect; 30 percent of the people who take something they believe in get a benefit, even if it's a water pill. For prescription HGH, there's a debate over its value. It has both risks and benefits, but it seems that it has more risks than benefits. That is, we see growth of all cells, not just muscle but cancer, as well as some bone and cartilage growth (which can promote carpal tunnel syndrome as well as fat loss). Our recommendation: Reduce your arterial aging to get younger, feel better, and have more energy. (See our tips for heart health, starting on page 31.)

Open Nose

Question: Do nose strips really work to improve breathing?—Layla, thirty

Answer: Although they're popular on NFL players and major-league snorers, scientific studies have failed to show any significant improvement in the amount of oxygen you receive by wearing them. But if your major issue is allergies, then using the strips to open up your nasal passages makes sense. If you are not overweight, a visit to the neighborhood ENT (that's ear, nose, and throat doc) may reveal a structural problem like mucous buildup, which can easily be cured with a minor procedure or Neti pot use. (See www.oprah.com/droz or RealAge.com for a demo of using a Neti pot.)

Hic Tricks

Question: What are hiccups, and how do you get rid of them?—Jennifer, thirty-six

Answer: Hiccups—whether they last for seventeen seconds or seventeen years—occur when the diaphragm becomes irritated by distention of the stomach by food, alcohol, tobacco, or air, as well as sudden changes in gastric temperature. The diaphragm gets out of sync and rapidly pushes air up in such a way that it makes an irregular sound. Hiccups can also be caused by excitement or stress. A lot of remedies have been tried, and they relate to stimulating nerves that innervate the back of your throat or your tongue or just startling you. Try sugar on the tongue, a spoon to your throat (do not let your spouse do this if she's mad at you), or just a real hard pinch at an unexpected time just below your jaw and near your ear.

Your Sleep

Sacrificial Sleep

Question: How do I make an intelligent choice between sleep and exercise? I usually sleep when time is tight and stress is high. Am I better off getting an extra hour of sleep or getting up to squeeze in my workout? Is there some other sleep-exercise combination that might be the best of both worlds?—Randi, thirty-three

Answer: For the most benefits, you should get at least seven to seven and a half hours of sleep a night, and you should be able to find twenty to thirty minutes a day to do walking (or another cardiovascular exercise), strength training, or flexibility training like yoga. If you must, we're okay with you going to six and a half hours of sleep to squeeze in exercise. But health isn't a version of *Let's Make a Deal,* where you pick one box (sleep) over another (exercise). What you have to do is figure out ways to make sure you get the right amounts of both. If that means reorganizing your life to schedule physical activity, good. If it means missing a *Sex and the City* rerun to squeeze in a workout, fine. If it means that you have to end your relationship with Messrs. Stewart and Leno to hit the pillow a little earlier, so be it. (Sorry, Jon and Jay.) Try recording and watching during your weekend.

Sleep Patterns

Question: Do men sleep more than women?—Andrew, forty-seven
Answer: Some people believe that women are biologically programmed to sleep better than men. Why? While you may write it off to women-do-everything-better reasons, it's actually a little more scientific. Estrogen—higher in women, of course—works on your brain's sleep center to decrease the number of awakenings after you fall asleep and increases total sleep time.

Tired Answers

Question: Why do you get dark rings or bags under your eyes when you are tired?—Jennifer, thirty-six
Answer: Your coworker isn't the only one who has thin skin. We all do—at least right there. The skin under your eyes is the thinnest anywhere on the body, and that allows dark venous blood to show through. So if you are standing or sitting upright, blood pools there more. In addition to being caused by lack of sleep, dark rings can be brought on by allergies or asthma. These conditions can cause more blood to pool in the tissues under the eye and can add puffiness to the area.

Your Guts

Burn Center

Question: What causes heartburn? How common is it? All my friends are taking purple pills. Am I missing out?—Marilyn, fifty-one

Answer: Heartburn is all about geometry and angles. The swallowing tube (esophagus) enters the stomach at a sharp angle that keeps food from regurgitating back up. When this angle is stretched by too much weight hanging off the stomach, as with a beer belly, or overly large meals or a hernia, the angle is made less sharp—more straight—and the acid can flow back up the esophagus. The result is a painful acid burn, which takes a few days to heal. For the 20 percent of Americans who suffer from heartburn, there are things they can do. Take the steps outlined below to help reduce problems.

Reflux Response

Question: Is it necessary to maintain a healthy esophagus by using prescription drugs, or is there a natural way to help prevent gastroesophageal reflux disease (GERD)?—Kris, forty-one

Answer: Throats are like mountains and sliding boards. It's much easier to have things go down them than to go up them. So, yes, we (as well as your spouse) would very much like you to avoid spewing fire across the table after you eat. These are the best steps to take for preventing GERD:

1. Make your meals smaller.
2. Lose weight if you are overweight (most important choice for those who are overweight, but it's the most time consuming).

3. Eliminate pepper, spicy foods, alcohol, and caffeine.

4. Take two baby aspirins a day with a glass of warm water to help prevent esophageal cancer from developing in GERD-burned area.

5. Do not eat within three hours of bedtime.

6. Stop smoking if you do.

7. Elevate your head six inches when lying on your back.

8. Talk to your doctor about OTC proton pump inhibitors like Prilosec. But do prevent the burn, because we don't want you to use your stem cells on GERD—you may need them to help repair your heart or brain.

Appendix Upended

Question: Why do you have an appendix if you can live without it?—Nancy H., forty

Answer: Many people think that your appendix is like e-mail spam—totally unnecessary. But it does have its purpose. A small pouch off the large intestine, the appendix has a wall that contains lymphatic tissue, making it part of the immune system that generates antibodies. But while it serves a function, your body will adapt if you lose it. That's because several other areas in the body contain similar tissue: the spleen, lymph nodes, and tonsils. (The spleen and tonsils can also be removed.)

The Food Shall Too Pass

Question: How long does it take to digest food?—Landon J., forty-eight

Answer: Your body can digest most food in less time than it takes hotshot celebrities to get engaged: about four to twelve hours. Fruits are the fastest travelers on the intestinal interstate, with meats driving like an oversized load in the right lane (they can take two to three days to be excreted or even longer as they rot inside your intestine). By the way, gum is processed as fast as most other foods—not the seven years that Mom had you believe.

Brown Out

Question: Not that I'm a color aficionado, but why is poop brown?—Paul B., thirty-seven

Answer: Blame it on bile. Bile secreted from the liver meets the food just past the stomach, then treats your waste like a wooden porch: It stains it greenish brown. If it's not that color, then treat your poop like a mood ring—a different color is an indicator of something else going on in your body. Green bowel movements signify rapid movement of food through the intestines or the digestion of blue or black foods. White-colored poop (yes, the poop actually looks this color) means that the bile from the liver is not entering your gut and you need to see a doctor. Red-colored poop usually means you ate beets, but it could also be blood from the large intestine. Black-colored poop means that you are taking iron pills or your stomach ulcer is bleeding.

Messy Matters

Question: Is diarrhea dangerous?—Marti F., forty-two

Answer: For the guy cleaning the latrine, it sure is. And sometimes it can be for infants and older people; the loss of water and salt that goes with diarrhea fells more infants worldwide than any other problem. But for most Americans or developed-world adults, the question isn't about danger, it's about hydration and whether we can keep enough water in when we get diarrhea. The large bowel's job is to reabsorb water, so during diarrhea these mechanisms are paralyzed. If you are having more than four episodes a day (or enough to disrupt your life) for more than three days, you probably should see a doctor. Bacteria and viruses will run their course, but taking chicken soup with rice helps by bringing sugar and salt to the bowel wall, where they can be absorbed at least a little. If the diarrhea lasts longer, you need to worry about parasites (like giardia) or allergies from the very rich network of immune cells in the bowel wall. Foods like milk, wheat, barley, oats, or rye can irritate the intestines, and you will diagnose this only by avoiding these foods for a week and seeing if you feel better.

Stomach Churn

Question: I just don't like vomiting—and am actually a little afraid of it. What can I do to overcome this?—**Barbara, twenty-seven**

Answer: You have a common phobia, but it is a miracle that humans *can* vomit. It gives us the ability to forage for food and cough it up if it doesn't agree with us. To do this, the stomach twists itself, and the swallowing tube (esophagus) starts contracting backward to propel the food up to your mouth. Animals that cannot burp or vomit are at great risk. So just brush your teeth to remove the bitter taste from the acid and forget about it.

Irritating Problem

Question: I've been told that I have irritable bowel syndrome. What is it?—**Nicole, thirty-seven**

Answer: To the surprise of most parents, irritable bowel syndrome isn't the fact that you can't get three minutes of peace in the bathroom. This is a very common ailment. It is a leading cause of belly pain and is probably due to subtle allergies, stress, or infections. Doctors need to customize the care of folks suffering from this condition and often start with soothing medications and elimination of culprit foods (especially dairy and wheat, oat, barley, and rye products). The solutions can be quite challenging. When the War of the Worlds is progressing through your intestines and enemy bacteria are taking over territory in your gut, you need allies. Many people are turning to probiotics in food or pill form, which have been useful (especially lactobacillus GG and *Bacillus coagulans*). Here's how they work: When the good bacteria in your gut become depleted by disease, stress, poor diet, or certain antibiotics, bad bacteria have room to spread like syrup over pancakes. Eventually they gain the upper hand in your intestines, thus causing the diarrhea, constipation, and inflammation in the intestines called colitis. Untreated, the gut wall can weaken and become "leaky," allowing undigested fats and proteins into the bloodstream to cause inflammation. Probiotics may prevent or reverse the problem by attaching to the intestinal wall and fighting the overzealous pathogens.

Tummy Trouble

Question: I have constant stomach pains, and I'm always tired. I've been to the doctor many times and have been told there was nothing wrong with me. Is there anything I can take for fatigue or stomach aches?—Crystal, twenty-three

Answer: If your doctor has cleared you, our guess is that your symptoms are being caused by one or more of the three things that are making you feel like a caterpillar on the wrong end of an army boot: stress, lack of sleep, or a surreptitious disagreement with a food you eat often. While you'll have to find the stress-reduction technique that calms and soothes you personally, we recommend two things that can be very effective for stress relief and overall health: a deep breathing technique and walking for thirty minutes with a friend at lunchtime every day. We recommend taking a multivitamin twice a day for insurance—that'll help guard against deficiencies that could be causing your sluggishness. As for finding a food that is causing you a problem, try the elimination plan on page 198.

Your Menstrual Cycle

Chocolate Mystery

Question: Why do women crave chocolate during their periods?—Heidi C., thirty-one

Answer: Any question that starts with "Why do women" may be a bigger mystery than a Roswell UFO case. The truth is, we don't know, and there's little scientific support for a link between Mars Bars and menstrual cycles. Some have suggested that Willy Wonka cravings during menstruation are related to a deficiency of magnesium or are linked to carbohydrate consumption as a way to self-medicate depression.

A Sensitive Period

Question: Why do your breasts get tender before your period?—Paula, thirty-seven

Answer: The same thing that causes increased hunger, mood swings, and all the other things associated with the menstrual cycle: hormonal fluctuations. They're what cause changes in the breast ducts and the breast lobules. The breast pain usually occurs during the second half of the menstrual cycle, when estrogen production increases, and peaks just prior to the middle of your cycle; it causes enlargement of the breast ducts, which then causes the pain. Simple anti-inflammatory medications like aspirin (with plenty of water) can help take the pressure off.

Flow Max

Question: I have a heavy menstrual flow. What can I do?—Kristen, thirty-six

Answer: Common causes of having a heavy period during your period include having a polyp, fibroids, or too thick an endometrial lining. Often these can be controlled with oral contraceptives, but if your bleeding lasts for more than seven days or you need to change tampons more than every two hours, you need a doctor. Same goes if your periods disappear for longer than three months. Clots are not rare, and you may have to change your tampons several times daily, but you need to thoroughly cleanse the lining of your uterus, so be thankful this self-cleaning oven system works.

Your Eyes

Vision Question

Question: I've never worn glasses or had a vision problem, but lately I'm having trouble reading. Do I need to go to the eye doctor, or can I just pick up those glasses at the drugstore? Are they okay for now?—Mary, forty-nine

Answer: It's normal for people to squint when they're looking at the sun, drug warning labels, or blood-heavy horror movies. But if you're having trouble making out these words right here or often opt for big-print editions of books and magazines, then yup, it's time you twirled the display rack to find which four-eyed frame looks best. Reading glasses are easy and inexpensive and can help make your reading material feel like billboards, but don't lose sight of the bigger problem: Even if a cheap pair of reading glasses clears the blur, your eyes could be sending you the message that something else is wrong, so see an ophthalmologist once a year (and go to the

ER with any sudden vision changes). Now, for those of you who still have time, try spending more time looking at the horizon: That will exercise your eyes in ways other than most of us are used to doing, and that can help protect against long-term vision loss. Either way, don't fret; most of us experience vision changes as we get older. Your new-fangled specs—and the fact that you knew enough to get some help—are merely signs of your old-fangled wisdom.

Low Light

Question: Does reading in dim light hurt my eyes?—Kyla B., twenty-seven

Answer: Dim lights are great for watching movies or having sex, and they're also fine for your eyes. What does hurt your eyes is being indoors a lot. People who grow up outdoors must accommodate their eyes to both close-up objects and the horizon; this exercise keeps their eyes limber and supple, so they can see better for longer. As a side note, our eyes are extremely sensitive to peripheral motion. When we focus ahead all day long, we don't take time to allow this peripheral vision to dominate. So if you work at a computer, take time to look at the person on the other side of the room (or even farther away). You'll be doing more than your eyes good, as achieving this peripheral vision is particularly useful for meditation.

Socket to Him

Question: At birth, are your eyeballs the size that they will be your whole life? —Len, forty-three

Answer: Newborns' eyes are about 18 millimeters in diameter, which is anywhere from two-thirds to three-quarters of the fully grown adult size. Most eye growth occurs in the first year of life, and by the time you're three, your eyes are mostly fully developed (unlike your vocabulary and manners).

Your Ears

Sounds Good

Question: I love my iPod but don't know if playing the music loudly can hurt my ears.—Janice, thirty-three

Answer: Huh? Come again? You say something? Of course loud sounds can hurt your ears! In fact, it's the most common culprit for causing deafness and typically is more prevalent in men because they have been traditionally exposed to more noise on the job. (This should dispel the myth that men are choosing *SportsCenter* over you; they just can't *hear* you.) Here's the scoop on iPods. Under environmental protection laws in the U.S., employers are not allowed to expose your ears to more than 90 decibels of sound for more than an hour at a time. This is the noise level of a busy city street. If you turn your iPod volume up to 70 percent to jam to Ludacris, you're at this same loudness. Now, if you're trying to block out the sounds on that same busy city street or crank Usher during a workout, it's your ears that are taking a pounding. We've got nothing against listening to music, those sexy headphones (which increase the sound another 10 decibels), or going bonkers downloading Sinatra's complete works, but we just want you to keep an eye on your dial—to keep your ears intact. So keep the iPod on less than 50 percent and take breaks from the music for five minutes every half hour.

Ring in the New Ear

Question: What causes ringing in the ears?—Craig, forty

Answer: If it sounds like a bad rendition of "Jingle Bells" in your ears, it can be caused by many things. Causes of the ear ringing called tinnitus include age-related hearing loss, trauma, medications, changes in ear bones, high blood pressure, head and neck tumors, temporo mandibular joint (TMJ) pain, ear infection, thyroid disease, increased blood flow to the ear, and wax buildup. That about got it covered?

Pop Till You Drop

Question: Why do your ears pop on an airplane?—Dan, thirty

Answer: When you take off, the air pressure in the cabin decreases as you ascend. The air trapped in your inner ear needs to escape and equalize the pressure between your inner ear and the atmosphere. How? The air escapes through your Eustachian tube, a small passage between the inner ear and the back of the nose and throat. This equalization of pressure is what makes your ears feel like Rice Krispies.

Clogged Pipes

Question: What is ear wax, anyway?—Cheri M., forty-four

Answer: It's a form of sweat (imagine *that* coming out of your pits) that's secreted by glands and mixed in with all the stuff it catches. Wax is like your high school principal: You think it's bad, but it's really not. Ear wax, sticky stuff that it is, traps anything foreign that flies, crawls, or is blown into the ear canals—like dirt, tiny bits of plant material, small insects, bacteria. Think of wax as the sticky stuff on a No Pest Strip. The primary purpose of ear wax is to protect your ear canal and eardrum from such foreign materials. So, unless it's dripping into your salad, your goal isn't to eliminate wax but just keep it from blocking your ear.

Wax Attacks

Question: Do you have to use mineral oil to clean out ear wax, or is there an alternate oil?—Laura, thirty-five

Answer: Hope you haven't got your eye on the WD-40 or Quaker State. We're not sure of other oils that break up the sticky wax, so we'd say that you ought to stick with mineral oil—Johnson's baby oil is just that. It's liquid at room temperature, and after sitting in your ear for about fifteen minutes, it works by dislodging the wax and then draining it when you tilt your ear to the other side.

Your Mouth

Question: Why do your teeth chatter when you're cold?—Rose O., fifty-one

Answer: Your body usually maintains a constant temperature of 98.6 degrees Fahrenheit; that's the temperature at which the cells of the body work best. So your body—like a lover trying to hang on to a relationship—will do anything it can to get back to that peaceful place. If there's any significant change in temperature, it's sensed by the area of the brain called the hypothalamus. When the body gets too cold, this center alerts the rest of the body to begin warming up. Shivering, the rapid movement of the muscles to generate heat, begins. Teeth chattering is simply localized shivering.

Spot On

Question: What are the white spots on my teeth?—Tina H., thirty-three

Answer: Polka-dotted teeth (the unintentional kind) are usually a sign of enamel breakdown and decalcification. Fluoride can be helpful in cleaning them up; they are often made worse by braces, which allow plaque to accumulate. If they're making you uncomfortable, see your dentist for cosmetic options.

Your Nose

Know Your Nose

Question: Why does my nose run in the winter?—Betty F., forty-six

Answer: You have small hairs called cilia that continually milk secretions up your nose toward the sinuses. The temperature in the nose is usually around 80°F (put down the thermometer; trust us on this one). But it can drop during cold weather, thus paralyzing these hairs. When the cilia cannot beat fast enough, the secretions drain down with gravity, and your nose "runs" faster than Forrest Gump on a country dirt road.

Sunny and Sneezy

Question: Why do you sneeze when you look at the sun?—Kim, thirty-two

Answer: The culprit is the photic sneeze reflex, which usually causes more than one sneeze and occurs in approximately 10 percent to 25 percent of the population. This genetic trait is thought to occur due to an accidental crossing of third-nerve signals in your brain at the fifth cranial nerve nucleus (remember that the next time you're playing Trivial Pursuit). If you have a parent who is a sun sneezer, you have a 50 percent chance of being a sun sneezer as well.

Plucky and Sneezy

Question: Why do I sneeze when I pluck my eyebrows?—Catherine, thirty-eight

Answer: The sneezing reflex is often considered more complex than a calculus problem. A sneeze—whether it's induced by pepper or allergies—starts with an irritation to your nasal passages, which excites your trigeminal nerve. The sneezing center then sends impulses back along the facial nerve to your nasal passages, mucus glands, blood vessels, and eyelids (which is the reason you close your eyes when you sneeze). Plucking a hair from your eyebrow stimulates a nearby branch of the nerve that services your nasal passages and thus can instigate the process that causes you to sneeze.

There She Blows

Question: Is it dangerous to hold in a sneeze?—Dina B., forty-seven

Answer: Holding in a sneeze is like holding down the top of a jack-in-the-box. Why not just let it out? The air expelled by sneezes is said to travel up to one hundred miles per hour; holding in a sneeze could cause fractures in the nasal cartilage, nosebleeds, burst eardrums, hearing loss, vertigo, or detached retinas. Therefore it is best to let your sneeze fly (shielded by a hankie, preferably). Plus, your body is trying to clear out your throat—and that's a good thing. To help the sneeze come out, look at a bright light. This stimulates the optic nerve, which crosses wires with the sneeze center (see "Sunny and Sneezy," above). The added irritation of an adjacent nerve will get the sneeze going.

Your Privates

Peeing Is Believing

Question: Why do women pee more than men?—Joan, forty-nine

Answer: Men have a larger bladder capacity and tend to pee in larger volumes; women have smaller bladders, so they pee less volume but more often.

Patient Procreation

Question: Should a man wait several days between sex to store up sperm if trying to impregnate his wife?—Tom, thirty-three

Answer: Like a circus show, the amount of times you have sex is a delicate balancing act (what you do with a trapeze is your own business). Studies agree that semen volume and sperm concentration increase with prolonged sexual abstinence. Studies also find that ejaculating several times per week will give you the highest number of fully functioning sperm.

Color Change

Question: Why do your nipples turn brown during pregnancy?—Robin, thirty-four

Answer: Many pregnant women of all complexions notice that their nipples have become somewhat darker. The increase in estrogen and progesterone levels causes the changes in your pigment. Your nipples, face, and belly are three areas where darkening of the skin can be most noticeable during (and often after) pregnancy.

Saddle Sore

Question: Can too much time on a bike lead to erectile dysfunction?—Henry, thirty-eight

Answer: While cycling is good for your heart and your legs, studies have shown that spending too much time sitting on a bicycle seat can affect your liftoff. People who spend a long time on a bike are at greater risk for erectile dysfunction. It's important to find an erectile-friendly seat and make sure that your bicycle fits properly to reduce the risk.

Private Practices

Question: **Is douching dangerous?—Gina, thirty**
Answer: The vagina is like a self-cleaning oven: Most times, it takes care of cleaning itself, so you don't need to douche. Vaginal douching has many risks and has been linked to a number of adverse health conditions, including bacterial and yeast infections, pelvic inflammatory disease, ectopic pregnancy, preterm birth, reduced fertility, and increased susceptibility to STDs.

Two Flows

Question: **What causes a split stream when you pee?—Ebony, twenty-nine**
Answer: While it may look like a city fountain, the split stream is the sign of a real condition that's caused by some residual debris in the urinary tube. It can also be caused by scarring of the urinary opening or damage to the urethra. In men, prostate infections or enlargement can also cause one's flow to have a second stream.

Good Morning Indeed!

Question: **Why do men wake up in the morning with an erection?—Dawn R., twenty-six**
Answer: Because, really, do we have anything better to do at 5:18 A.M.? Actually, the penis is like a bat—it's a very nocturnal creature (that, and there's no telling where you'll find it flying around). The reason why men have an erectile alarm clock? These nighttime erections occur in the REM (rapid eye movement) phase of sleep, and REM sleep is more frequent just before waking up. On a side note, erections can also happen at other times without any stimulus. So just because a man may stiffen anywhere anytime doesn't mean it's something he can control.

SOS for PCOS

Question: A friend of mine mentioned that she has polycystic ovarian syndrome (PCOS). What is it?—Jennifer, thirty-eight

Answer: The hormonal and reproductive disease affects 10 percent of women. It causes obesity, irregular periods, acne, the need to wax your mustache, and/or elevations in blood sugar, lousy cholesterol (and low healthy cholesterol), or blood pressure (metabolic syndrome). Oral contraceptives are very effective at treating symptoms, but if you're trying to get pregnant, the medications metformin and Clomid (clomiphene) can help.

Lose the Hair?

Question: I have so many ingrown hairs in my bikini line region, and sometimes they get infected and pus up and get hard and painful. The other night I had the largest pus pocket I've ever seen, and I had to pop it to get rid of it. Should I get a Brazilian wax?—Brittney, twenty

Answer: The purpose of hair is to reduce chafing and preserve odor from the genital area, since it attracts mates. But health-wise, there are no long-term issues with a Brazilian wax, so it's merely a personal choice of comfort—and what feels best for you.

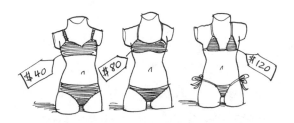

Your Skin

Wash Off

Question: Do hand-washing alcohol-based lotions dry out the skin?—Regina, forty-four

Answer: The Purell or Cal Stat that our hospitals use work even better than hand washing. The newer ones we carry in our pockets have a moisturizer in the mixture to reduce making hands dry and crinkly. If you still have dry skin after use, add Vaseline or petroleum jelly at night and slip on a pair of clear plastic gloves.

Thicker Skin

Question: I'm a senior citizen, and my skin is thin and tears easily. How can I heal my skin?—Cheryl A., seventy

Answer: Thin skin is more than just the inability to deal with a public beating by the boss. It's actually caused by not enough protein in your diet, not enough blood flow, not enough healthy fat, or too much of one hormone or another. Technically, you're not losing skin—it's decreased thickness of each cell that causes thinness and tearing (most often on the forearms). Our patients tell us that eating an ounce of walnuts (about twenty-four half walnuts) (good protein and good fat) a day or taking a DHA omega-3 supplement helps, as does using Vaseline on the forearms.

Fat Chance

Question: Why do some women have cellulite and others don't?—Beth, forty-six

Answer: Skinny women can have it, and heavy women can have it. There's no cure for cellulite, so stop wasting your money on methods that claim to remove it permanently.

Irritable Itch

Question: Is shingles contagious? How do you get it, and how long does it last after taking medicine?—Patty K., thirty

Answer: Shingles is caused by the chicken pox virus, which is localized to a collection of nerves just outside your spinal cord or outside the brain stem. Once the skin lesions are gone, we do not think shingles is easily contagious. The painful condition of shingles makes most suffers feel like they are being stabbed repeatedly. Shingles treatment is carried out on two fronts. In addition to curing the bothersome rashes, we aim to prevent the chronic shooting pains that parallel the way that a nerve travels through your body. Therapy is most effective when initiated early in the course of the disease. For the treatment—of the shingles rash and to prevent the development of long-lasting shooting pains that parallel the way a nerve travels through your body—you have to apply the old "the earlier, the better" standard. Using a medication that blocks the nerve or an antiviral for herpes (Valtrex, for instance) means there's less chance the pain will persist after the lesions heal. By the way, there is now a shingles vaccine. It's recommended for all people with normal immune systems who have had chicken pox and are over age sixty. (Talk to your doc if you have not had chicken pox, because you probably should get a vaccine for that.) It's preventive in 60 percent of patients and lessens the post-shingles pain in many of the other 40 percent.

Emergency Situations

Question: I fell in my boat, and my leg was really bleeding. I stopped the blood with a towel, but it made me realize that I need a first-aid update. What should I have done?—Jason, thirty-five

Answer: Seeing blood unrelated to horror movies or biology class can be a scary thing, so it's no wonder that people don't always remember what to do after a cut, gouge, or gaping skin split. You did the right thing by using a towel (as long as it was clean and not covered in fish goop); there's no need to use a tourniquet unless that's the only way to stop the geyser. Once the bleeding has stopped, wash out any bits of material that don't belong to you—you know, things like dirt and tuna teeth. Then, whether the wound hurts or not, go to an ER, so docs can determine whether you need antibiotics or a tetanus booster shot. To relieve the pain, try aspirin (with water). See below for what to use for a wound.

Cutting Question

Question: What's the best solution to put in a wound?—Gerardo L., thirty-nine
Answer: Put nothing in a cut that you would not put in your eyes. If you do, you will kill millions of your loyal defender cells in order to knock off a few bacteria. Wounds will heal the safest and fastest by letting nature run its course with a scab formation. Just make sure that you clean out any gross debris (rocks, glass, and so on) with water or saline. And be sure to have a tetanus shot every ten years.

Button Up

Question: Why are some belly buttons innies and others are outies?—Laura, forty
Answer: When the doctor cuts your umbilical cord at birth, a scar can form that pushes up the belly button. Occasionally, a small hernia, or hole in the leather lining called the fascia, can be found, and these have a small risk of letting the bowel push through. This hernia is found particularly in pregnant women, since the baby stretches the belly button hole larger. This bulge usually goes away after the delivery and often will not be a problem unless the mother puts on lots of weight.

Ba-Bump

Question: The backs of my arms have these red bumps that don't go away. I've read about this, and it seems like there's not much I can do about it—something about dead cells not going away? But I hate to believe that I'm stuck with bumpy arms, particularly in the summer.—Arline, fifty-three

Answer: Since there must be more forms of red bumps than car brands, it can be hard to tell. It might be keratosis pilaris, which gets better with glycolic acid and tanning, but will return if you stop. Some red bumps are from insect bites, common in mornings, and can be treated with skin creams and hot washing and changing your bed stuff (yes, sometimes even *him*). Some bumps can be allergic reactions to your soap or laundry detergent that you use to wash clothing. Some are due to skin conditions that are responsive to 1 percent hydrocortisone cream, and some from rarer skin conditions. But it does sound like something you may want to see a dermatologist about.

Your Family

Digital Issues

Question: It seems like all my daughter does is play video games. Should I worry?—Gerri, forty-three

Answer: It may seem like Mario and his brothers are as healthy as coconut cream smoothies, but video games are good not just for your daughter's digital dexterity. For one, video games have social benefits, as long as you're making sure that she's swapping her laser fire with wholesome playmates. And your daughter may even be developing motor skills that could come in handy when she's robotically operating on hearts in a couple of decades. Most important, though, those controllers serve this valuable purpose: They're going to help keep her thin. How? With two hands on buttons, there are no hands in the chip bags and cheese dips. Many studies show that watching TV is associated with obesity, while playing video games is not. Just make sure that your daughter gets at least thirty minutes of physical activity a day or that she plays a game like Dance Dance Revolution, which has foot controls and will keep her moving. That way she'll get the best of both worlds.

Staying Sore

Question: I have a fifteen-year-old who has chronic muscle pain. We have been to numerous doctors, who have run blood tests and even an MRI, but everything seems to be normal? Do you recommend any vitamins?—Shelley, forty-seven

Answer: Assuming that no genetic, infectious, or other disease is found, your child may have chronic fatigue syndrome. Most doctors feel that this type of chronic muscle pain is due to a viral infection in nerve cells. Recent data show that most such people have abnormal genetic functioning in their white cells, indicating a viral infection. Until we learn more about how to treat the infection, the best therapies are: seven and a half hours of sleep a night; avoid foods high in saturated and trans fats; eat healthy fats, like an avocado with veggies (these are feelings, not based on solid data); 800 micrograms of folate, 4 to 6 milligrams of B6 and 800 micrograms of B_{12} a day; D-Ribose (5 grams twice a day) and force yourself to walk and exercise—even if pain pills or aspirin are necessary—to maintain or increase stamina, strength, and immunity.

Family Matters

Question: My mother passed away two years ago, and since then my father has become very withdrawn. I try to get him to socialize with friends, but he only wants to watch TV. How do I get him out of his shell? Mom was always the social one, but I think Dad needs people in his life too.—Jennifer, forty-eight

Answer: Loss of a significant other is a major life stress and cause of depression. His withdrawal makes it more likely that he ages more from the loss of a significant other. So in addition to making sure he gets adequate food (appetite often goes, and that makes the depression worse due to lack of essential omega-3 fats and probably key vitamins), keep exploring ways to get other friends, even distant ones, to engage him. As for you, spend extra time dragging Dad to eat fish, or DHA supplements from algae, or walnuts, and getting him to walk with you.

Your Immune System

V for C

Question: I've heard there is a vaccine for cancer. When will it be available, and what cancers will it prevent?—Maureen C., thirty-nine

Answer: The kinds of shots that usually get the most attention are basketball shots, tequila shots, and high-dollar paparazzi shots. But it seems that the biggest shot yet could be the small one that prevents the "big C." You heard correctly. The vaccine for human papillomavirus (HPV), the virus associated with cancer of the cervix (in women) and much cancer of the head and neck region in both genders, can prevent 70 percent of such cancers. The vaccine may even be helpful in treating such cancers. It is available now and recommended for all girls aged nine to eleven; we think you should talk to your doc about it no matter what age you are. Soon men may be eligible, because some male cancers may also be related to HPV. The FDA has fast-tracked it, and its manufacturer, Merck, has been gearing up for production, so the best estimate is that men may be able to get it if found effective in 2009 or 2010.

Hot Topic

Question: Call me paranoid, but I refuse to use a microwave. Do they cause cancer?—Lucy B., sixty-two

Answer: No, but they do cause more than extreme pizza sogginess. About 90 percent of Americans have plastic residue in their urine because they microwave in plastic (that residue is called phthalates, for you spelling-bee champs). This is potentially harmful because some additives used in the manufacturing of plastic, particularly those that make it pliable, may migrate into food, especially at high temperatures. Only plastic containers that have been specifically designed for microwave cooking should be used, and they should be discarded when the surface shows any signs of breaking down.

Grill Drill

Question: How can barbecuing cause cancer?—Doug, thirty-five

Answer: Sorry, burger boy, but studies have shown that two types of cancer-causing agents can be formed during barbecuing. PAHs (polycyclic aromatic hydrocarbons) and HCAs (heterocyclic amines) are formed in smoke and are found on the surface of meat. Marinating for fifteen minutes in an olive oil–balsamic vinegar mix before barbecuing decreases PAHs and HCAs by more than 90 percent.

Supplemental Coverage

Question: Are there supplements or herbs that will help cure or treat hepatitis B?—Beverly T., thirty-six

Answer: Just as we wish there were flying cars and no-calorie doughnuts, we also wish there were supplements that could suppress a virus. But there are no supplements—

or even real medicine—that can do that. The best course is prevention through the hepatitis B vaccine. Who should get it? Everyone who's sexually active in a non-monogamous relationship and every teenager who hasn't been vaccinated.

Contagious Cat

Question: Is it true that women should avoid cats and kitty litter during pregnancy?—Lauren, thirty

Answer: You're probably referring to toxoplasmosis, an infection caused by a parasite. Yes, cat feces and kitty litter are major sources of toxoplasmosis. The Centers for Disease Control and Prevention estimates that only about 1 percent of women of childbearing age are immune to toxoplasmosis. An estimated 100 to 1,450 (yes, we know that's a wide range and a small percentage of the 4 million births) cases of congenital toxoplasmosis occur in the U.S. each year, which can cause miscarriage, stillbirth or death shortly after birth, and blindness and mental retardation.

Infection Detection

Question: Why do women always get urinary tract infections?—Yvonne, thirty-two

Answer: The urethra (where urine comes out of) is shorter in women than it is in men—thus making it easier for bacteria to travel the wrong way up a one-way street back to the bladder. It's also located closer to the rectum in women, and there are more bacteria in this area that can find their way into the bladder. Sexual activity can also push bacteria into the sterile urine. The best solution is a single dose of the antibiotic Bactrim, but cranberry juice is also effective if taken in high doses. It helps by increasing the acidity of the urine, which kills most bacteria. Make sure to wipe from front to back to avoid further infections.

Toilet Trouble

Question: Can you get an infection from a toilet seat?—Freda K., sixty-four

Answer: About as likely as your winning a $5 million lottery—without buying a ticket. Most dried secretions lose their ability to infect you. To gain access to your body, the bacteria or viruses usually have to get into one of your holes (mouth, anus, urethra). The bad boys cannot jump from the toilet, so you're safe. A much more dangerous enemy is saliva, since people can contaminate you while coughing or by getting infections on their hands during a sneeze, then passing it along to you during a friendly handshake.

Your Hormones

Waterlogged

Question: Can you drink too much water? I heard that a woman died from this because of a hormone problem.—Mary, forty-nine

Answer: Water intoxication, or sickness from drinking too much water, occurs when you exceed your capacity to get rid of water. Your capacity to excrete water is normally about 1,000 milliliters per hour (which is about four glasses), so if you drink more than this, you will dilute your body salts. If the capacity to excrete water is impaired, then even lesser rates of consumption will result in low-sodium concentration in your blood. Kidney failure is one reason for such an impaired capacity. The other major reason for a failure to excrete water is the presence of a hormone called vasopressin—the antidiuretic hormone. This explains the frequency of low sodium concentration in the blood of marathon runners: they sweat and become volume depleted, vasopressin rises, thirst increases, and due to the vasopressin, the water load cannot be adequately excreted and salt concentration falls.

Drink Tank

Question: Whenever I drink, even if it's just a few drinks, I always have the worst hangovers. Are hormones responsible for hangovers?—Tonya S., thirty

Answer: Besides the tornado of tequila you used to celebrate your new raise? Hangovers happen when fluid shifts across the blood-brain barrier with toxins included in the alcohol. Darker drinks have more of these toxins, which is why vodka and gin cause these symptoms less frequently. Combat hangover symptoms by drinking water to help excrete the toxins and reduce brain irritation. Aspirin (if you don't have ulcers) can be helpful but should be taken with lots of water. Caffeine is helpful, since it counterbalances the depressant effect of alcohol on the brain.

Your Diet and Supplements

A Real Nutty Question

Question: You recommend eating a handful of walnuts daily; I am taking an omega complex supplement. Is it necessary to do both?—D.W., forty-eight

Answer: No, not for the healthy fat; but you can enjoy the walnuts more than taking a liquid, and you will get the rest of the nut—healthy protein. But the omega complex (2 grams of distilled fish oils or 600 milligrams of DHA from algae) daily is a perfect fat, and many people like it because they do not have to worry about toxins in fish (the liquid is distilled or from algae).

Rule the Roast

Question: I heard that we shouldn't eat roasted nuts. But I don't like the taste of raw. What should I do?—Zoe, thirty-four

Answer: As evidenced by snake charmers and *Survivor* contestants, the world has all kinds of nuts. Though they're certainly a healthier snack than chips, candy, or pepperoni logs, nuts do have their own hierarchy. You want nuts to be raw, fresh, and unsalted. That's because nuts lose up to 15 percent of their healthy oils when they're roasted (roasting at high temperatures may even cause the formation of chemicals that promote aging). If you want to roast them, put them in the oven at 350 degrees for nine minutes. If you do it yourself, it won't cause any bad fats or dangerous chemical acrylamides to form.

Are we driving you nuts? We hope to drive you *to* nuts. Here's our pecking order, from best to worst:

★   Fresh and freshly refrigerated

★   Freshly toasted and dry roasted (in your oven); we like the taste of these best too

★   Roasted in their own fat and salted (packaged)

★   Roasted in partially hydrogenated fat (especially if sugared)—we avoid this totally

Oil Change

Question: Is it okay to cook with olive oil? Or does any heating make the good fat turn bad?—Ashley, thirty-eight

Answer: Olive oil has been well studied. It's more than okay; it is probably better than other oils, but not pomace olive oil, which has been extracted with the toxin hexane.

The level of oxidation in olive oil probably depends on the duration of heat exposure and the heat temperature. Deep frying should be at 350 degrees or less. Most of these studies are about the commercial use of deep frying in olive oil: it takes ten to fifteen reheatings to produce the really bad chemicals.

Living in the Red

Question: I understand I should eat ten tablespoons of tomato sauce a week, but does something like V8 juice count? I'm not wild about tomato sauce, but if juice works, I can do that.—Paula, forty-four

Answer: V8s don't just do wonders for sports cars. They will also give your bodily engine lots of cancer-protecting power. V8 juice counts the same as tomato sauce because it's pasteurized, but you do have to drink it with a little healthy fat for it to be absorbed. So drink it after having a few nuts (six walnuts, or twelve almonds, or twenty peanuts, for example) or after having fish oil or avocado, peanut, walnut, or almond spread (a half tablespoon does the trick). One eight-ounce can is the same as one tablespoon of tomato sauce.

The Dark Side

Question: When you give advice to "snack on dark chocolate made from real cocoa," what should I look for on the label? When I look at the contents of what seems to be dark chocolate candy, it refers only to "cocoa butter."—Denise, fifty-seven

Answer: Good work. You found it. Cocoa butter *is* cocoa—or real chocolate. For your chocolate to be healthy, you want to make sure it doesn't have milk fat or solids and no trans fat. By the way, dark chocolate looks dark; many American bars are made with milk chocolate and therefore are lighter in color. By European standards, dark chocolate must contain a minimum of 43 percent cocoa to be called dark. A 70 percent cocoa chocolate is considered quite dark, while 85 percent and even 88 percent cocoa dark chocolates have become quite popular for dark-chocolate lovers. Look for 70 percent or more.

Think about Drinks

Question: I'm moved from drinking water and Gatorade for my workouts to those new energy drinks, and my friends all say there's nothing to them. But I definitely feel more energetic after drinking them. Are they bad for you?—Tom, forty-five

Answer: Energy, whether it's for your house, your body, or the bedroom, is a good thing. However, with energy drinks, you're not getting the boost from the vitamins they may be touting but from the caffeine and a temporary high from too much sugar. Drinking them could be dangerous to the heart because of the amount of caffeine. If you were to drink multiple glasses of this mixture or concoctions and a few cups of coffee, we think there would be a potential for significant danger—in the form of a racing heartbeat, elevated blood pressure, and even potentially a heart attack. And too much sugar can make your arteries age, sapping your energy in the long run. One eight-ounce bottle after a long workout (more than one hour of exercise) is fine, but limit it to no more than that.

Going Bananas

Question: What's the recommended dose for a potassium supplement?—Patricia K., forty-nine

Answer: We don't recommend the potassium that comes in a bottle; we recommend the kind that can be peeled. That's because potassium in pills can be dangerous if you have kidney problems. So it's best to get your potassium through your diet. While bananas serve as the symbolic icon of potassium (with 400 milligrams each), most servings of fruits and vegetables contain 400 milligrams of potassium. If you eat our recommended nine servings of fruits and vegetables a day, you'll reach the optimum number of more than 3,000 milligrams.

A Question

Question: You once mentioned on your XM Radio show that one shouldn't take more than 2,500 IU of vitamin A, or it ceases being effective as an antioxidant. I take Lipitor together with a multivitamin that has 5,000 IU of vitamin A. What would you suggest?—Gail, forty-two

Answer: The risk of vitamin A in high doses is that it can demineralize your bones, making them weaker. Your doc may know the results of a bone scan. If that shows no demineralization, the vitamin A may not be a significant risk to you. But more than 2,500 IU of vitamin A also slightly increases the risk of liver and lung cancer. The Lipitor pertains more to your vitamin E and vitamin C doses than A doses. Lipitor has three benefits for your arteries: It decreases the lousy LDL significantly, increases the healthy HDL cholesterol slightly, and inhibits inflammation. (The inflammation effect appears to be 40 percent or so of the benefit of Lipitor or most statins in a typical person—the cholesterol effects account for 60 percent of the benefit.) Vitamin C greater than 100 milligrams a day in supplements and vitamin E in doses greater than 100 IU a day inhibit the anti-inflammatory effect of Lipitor. So check your vitamin pills for these.

Salt a Deadly Weapon?

Question: Is salt really a problem?—Paulette, forty-five

Answer: Yes, it's a big problem for a few people: those who are salt-sensitive. And it's less of a problem for most of us. The average person takes in 4,000 milligrams of sodium a day. That raises blood pressure by 40/20 in some, making their RealAges nine to twelve years older from salt. For the rest of us, decreasing sodium to 2,300 milligrams for young whites and 1,500 milligrams for all others (minorities and older whites), would save 150,000 lives in the United States—and make your blood pressure 7/4 lower. To put this in perspective, if we cut trans fats completely, we would save 50,000 lives per year. Even bread has lots of salt. Sea salt is not safer, but since the taste is stronger, people tend to use less of it.

Flour Power

Question: You stated that enriched flour should be avoided. We have been using a brand of unbleached enriched flour. We assumed that as long as the flour was unbleached, it wasn't bad for you in moderation. We read the label, and it states, "enriched with vitamins." Please clarify.—Edwin C., forty-four

Answer: Anything other than 100 percent whole grains means they took the good stuff out. *Enriched* means they took all the good stuff out and put a little of it back. Stick with 100 percent whole grains only. Enriched flour is not much better for you than straight sugar.

Your Embarrassing Questions

Breast Issue

Question: Call me crazy, but I feel like I'm extrasensitive about what I wear because of my chest. Why do nipples get erect?—Jackie A., thirty-seven

Answer: The original nipple erections (isn't that the name of a college band?) stemmed from our need to feed our babies. Smooth muscles around the nipple plump up the nipple during stimulation from a child to facilitate breast feeding. But milk doesn't necessarily have to flow for your nipples to feel stiffer than a twice-starched Oxford. The conditioned response can also occur in response to other stimuli, like sexual arousal and fear.

Natural Gas

Question: I seem to have an extraordinary amount of gas—to the point where I'm squirming around in my office chair to stifle it. What causes all this gas?
—Denise B., forty

Answer: We have two main sources for nature's rear-propulsion system. Flatus comes from the air we swallow (20 percent) and the digestion of foods by bacteria in our intestines (80 percent). We have trillions of bacteria in our intestines and five hundred species that are so lethal that any one could kill us. These bacteria love digesting sugars, fiber, or milk; if you are missing the enzyme that digests milk sugar (lactase), or you are lactose intolerant, then you cannot cannot digest them quickly. The result is lots of gas made up of carbon dioxide, nitrogen, and methane (which is flammable). Unfortunately, you need to read labels and try an elimination diet by getting rid of specific foods in your diet for three days at a time until you find what's triggering your discomfort. You can reduce swallowing air by avoiding cigarettes, gum, and carbonated beverages, and by slowing down when eating or drinking.

Smelly Situation

Question: My wife claims her gas doesn't smell, but she kicks me out of the bedroom because mine is worse than a landfill, she says. Why does gas smell?
—Peter Z., fifty-seven

Answer: Think of your body as a refrigerator. If you let food sit in there, it's going to smell after a while. In your body, sulfur-rich foods like eggs, meat, beer, beans, and cauliflower are decomposed by bacteria to release hydrogen sulfide—a smell strong enough to flatten a bear. Avoiding these foods is the ideal solution, but when stinky gas persists, the best solutions are leafy green vegetables and probiotics (specifically lactobacillus GG and *Bacillus coagulans*; these can be found in some yogurts or digestive aid tablets). Beano can sometimes work with beans, but soaking the beans ahead of time is useful as well.

The Price of Gas

Question: Why do older people fart more than younger people?—Lena, sixty-five
Answer: The amount of gas produced a day is the same. The difference? A loss of muscle tone occurs as people age, and this includes the muscles around the anal sphincter. Therefore, an older person simply has less ability to hold in the gas.

Sting Operation

Question: Does urinating on a jellyfish sting really stop the pain?—Wendy, fifty-three
Answer: It's a myth and potentially painful (not to mention that it could land someone you love dearly on YouTube). Tests show that urine, ammonia, and alcohol have caused active stinging. You need to use an acidic compound like vinegar to reduce the sting.

Pee Problems

Question: When I sneeze, I pee. I walk, I pee. I laugh, I pee. I talk, I pee. I cough, I pee. I exercise, I pee. If I don't run to the bathroom just after sex, I pee. Sometimes I barely make it to a bathroom, and before I can unzip my pants, I am peeing. I feel like I am ready for diapers. It is distressing, embarrassing, and a complete disruption in my life. Will Kegel exercises work?—Marcy S., forty-four
Answer: While it may seem like you have less bladder control than a week-old puppy,

there are things you can do to slow down this trickle effect. If you're having incontinence during or right after pregnancy, Kegel exercises (that is, exercises that strengthen your pelvic muscles) can work. But you have to do them the right way. Tighten your butt muscles up toward your belly button and hold for as long as you can (for added effect, put some hip-hop on in the background). What you're really doing is tightening the muscles of the pelvic floor. Repeat until you cannot take the pain anymore (around ten times). The best way to learn—get on the throne, start to pee, then stop your stream mid-pee, and repeat as many times as you can. But if your youngest kid just joined Medicare, you'll often need more than exercises and a Depend coupon; you'll need an aggressive solution for urinary incontinence, like collagen injections or surgery to resuspend your bladder. As women age and their estrogen levels decline, the bladder neck falls beneath the support muscles of the pelvis and loses the angle that helps prevent the bladder from running like an open faucet.

Drip Dry

Question: I sweat all the time—no matter what I'm wearing, no matter what the temperature, no matter whether I'm sitting still or walking around the house. What's happening?—Cristina Y., forty-five

Answer: If you sweat more than a sumo wrestler in the Sahara, then you may have a condition called hyperhidrosis, which arises from overproductive sweat glands of the hands or feet. (The major causes of sweat problems are thyroid or testosterone abnormalities.) Botox has been used for this ailment. For hand sweat, surgery that cuts the offending nerves can work. This is actually a very common condition among Asians and may explain why Asians often bow or wear white gloves—they do not want you to shake a wet hand when they greet you.

Sweat Shop

Question: I'm literally the butt of all jokes. I suffer from excessive sweating from my butt when I'm nervous. When I was supposed to give my brother's eulogy, I was sweating so much I had to put my butt next to the air vents of my car to dry off. Nothing works.—Tracy A., forty-two

Answer: We think it would be unfair of us to *crack* a joke here, so let's agree to get right to the *bottom* of your problem. Really, we don't mean to be *cheeky* about it; you do have a real medical condition. You could have a problem with just too much sweating there and need to consider an expert who could dry that condition with Botox or another method to decrease specific nerve firing. But more likely it is an infectious condition: The buttock crease above your anus is a moist nesting ground for infections that can penetrate into hair follicles and cause deep infections. Those infections can drain clear secretions with little odor to reddish secretions with an odor. (It's most commonly found in hairy men in the hot summer; now, *there's* a pretty picture.) Improved hygiene will help: Wash the area with a cloth and apply antimicrobials like tea tree oil directly in the crease periodically. Waxing isn't just for sex appeal; it will remove hairs that trap debris—and can ultimately make you feel cleaner than an Osmond family concert.

Smelling Assault

Question: I've always had bad BO. I start sweating between my thighs, and before you know it, I smell. I can't find a deodorant to hold my musk.—Cynthia, thirty-four

Answer: If you smell funkier than a Rick James album, then there's probably a good explanation. Our major sweat glands (they're called eccrine glands, in case you're ever on *Jeopardy!*) release a sterile solution that attracts smelly bacteria in some people. These secretions are stored in coiled circular glands four feet long and cover our entire skin surface. But the actual composition of your sweat is based on your genes and your diet. Garlic will quickly pass into your skin and quickly share itself with others. Washing frequently helps, but sometimes a quick course of topical antibiotics from your doctor is the best anti-smell solution.

Pelvic Pain

Question: Two years ago I ruptured the base of my penis when the girl I was seeing excitedly sat on my lap. I heard a painful pop and immediately felt intense pain. I now have five scarred rings at the base and am unable to achieve the full erection that I used to. Do you know of anything that might help this dilemma?—Frank F., thirty-six

Answer: You don't have to be an Olympic archer to know that you've got big problems when your arrow won't fly. To understand how to fix it, you need to get a little more familiar with your penis (though it seems you know it pretty darn well at this point). The penis shaft is contained within a leathery wrap. When the wrap is under pressure during an erection and is suddenly kinked, that wrap can crack (it most often happens in the woman-on-top position). The healing process causes a scar, thus breaking the arrow by causing the penis to become deformed and angular. This change in shape is pretty darn painful, so your body rebels by not giving you as many erections (or making them as fun). You'll need surgery to remove the scar and make you a straight shooter again.

Index

pineal gland, 261
pineapple(s), 142
  -Banana Frappé, 379
pituitary gland, 317–18, *319*
Pizza, Smoked Mozzarella and
  Veggie-Stuffed, 418
plants, 165
plaque:
  arterial, *39*, 40, 41, 60, 177, 288
  dental, 177
platelets, 41, 57, 60, 62
Plums and Prunes, Maple
  Oatmeal with, 381
PMS, 251
pneumonia, 158
pollution, 165–66, 221
polychlorinated biphenyls (PCBs),
  60
polycystic ovarian syndrome
  (PCOS), 487
polyps, 152, 191, 193, 361
pomace olive oil, 499
Portuguese Bean Soup, 397
positive attitude, 464–65
postpartum depression, 94
postsynaptic cell, *72*
posture, 143
potassium, 63, 335, 500–501
Potatoes, Wasabi Mashed, Grilled
  Chicken or Fish with
  Caramelized Sweet Onions
  and, 415
Power Quesadillas, 409
PP (pancreatic polypeptide) cells,
  219
pregnancy, 236, 239
  cats and kitty litter, 495
  and middle ear, 266
  and nipple color, 485
presynaptic cell, *72*
Prevachol, 63, 96
primrose oil, 251
probiotics, 186, 476, 504
progesterone, 236, 237, 327
progestin, 238
prolactin, 315, 318
Prometheus, 207
Prometrium, 238

proofreader gene, 348–49, 354
proprioception, 87, 270
prostate, 92, *234*, 239, 240, *241*, 242
prostate cancer, 238, 240, 252, 326,
  356, 360, 361
prostate exams, 254, 360
protein:
  and amino acids, 215
  and calcium, 140
  C-reactive, 55
  high-protein diets, 140
  and homocysteine, 54
  produced by the liver, 210
prune(s), 191
  Maple Oatmeal with Plums
  and, 381
psyllium, 191, 199
pulmonary embolism, 238
pulse, 34
pumpkin seeds, 309
pus, 311
push-ups, 453
pyroglutamate, 463

Q-tips, 262, 271
quadriceps, exercises for, 440
Quesadillas, Power, 409

radon, 166, 351
Rainbow Shrimp Moo Shu Roll-
  ups, 423
Raisin Curry Chicken, 428
rashes, 159, 272
Raspberry-Orange Smoothie, 383
reactive depression, 84
RealAge.com, 459
recipes, *see* Owner's Manual Diet
recovery time, 56
rectum, *188*, 189, 192
red clover, 239
Reds and Greens Parade, 408
Red Snapper, Barbecued, with
  Spicy Red Beans and Rice,
  416
red wine, 97
reflux disorder, *181*, 182, 183, 195,
  472–73
regurgitation, 180, 181

REM (rapid eye movement) sleep,
  155, 156
reproduction, 242, *243*, 244
reptilian functions, 69
resistance exercises, 124–28, 135,
  364
respiratory system, *see* lungs
resveratrol, 97
retina, 258, *259*, 260, 261, 263, 278,
  284–85
rheumatoid arthritis, 119
rice:
  chicken soup with, 184
  Spicy Red Beans and,
  Barbecued Red Snapper
  with, 416
  Whole-Grain Jasmine, Teriyaki
  Tofu with Red Bell Pepper
  and Shiitakes over, 422
right hemisphere, 71
Roasted Red Pepper and Kalamata
  Olive Sicilian Salad, 395
Roasted Tomato Basil Soup, 403
ROBE (routine operative breast
  endoscopy), 351–52
rock concert, and hearing loss, 278
rods and cones, 263
rotator cuff, 114, *115*
  exercises for, 435, 456
routine, avoiding, 89, 90–91
runny nose, 159, 483

SAD (seasonal affective disorder),
  84
salads:
  Asian, Edamame with, 391
  Non-Caesar Caesar (no egg),
  396
  Roasted Red Pepper and
  Kalamata Olive Sicilian, 395
  Texas Slaw, 407
  Warm Spinach, with Chicken,
  Apples, and Toasted
  Almonds, 413–14
saliva, 200, 496
salmon, 284
  Canned, Avocado Stuffed with,
  389